THE KIDNEY IN PREGNANCY

TOPICS IN RENAL MEDICINE

Vittorio E. Andreucci, Series Editor

THE KIDNEY IN PREGNANCY

EDITED BY

VITTORIO E. ANDREUCCI

MARTINUS NIJHOFF PUBLISHING
A MEMBER OF THE KLUWER ACADEMIC PUBLISHERS GROUP
BOSTON DORDRECHT LANCASTER

Distributors

for the United States and Canada: Kluwer Academic Publishers, 190 Old Derby Street, Hingham, MA, 02043, USA

for the UK and Ireland: Kluwer Academic Publishers, MTP Press Limited, Falcon House, Queen Square, Lancaster LA1 1RN, UK

for all other countries: Kluwer Academic Publishers Group, Distribution Centre, P.O. Box 322, 3300 AH Dordrecht, The Netherlands

Library of Congress Cataloging in Publication Data
Main entry under title:

The Kidney in pregnancy.

(Topics in renal medicine)
1. Pregnancy, Complications of. 2. Kidneys—Diseases. I. Andreucci, Vittorio E. I. Series.
[DNLM: 1. Kidney—physiology. 2. Kidney—physiopathology. 3. Pregnancy Complications. WJ 301 K46]
RG580.K5K523 1985 618.3 85-11437
ISBN 0-89838-741-8

To my mother, wife, and daughter

and

to all pregnant and nonpregnant women

CONTENTS

Contributing Authors

Vittorio E. Andreucci, MD
Professor of Nephrology
and Chairman,
Department of Nephrology
Second Faculty of Medicine
University of Naples
80131 Naples
ITALY

Gavin J. Becker, MD
Department of Nephrology
The Royal Melbourne Hospital
Parkville 3050, Victoria
AUSTRALIA

Michael Broyer, MD
Professor of Paediatrics
Necker-Enfants Malades Hôpital
149 rue de Sèvres
75730 Paris Cedex 15
FRANCE

Piero Capetta, M.D.
II Clinica Ostetrico-Ginecologica
University of Milan
Via Commenda, 12
I-20122 Milano
ITALY

Sabri Challah, MA, BM, BChir, MSc
Director, EDTA Registry
Lecturer in Community Medicine
St. Thomas' Hospital
London SE1 7EH
UNITED KINGDOM

Maria Matilde Cossu, MD
Centro Trasfusionale e di Immunoematologia
Instituti Clinici di Perfezionamento
Via Commenda 12
20122 Milano
ITALY

Antonio Dal Canton, MD
Cattedra di Nefrologia Medica
Seconda Facoltà di Medicina
Università di Napoli
Via S. Pansini 5
80131 Napoli
ITALY

John M. Davison, MD
Medical Research Council
Human Reproduction Group
Princess Mary Maternity Hospital
Newcastle upon Tyne NE3 4JQ
ENGLAND

Edward N. Ehrlich, MD
Department of Medicine
University of Wisconsin and
Endocrine Research Laboratory
Madison General Hospital
Madison, Wisconsin 53792
USA

Kenneth F. Fairley, MD
Department of Nephrology
The Royal Melbourne Hospital
Parkville 3050, Victoria
AUSTRALIA

Dominique Ganeval, MD
Department de Nephrologie
Hopital Necker
161 rue de Sèvres
75743 Paris Cedex 15
FRANCE

Norman F. Gant, MD
University of Texas Southwestern
Medical School at Dallas
Department of Obstetrics and Gynecology
5323 Harry Hines Boulevard
Dallas, Texas 75235
USA

Gina Gregorini, MD
Division of Nephrology
"Spedali Civili" di Brescia
Brescia
ITALY

Jean-Pierre Grünfeld, MD
Department de Nephrologie
Hopital Necker
161 rue de Sèvres
75743 Paris Cedex 15
FRANCE

Priscilla S. Kincaid-Smith, MD
Director, Department of Nephrology
The Royal Melbourne Hospital
Parkville 3050, Victoria
AUSTRALIA

Iain R. McFadyen, FRCOG
Section of Perinatal and Child Health
MRC Clinical Research Centre
Watford Road, Harrow

Middlesex HA1 3UJ
UNITED KINGDOM

Wolfram E. Nolten, MD
Department of Medicine
University of Wisconsin and
Endocrine Research Laboratory
Madison General Hospital
Madison, Wisconsin 53792
USA

Robyn A. North, MD
Department of Nephrology
The Royal Melbourne Hospital
Parkville 3050, Victoria
AUSTRALIA

Israel Penn, MD
Department of Surgery
University of Cincinnati Medical Center
and Cincinnati Veterans Administration
Medical Center
3200 Vine Street
Cincinnati, Ohio 45220
USA

Norberto Perico, MD
Mario Negri Institute
for Pharmacological Research
Via Gavazzeni 11
24100 Bergamo
ITALY

Nathalie Pertuiset, MD
Department de Nephrologie
Hopital Necker
161 rue de Sèvres
75743 Paris Cedex 15
FRANCE

Jack A. Pritchard, MD
University of Texas Southwestern
Medical School at Dallas

Department of Obstetrics and Gynecology
5323 Harry Hines Boulevard
Dallas, Texas 75235
USA

Giuseppe Remuzzi, MD
Mario Negri Institute
for Pharmacological Research
Via Gavazzeni 11
24100 Bergamo
ITALY

Gianfranco Rizzoni, MD
Associate Professor of Paediatric Nephrology
Clinica Pediatrica dell'Universita'
Ospedale Civile di Padova
Padova
ITALY

Edoardo Rossi, MD
Centro Trasfusionale e di Immunoematologia
Instituti Clinici di Perfezionamento
Via Commenda 12
20122 Milano
ITALY

Domenico Russo, MD
Department of Nephrology
Second Faculty of Medicine
University of Naples
80131 Naples
ITALY

Benjamin H. Spargo, MD
Department of Pathology, Box 327
University of Chicago
Pritzker School of Medicine
5841 Maryland Avenue
Chicago, Illinois 60637
USA

James R. Taylor, MD
Department of Pathology, Box 327

University of Chicago
Pritzker School of Medicine
5841 Maryland Avenue
Chicago, Illinois 60637
USA

Antony J. Wing, MA, DM, FRCP
Chairman, EDTA Registry
Consultant Physician
St. Thomas' Hospital
London SE1 7EH
UNITED KINGDOM

LIST OF ABBREVIATIONS USED IN THIS BOOK

AA, arachidonic acid
ACE, angiotensin-converting enzyme
AFLP, acute fatty liver in pregnancy
AI, angiotension I
AII, angiotension II
ARF, acute renal failure
ATN, acute tubular necrosis
AVP, arginine vasopressin
BRCN, bilateral renal cortical necrosis
CAPD, continuous ambulatory peritoneal dialysis
CBG, corticosteroid-binding globulin
CHP, chronic hypertension in pregnancy
CO, cardiac output
CSU, catheter specimen urine
Ca, calcium
DHEA, dehydroepiandrosterone
DIC, disseminated intravascular coagulation
DOC, desoxycorticosterone
DOCA, desoxycorticosterone acetate
ECV, extracellular volume
EDTA–ERA, European Dialysis and Transplant Association—European Renal Association

EFA, essential fatty acid
EPH, edema proteinuria hypertension
ERPF, effective renal plasma flow
FDP, fibrin(ogen) degradation products
FF, filtration fraction
FPA, fibrinopeptide A
GBM, glomerular basement membrane
GFR, glomerular filtration rate
GPF, glomerular plasma flow
HDL, high-density lipoprotein
HMWFC, high molecular weight fibrin(ogen) complex
HRG, histidine-rich glycoprotein
HUS, hemolytic uremic syndrome
IVP, intravenous pyelography
K_f, ultrafiltration coefficient
LDL, low-density lipoprotein
L/S, lecithin–sphingomyelin
LT3, leucotrienes of the 3 series
MSU, midstream urine
Mg, magnesium
P_G, glomerular pressure
PAH, para-amino hippurate
PCK, polycystic kidney
PET, preeclamptic toxemia
PG, prostaglandin
PGE, prostaglandin E
PGI_2, prostaglandin I2 or prostacyclin(e)
PIH, pregnancy-induced hypertension
PRA, plasma renin activity
PRC, plasma renin concentration
PSF, plasmatic stimulating factor
PT, prothrombin time
PTT, partial thromboplastin time
RBF, renal blood flow
RPF, renal plasma flow
SIgA, secretory immunoglobulin A
SLE, systemic lupus erythematosus
SNGFR, single nephron glomerular filtration rate
SPA, suprapubic aspiration (specimen)
SV, stroke volume
THDOC, tetrahydro-DOC
TTP, thrombotic thrombocytopenic purpura
UTI, urinary tract infection
VLDL, very low density lipoprotein

PREFACE

The behavior of the kidney in normal pregnancy, as well as in complicated pregnancy, is a very interesting, but still in many ways an unknown topic in renal medicine.

It is undoubtedly difficult to determine, even in normal women, the behavior of renal hemodynamics throughout gestation, since the fear of impairing a new life (i.e., the fetus's life) will limit, for ethical reasons, the use or the frequent repetition of diagnostic tests on the mother. On the other hand, the study of complicated pregnancy even for diagnostic purposes (for planning adequate treatment), except in a few countries that are known for the advanced health education of the population, has to face serious difficulties.

First of all, pregnant women usually seek the help of an obstetrician when gestation is already in an advanced stage. This makes it difficult to determine when and how asymptomatic signs of any disease discovered during pregnancy have first occurred. A second difficulty is that frequently the patient does not know whether a given disease has preceded pregnancy. Pregnancy is a condition of young women, and a young woman frequently has never seen a physician; thus, no urine analysis or blood tests have been performed before the gestation. Not infrequently, even blood pressure has never been measured. This will make it difficult to classify hypertension discovered in late pregnancy as pregnancy-induced hypertension or as chronic hypertension in pregnancy.

It is also unusual that a pregnant woman seeks the advice of a nephrologist during pregnancy, even when a renal disease has been discovered. Neither does the obstetrician consult the nephrologist when signs of renal involvement are evident during gestation, unless severe renal failure occurs. This lack of collaboration between obstetricians and nephrologists may explain the present situation: most nephrologists do not have any experience of renal disease in pregnancy.

For these reasons, in deciding on a program for a series of books on "Topics in Renal Medicine," I have chosen "The Kidney in Pregnancy" as the first volume of the series. Experts on the different aspects of this topic have been invited to write the chapters of this volume, which represents the most up-to-date review of both normal and complicated pregnancy.

Topics such as treatment of hypertension preceding pregnancy during gestation (usually disregarded both in books for obstetricians and in those for nephrologists), urinary tract infection during pregnancy (frequently disregarded in-depth reviews of renal involvement during pregnancy), and pregnancy following renal transplantation (a new interesting experience) have been included.

The Editor hopes that this volume will be of great benefit to those concerned with the care of pregnant women and will create a better "liaison" between obstetricians and nephrologists. Only by working together, in fact, will obstetricians and nephrologists clarify the still numerous controversial aspects of the behavior of the kidney in normal and complicated pregnancy, for the benefit of both mothers and fetuses.

All the contributors to this volume have provided clear, complete, and up-to-date chapters. I am deeply grateful to them all.

Special thanks to Martinus Nijhoff Publishers for the excellent and rapid publication of the volume.

Vittorio E. Andreucci
Editor

1. RENAL HEMODYNAMICS IN PREGNANCY

ANTONIO DAL CANTON and VITTORIO E. ANDREUCCI

1. CHANGES IN CENTRAL HEMODYNAMICS

1.1. Normal pregnancy

In normal pregnant women, plasma volume begins to rise after six weeks of amenorrhea [1] and attains the maximum increment toward the end of the second trimester. This increase is sustained to term [2]. The maximum amount by which plasma volume increases is extremely variable, ranging from 0.6 to 2.0 liters in different women, and is chiefly related to the size of the product of conception [1]. In pregnancy, the red cell mass also increases, but to a lesser extent than plasma volume, leading to a fall in hematocrit [3]. The increase in blood volume is associated with a rise in cardiac output (CO) [4]. Opinions differ as to whether CO is increased throughout gestation [5] or declines in late pregnancy [6]. Recently, serial measurements of CO in normal pregnant women have been performed by noninvasive technique [7]. These studies have confirmed a 20% increase in CO at week 15. CO rises further to a peak increment of 40% at weeks 25–28 of gestation, and then declines to near postpartum levels in the final weeks. In early pregnancy, the increase in CO is mainly due to an increased stroke volume (SV). As pregnancy advances, the rise in SV diminishes and increased heart rate becomes significantly contributory in maintaining the elevated CO. Echocardiographic studies have shown that the high-output hemodynamic condition in pregnancy is associated with a significant increase in left ventricular mass [8]. In normal pregnancy, despite the rise in blood volume and CO, blood pressure is unchanged or even slightly reduced, owing to a fall in peripheral vascular resistance [7, 9].

Similar changes in central hemodynamics as in man have been observed during pregnancy in several animal species [10–13]. Animal studies have provided evidence that the rise in CO is almost entirely devoted to meet the huge increase in blood flow to reproductive organs [10]. The low-resistance system of the uteroplacental bed, in parallel with the general circulation, accounts for much of the reduction in peripheral resistance. A decrease in vascular resistance, however, occurs also in nonreproductive organs, such as the kidney [10] (see section 2).

1.2. Pregnancy and hypertension

Hypertension may either precede pregnancy (chronic hypertension in pregnancy, CHP) or result, in a previously normotensive woman, from a disorder of pregnancy itself (pregnancy-induced hypertension, PIH). PIH usually occurs after week 24 of gestation and often, even if not always, is associated with proteinuria and/or edema. When these associations obtain, the syndrome is defined as *toxemia of pregnancy, preeclampsia,* or *EPH gestosis* (E, edema; P, proteinuria; H, hypertension) [14]. The last definition has been proposed and recommended by the Gestosis Organization [15].

In this chapter, CHP and PIH are discussed as definite entities. The reader, however, should always bear in mind that neither of these definitions indicates a single nosologic unit, but rather encircles a group of disorders.

1.2.1. Chronic hypertension in pregnancy (CHP)

Plasma volume has been found to be lower during pregnancy in patients with chronic hypertension than in normotensive patients [16, 17]. The effects of hypertension on plasma volume in pregnancy depend on the level of blood pressure. In pregnant women with CHP, in fact, plasma volume is negatively correlated with blood pressure [18]. Sibai et al. detected no plasma volume depletion in pregnant women with mild hypertension, but the same authors observed volume depletion in severely hypertensive patients [19, 20]. Similarly, Lim and Walters [21] found no difference in average plasma volume of normotensive and mildly hypertensive patients, but in the latter a relative volume depletion was suggested by increased hematocrit.

The effects of CHP on CO are not as clear as those on plasma volume. Lim and Walters [21] found a greater CO in patients with mild hypertension than in normotensive subjects. On the other hand, others either found a considerable reduction in CO in patients with CHP or did not detect any difference in CO between normotensive and hypertensive gravidas [8, 22]. These discrepancies probably reflect the heterogeneity of the pathogenic conditions included in the definition of *chronic hypertension.* More convincing information on the changes occurring in central hemodynamics with pregnancy in chronically hypertensive subjects would be obtained with serial studies. Until these become available, however, some useful information may be derived from animal studies with a reproducible type of chronic hypertension. Thus, in rats with either spontaneous (SRH strain) or renal hypertension, the increased blood pressure has been shown to prevent partially or completely the normal rise in CO during gestation [11, 22]. Recently we have shown that a salt-losing tendency in pregnant rats with renal hypertension is associated with decreased salt retention and weight gain [23]. These findings suggest that, in rats with chronic hypertension, the reduced plasma volume and CO reflects extracellular fluid volume depletion.

1.2.2. Pregnancy-induced hypertension (PIH)

Even if some anecdotal exceptions have been reported [24], there is general agreement that plasma volume in patients with PIH is decreased as compared with that in normal pregnant women [25]. The reduction in plasma volume occurs early in patients with PIH, some evidence even existing that volume depletion precedes the development of hypertension [18, 26]. A matter of debate is the degree of volume depletion. Goodlin [27], in fact, has characterized severe preeclampsia as being a state of "chronic shock," while Assali and Vaughn [28] have minimized the reduction in blood volume as being a simple adjustment to reduced vascular capacity ensuing from increased peripheral vascular resistance. Probably, there is some truth in both of these extremes. In a series of studies reported by Assali and Vaughn [28], average volume depletion ranged from 5% to 29%, and this great variability should undoubtedly reflect even larger individual variations. The variable changes in plasma volume probably account for the variable changes observed in CO [8, 29]. Whatever the effects of PIH on plasma volume and CO are, this disorder is definitely associated with a rise in peripheral vascular resistance [29]. This hemodynamic change, therefore, entirely accounts for the increase in blood pressure.

It is of great interest that in PIH there is no apparent relation between the degree of plasma volume depletion and the overall status of extracellular fluid volume (ECV). Similar reductions of plasma volume, in fact, have been found in nonedematous patients as in patients with gross peripheral edema, indicating large ECV expansion [18]. Clearly, in the latter condition, fluid has to be redistributed out of the intravascular compartment into the interstitial space.

1.3. Conclusions

In conclusion, plasma volume and cardiac output increase in normal pregnancy. Present data indicate that plasma volume depletion (compared with the expected volume expansion) is a common condition in both CHP and PIH. While in CHP the reduced plasma volume seems to reflect reduced ECV and salt depletion, however, in PIH the primary mechanism for decreased plasma volume seems to be a redistribution of fluid out of the intravascular compartment (table 1-1).

Table 1-1. Effects of pregnancy on systemic hemodynamics and extracellular fluid volume

	Normal pregnancy	CHP[a]	PIH[b]
Blood pressure	↓=	↑	↑
Total peripheral resistance	↓	↑	↑
Blood volume	↑	↓	↓
Extracellular fluid volume	↑	↓?	↑

[a]Chronic hypertension in pregnancy.
[b]Pregnancy-induced hypertension.

2. CHANGES IN RENAL HEMODYNAMICS

2.1. Normal pregnancy

The effects of normal human pregnancy on renal plasma flow (RPF) have been exhaustively reviewed by Davison and Dunlop [30], who have emphasized that defects in methodology account for some discrepant results found in the past. In normal pregnancy, RPF rises after week 9 of gestation; it increases by a maximum of 50%–85% until week 20 and then declines after approximately week 30, remaining higher than before pregnancy until term.

The rise in RPF is associated with a rise in glomerular filtration rate (GFR). GFR increases as early as five weeks after the last menstruation [31], reaches a maximum increment of 50% by week 16 of gestation, and remains at this level later in pregnancy [32].

2.1.1. Intrarenal mechanisms

The intrarenal mechanisms responsible for the changes in RPF and GFR have been studied by micropuncture technique in the rat. Also in this animal species, in fact, RPF and GFR increase during gestation. The rise in both total GFR and GFR in single nephrons (SNGFR) has been shown to occur as early as after 5–6 days of gestation [33–35] (gestation in rats lasts 21–22 days). Baylis [36] has found a 29% increase in SNGFR in nine- to 12-day pregnant rats. At this stage of pregnancy, the rise in SNGFR is entirely due to an increase in glomerular plasma flow (GPF), the other determinants of ultrafiltration (i.e., filtration pressure and the ultrafiltration coefficient) being unmodified. The increase in SNGFR and GPF is strictly proportional, as is expected since the rats are in the condition of filtration pressure equilibrium. By definition, this means that the transcapillary pressure gradient is zero at the efferent end of glomerular capillaries, a condition in which the rate of ultrafiltration is directly dependent on GPF [37].

Further modifications in glomerular dynamics have been shown by us to occur later in gestation [38]. In 15- to 16-day pregnant rats, in fact, a significant rise in glomerular hydrostatic pressure (PG) is associated with a rise in GPF that is even greater than in early gestation (+65%). Both changes are secondary to a marked fall in the resistance of the afferent arteriole, which is almost halved. Unfortunately, data on arteriole resistance have not been reported in 12-day pregnant rats. The rise in PG and the greater increase in GPF occurring in 15-day pregnant rats, however, probably reflect a more pronounced afferent arteriole dilatation in 15-day than in 12-day pregnant animals.

The 15-day pregnant rats differ from those at 12 days of gestation in other respects. In 15-day pregnant rats, in fact, filtration pressure equilibrium is not achieved, allowing more precise calculation of the ultrafiltration coefficient (K_f). The ultrafiltration coefficient represents the product of the filtering area surface and the capillary hydraulic permeability, and is significantly decreased in 15-day pregnant rats. This decrease is moderate (-14%) and, in normal rats, its effect in lowering SNGFR is counterbalanced by the rise in filtration pressure resulting from increased PG. The low K_f in 15-day pregnant rats, however, prevents the rise in SNGFR that is normally caused by ECV expansion with saline [38]. This occurs because ECV expansion raises SNGFR by increasing GPF. The dependence of SNGFR on GPF, however, declines as GPF rises and is greatly attenuated at the huge values of GPF occurring with volume expansion in pregnant rats. In this condition, therefore, the influence of other determinants of ultrafiltration, such as K_f, on SNGFR becomes fully evident.

2.1.2. Relations of intrarenal changes with hormonal factors

The modifications in renal hemodynamics occurring in pregnancy may be, at least in part, secondary to changes in hormone activity. Thus, the marked renal vasodilatation may be due to increased prostaglandin(s) (PG) secretion. In fact, both plasma concentration and urinary excretion of PGE, which is known to have potent renal vasodilatory effect, are increased in human pregnancy [39, 40]. Increased activity of prostacyclin (PGI_2) might also contribute to renal vasodilation [41]. Pregnancy is associated with a rise in plasma renin activity, plasma renin concentration, plasma renin substrate concentration, and plasma concentration of aldosterone and angiotensin II [42, 43]. The reasons for this resetting of the renin–aldosterone system are not well understood, even if these changes are related to both the complex circulatory adjustments and the modifications in salt balance taking place during gestation. It is possible, however, that the rise in plasma angiotensin-II concentration is mainly responsible for the decrease in ultrafiltration coefficient detected in pregnant rats [38]. In pregnant women, plasma parathyroid hormone concentration increases in the second trimester [44]. Should this occur also in rats, it might contribute to the reduction of the ultrafiltration coefficient [45]. Among sexual hormones that increase during pregnancy, prolactin is able to increase SNGFR, while there is evidence that progesterone is not able to do so [46].

2.2. Pregnancy and hypertension

2.2.1. Chronic hypertension in pregnancy (CHP)

To our knowledge, no serial study of renal hemodynamics has been performed in pregnant women with chronic hypertension. The information available is limited, therefore, to uncontrolled measurements of GFR and RPF in third-trimester patients. Lindheimer and Katz [47], in patients with mild to moderate hypertension, found an average GFR of 180 ml/min (range, 166–211) and an average RPF of 841 ml/min (range, 511–914). Both of these average values are within the range of normality, close to its upper limit [30]. In contrast with these findings, Sarles et al. [48] found that both GFR and RPF were consistently lower in patients with CHP than in normal subjects. This discrepancy is not surprising, however, if one considers that renal function may be affected by chronic hypertension to a variable degree; hence the need for investigation of the changes in GFR and RPF as gestation starts and progresses in hypertensive patients.

Unfortunately, our poor information in the human does not receive adequate compensation from animal studies. At present, some information is available only in the rat. Lindheimer et al. [49] have studied kidney function in pregnant rats with spontaneous hypertension (SHR), using normotensive rats of the same strain (WKY) as control. Total kidney GFR did not increase with pregnancy in SHR, while it did in WHY. Filtration fraction was unchanged during pregnancy in SHR, while it increased in WHY. Some caution is necessary, however, in interpreting these results, since GFR is basically (that is, independently of pregnancy) lower in SHR than in WHY rats, and the lower GFR in SHR may be a primary characteristic with a pathogenetic role in the development of hypertension. In addition, pregnancy did not increase plasma renin activity in SHR or in WHY rats, in contrast with what occurs normally in this as well as in other animal species. Preliminary micropuncture data on glomerular hemodynamics have been recently obtained by us in pregnant rats with renal hypertension [50]. Munich-Wistar rats were rendered hypertensive by placing a clip on one renal artery. The untouched kidney was studied five weeks after this maneuver, at day 15 of gestation. Rats that remained normotensive despite insertion of the clip were used as controls. In hypertensive rats, SNGFR was moderately, but not significantly, higher than in controls, while GPF was greatly increased, thereby accounting for a fall in filtration fraction. The rise in GPF was clearly secondary to impaired autoregulation, i.e., to a rise in afferent arteriole resistance that was inadequate to counterbalance the increased arterial perfusion pressure [50].

2.2.2. Pregnancy-induced hypertension (PIH)

Our information on the effects of PIH on renal hemodynamics is not satisfactory and is almost entirely confined to humans, owing to the difficulty of reproducing PIH in most animal species. It is clear, however, that the renal hemodynamic changes caused by PIH encompass a wide range of variations, from a mild to moderate decrease in GFR and RPF [51, 52] to a picture of acute renal failure [53]. The reduced GFR and RPF are secondary to a rise in renal vascular resistance, which seems to be located in the afferent vascular segment [54]. The renal changes are related to the levels of hypertension. When PIH is severe, irreversible defects in renal cortical perfusion may occur [53].

2.2.3. Hormonal factors

In vitro studies have detected decreased production of prostacyclin (PGI_2) by maternal blood vessels in women with PIH [55], suggesting a PGI_2 deficiency as a possible vasoconstrictive mechanism in the renal circulation. Ylikorkala [41], however, did not find any decrease in the circulating levels of 6-cheto-PGF_1 (the stable metabolite of PGI_2), and Fievet et al. [56] found a normal urinary excretion of 6-cheto-$PGF_{1\alpha}$ in patients with PIH. Even in the presence of normal PGI_2 production, an increased ratio of thromboxane A_2 (the vasoconstrictor prostaglandin) to PGI_2 has been suggested to account for vasoconstriction in PIH [57]. Urinary excretion of PGE is normal in patients with PIH [40, 56]. Since urinary levels reflect renal synthesis of PGE, decreased intrarenal production of this vasodilator prostaglandin seems not to be responsible for the rise in renal vascular resistance occurring in PIH. Urinary excretion of PGE has been found to be inversely related to level of hypertension in a group of patients with chronic hypertension in pregnancy [40]. The renal impairment in PGE production, however, probably reflected in these patients the renal damage secondary to chronic hypertension.

3. RENAL HEMODYNAMICS AND SALT EXCRETION

As discussed in chapter 5, during pregnancy a new salt balance develops that allows salt retention. This new equilibrium, however, appears labile, to the point that pregnancy has been compared with a condition of subtle salt wasting (see chapter 5). There is some evidence that this salt-losing tendency is greater in hypertensive pregnant subjects. Thus, Sarles et al. [48] have found a higher baseline sodium excretion in pregnant patients with essential hypertension than in normotensive pregnant subjects. To our knowledge, however, no adequately controlled balance study has been performed in man as yet. We have carried out balance studies in rats with renal hypertension [50]. This model has some advantages, such as the possibility of knowing exactly the duration and severity of hypertension; furthermore, the effects of this model of hypertension on salt balance in nonpregnant rats are already well known [58]. The results of our studies are summarized in figure 1-1. As shown in the figure, (a) pregnant rats excrete more salt than do nonpregnant rats, whatever the level of blood pressure is, and (b) in pregnant rats, the higher blood pressure is, the greater is salt excretion.

These results indicate clearly that hemodynamic factors are important determinants of salt excretion in pregnancy. It is our opinion that the renal hemodynamic changes characteristic of pregnancy contribute to the subtle salt-losing tendency in this condition and account for the increased salt excretion caused by hypertension. Both the increase in GFR and the reduction in filtration fraction (which was found in single nephrons in hypertensive rats) [50], in fact, predispose the subject to increased salt excretion by respectively increasing the filtered load of salt and decreasing peritubular oncotic pressure and consequently salt reabsorption in the proximal tubule. Another mechanism, however, may be even more important in

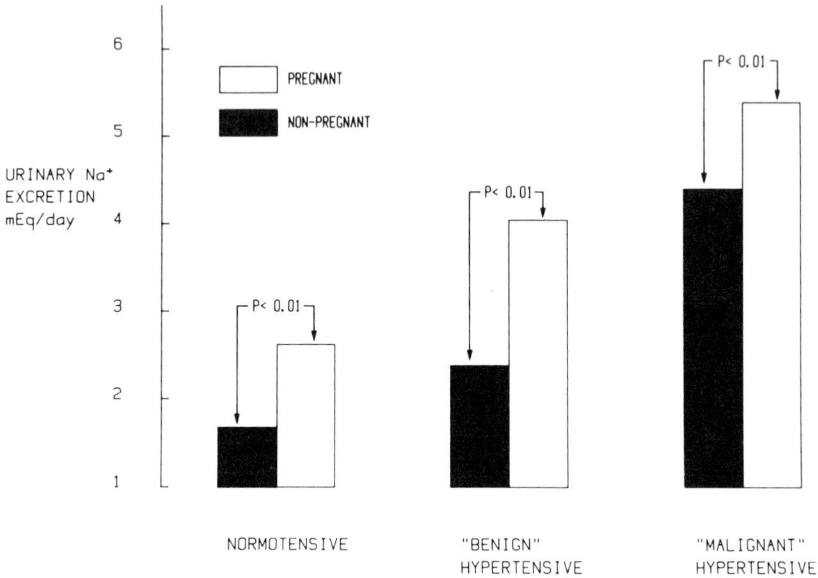

Figure 1-1. Average urinary sodium excretion in pregnant and nonpregnant rats. Systolic blood pressure was < 130 mm Hg in *normotensive* rats, 140–180 mm Hg in *"benign" hypertensive* rats, and > 180 mm Hg in *"malignant" hypertensive* rats.

eliciting increased salt excretion in hypertensive pregnant rats; that is, the transmission of increased hemodynamic pressure to the vasa recta. This mechanism is made possible by the potent renal vasodilatory effect of pregnancy that blunts renal autoregulation. In pregnant rats with renal hypertension, in fact, total arteriolar glomerular resistance is much lower than in nonpregnant rats with a similar degree of high blood pressure (figure 1-2). Inhibition of salt reabsorption in the Henle loop by increased hemodynamic pressure in the vasa recta is considered to be responsible also for the exaggerated natriuresis of hypertension [59]. Exaggerated natriuresis is the phenomenon (independent of pregnancy) by which hypertensive patients excrete a salt load more rapidly than do normotensive subjects [60]. In exaggerated natriuresis, renal vasodilatation is evoked by rapid ECV expansion. Increased perfusion pressure and renal vasodilatation, therefore, occur in exaggerated natriuresis as in CHP.

In conclusion, we propose that renal vasodilatation is responsible for the increased salt excretion observed in hypertensive pregnant rats. The mechanism by which this occurs is similar to that elicited by salt loading in hypertensive nonpregnant subjects.

ACKNOWLEDGMENT

This work was supported by CNR (*Consiglio Nazionale delle Ricerche,* Italy), contract 78.01958.04.

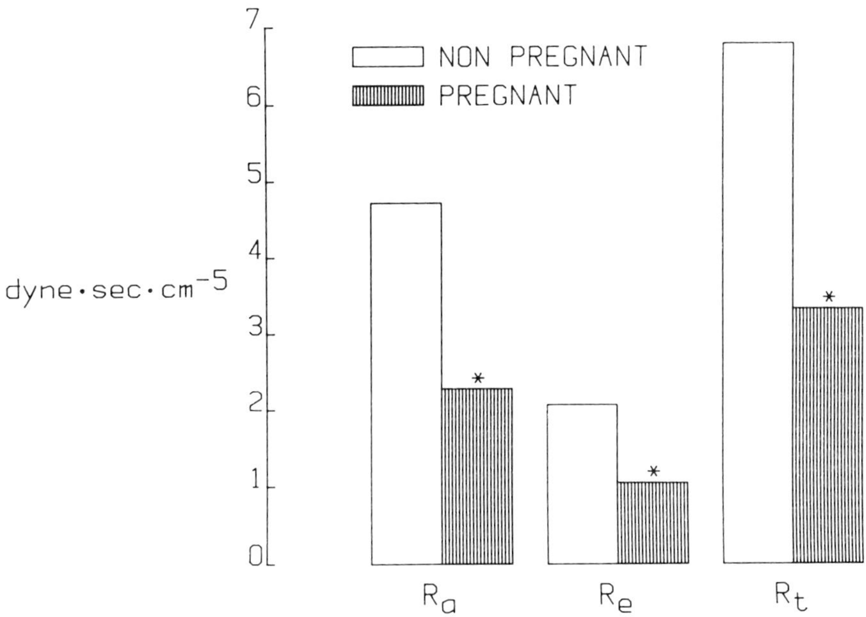

Figure 1-2. Effect of pregnancy on glomerular resistances in hypertensive rats: R_a, *afferent arteriole resistance;* R_e, *efferent arteriole resistance; and* R_t, *total glomerular resistance* (* $p < 0.01$).

REFERENCES

1. Hyhen FE, Paintin DB: Increase in plasma volume during normal pregnancy. Br J Obstet Gynaecol 70:402–407, 1963.
2. Pirani BBK, Campbell DM, MacGillivray I: Plasma volume in normal first pregnancy. J Obstet Gynaecol Br Commonw 80:884–887, 1973.
3. Pritchard T: Changes in blood volume during pregnancy and delivery. Anesthesiology 26:-393–399, 1965.
4. Bader ME, Bader RA: Cardiovascular hemodynamics in pregnancy and labor. Clin Obstet Gynecol 11:924–939, 1968.
5. Lees MM, Taylor SH, Scott DB, Kerr MG: A study of cardiac output at rest throughout pregnancy. J Obstet Gynaecol Br Commonw 74:319–328, 1967.
6. Ueland K, Novy MJ, Petersen EN, Metcalfe J: Maternal cardiovascular dynamics. IV. The influence of gestational age on the maternal cardiovascular response to posture and exercise. Am J Obstet Gynecol 104:856–864, 1969.
7. Myhrman P, Granerus G, Karlsson K, Lundgren Y: Cardiac output in normal pregnancy measured by impedance cardiography. Scand J Clin Lab Invest 42:513–520, 1982.
8. Larkin H, Gallery EDM, Hunyor SN, Gyory AZ, Boyce ES: Cardiac and haemodynamic measurements in hypertensive pregnancy. Clin Sci 59:357s–360s, 1980.
9. Lees MM: Central circulatory responses in normotensive and hypertensive pregnancy. Postgrad Med J 55:311–314, 1979.
10. Nuwayhid B: Hemodynamic changes during pregnancy in the rabbit. Am J Obstet Gynecol 135:590–596, 1979.
11. Lundgren Y, Karlsson K, Ljungblad U: Circulatory changes during pregnancy in spontaneously and renal hypertensive rats. Clin Sci 57:337s–339s, 1979.
12. Baylis C: Effect of early pregnancy on glomerular filtration rate and plasma volume in the rat. Renal Physiol 2:333–339, 1980.

13. Atherton JC, Dark JM, Garland HO, Morgan MRA, Pidgeon J, Soni S: Changes in water and electrolyte balance, plasma volume and composition during pregnancy in the rat. J Physiol 330:81–94, 1982.
14. Dal Canton A, Dall'Aglio P, Olivetti G, Gardini F, Benassi L, Migone L: EPH-gestosis isolated and complicating a pre-existing renal disease. Panminerva Med 19:415–422, 1977.
15. Rippmann ET: The organization gestosis. In: Hommel AG (ed) EPH-gestosis. Zurich: Bühler, 1972, pp 24–26.
16. Arias F: Expansion of intravascular volume and fetal outcome in patients with chronic hypertension and pregnancy. Am J Obstet Gynecol 123:610, 1975.
17. Soffronoff EC, Kaufman BM, Connaughton JF: Intravascular volume determinations and fetal outcome in hypertensive disease of pregnancy. Am J Obstet Gynecol 127:4–9, 1977.
18. Gallery EDM, Hunyor SN, Györy AZ: Plasma volume contraction: a significant factor in both pregnancy-associated hypertension (pre-eclampsia) and chronic hypertension in pregnancy. Q J Med 48:593–602, 1979.
19. Sibai BM, Abdella TN, Anderson GD, Dilts PV: Plasma volume findings in pregnant women with mild hypertension: therapeutic considerations. Am J Obstet Gynecol 145:539–544, 1983.
20. Sibai BM, Abdella TN, Anderson GD, McCubbin JH: Plasma volume determination in pregnancies complicated by chronic hypertension and intrauterine fetal demise. Obstet Gynecol: 174–178, 1982.
21. Lim YL, Walters WAW: Haemodynamics of mild hypertension in pregnancy. Br J Obstet Gynaecol 86:198–204, 1979.
22. Lundgren Y, Karlsson K, Ljungblad U: Changes in central hemodynamics during pregnancy in renal hypertensive rats. Clin Exp Hypertens [B] 1:441–453, 1982.
23. Dal Canton A, Sabbatini M. Esposito C, Altomonte M, Romano G, Uccello F, Andreucci VE: Renal function in pregnant rats with 2-kidney Goldblatt hypertension. Proc Eur Dial Transplant Assoc 20:499–506, 1983.
24. Goodlin R, Holdt D, Woods R: Pregnancy-induced hypertension associated with hypervolemia: case report. Am J Obstet Gynecol 142:114–115, 1982.
25. Sehgal NN, Hitt JR: Plasma volume expansion in the treatment of pre-eclampsia. Am J Obstet Gynecol 138:165–168, 1980.
26. Blekta M, Hlavaty V, Trukova M, Bendl J, Bendova L, Chytil M: Volume of whole blood and absolute amount of serum proteins in the early stage of late toxemia of pregnancy. Am J Obstet Gynecol 106:10–13, 1970.
27. Goodlin RC: Severe pre-eclampsia another great imitator. Am J Obstet Gynecol 125:747–753, 1976.
28. Assali NS, Vaughn DL: Blood volume in pre-eclampsia: fantasy and reality. Am J Obstet Gynecol 129:355–359, 1977.
29. Assali NS, Holm LW, Parker HR: Systemic and regional alterations in toxaemia. Circulation [Suppl 11] 29 and 30:11–53, 1964.
30. Davison JM, Dunlop W: Renal hemodynamics and tubular function in normal human pregnancy. Kidney Int 18:152–161, 1980.
31. Davison JM: Changes in renal function and other aspects of homeostasis in early pregnancy. J Obstet Gynaecol Br Commonw 81:1003, 1974.
32. Dunlop W: Renal physiology in pregnancy. Postgrad Med J 55:329–332, 1979.
33. Atherton JC, Pirie SC: The effect of pregnancy on glomerular filtration rate and salt and water reabsorption in the rat. J Physiol 319:153–164, 1981.
34. Atherton JC: Glomerular filtration rate and salt and water reabsorption during pregnancy in the conscious rat. J Physiol 334:493–504, 1983.
35. Garland HO, Green R: Micropuncture study of changes in glomerular filtration and ion and water handling by the rat kidney during pregnancy. J Physiol 329:389–409, 1982.
36. Baylis C: The mechanism of the increase in glomerular filtration rate in the twelve-day pregnant rat. J Physiol 305:405–414, 1980.
37. Brenner BM, Troy JL, Daugharty TM, Deen WM, Robertson CR: Dynamics of glomerular ultrafiltration in the rat. II. Plasma flow dependence of GFR. Am J Physiol 223:1184–1190, 1972.
38. Dal Canton A, Conte G, Esposito C, Guasco R, Russo D, Sabbatini M, Uccello F, Andreucci VE: Effects of pregnancy on glomerular dynamics: micropuncture study in the rat. Kidney Int 22:608–612, 1982.

39. Bay WH, Ferris TF: Factors controlling plasma renin and aldosterone during pregnancy. Hypertension 1:410–415, 1979.
40. Montquin JM, Leblanc N: A prospective study of urinary prostaglandins E in women with normal and hypertensive pregnancies. Clin Exper Hypertens [B] 1:539–552, 1982.
41. Ylikorkala O: Prostacyclin and thromboxane during human pregnancy. Acta Obstet Gynecol Scand [Suppl] 113:51–53, 1983.
42. Geelhoed GW, Vander AJ: Plasma renin activities during pregnancy and parturition. J Clin Endocrinol Metab 28:412–415, 1968.
43. Weir RJ, Jehoiada, Brown J, Fraser R, Lever AF, Logan RW, Mellwaine GM, Morton JJ, Robertson JIS, Tree M: Relationship between plasma renin, renin substrate, angiotensin II, aldosterone and electrolytes in normal pregnancy. J Clin Endocrinol Metab 40:108–115, 1975.
44. Conforti A, Biale Y, Levi M, Shany S, Shainkin-Kestenbaum R, Berlyne GM: Changes in serum calcitonin, parathyroid hormone and 25-hydroxycholecalciferol levels in pregnancy and labor. Minerva Electrol Metab 3:323–328, 1980.
45. Ichikawa J, Humes HD, Dousa TP, Brenner BM: Influence of parathyroid hormone a glomerular ultrafiltration in the rat. Renal Fluid Electrol Physiol 3:F393–F401, 1978.
46. Elkaril AO, Garland HO, Green R: Acute and chronic effects of progesterone and prolactin on renal function in the rat. J Physiol 337:389–400, 1983.
47. Lindheimer MD, Katz AI: Effects of hypotonic expansion on sodium and water excretion in hypertensive non-preeclamptic gravidas. Am J Obstet Gynecol 111:1053–1058, 1971.
48. Sarles HE, Hill SS, Le Blanc AL, Smith GH, Canales CO, Remmers AR: Sodium excretion patterns during and following intravenous sodium chloride loads in normal and hypertensive pregnancies. Am J Obstet Gynecol 102:1–7, 1968.
49. Lindheimer MD, Katz AI, Koeppen BM, Ordoner NG, Oparil S: Kidney function and sodium handling in the pregnant spontaneously hypertensive rat. Hypertension 5:498–506, 1983.
50. Dal Canton A, Sabbatini M, Esposito C, Altomonte M, Romano G, Uccello F, Conte G, Fuiano G, Russo D, Andreucci VE: Effects of hypertension on renal function in pregnant rats. Contrib Nephrol 37:179–181, 1984.
51. Gallery EDM, Györy AZ: Glomerular and proximal renal tubular function in pregnancy-associated hypertension. Eur J Obstet Gynaecol Reprod Biol 9:3–12, 1979.
52. Topporada M, Ghoneim A, Habib YA, El-Ziadi L, El-Damarawy H: Effect of prostaglandin A on renal hemodynamics in pregnancy toxemia. Am J Obstet Gynecol 135:581–585, 1979.
53. Burden RP, Boyd WN, Aber GM: Structural and functional changes in the renal circulation after complicated pregnancy. Nephron 24:183–192, 1979.
54. Assali NS, Kaplan SA, Fomon J, Douglass RA Jr: Renal function studies in toxemia of pregnancy. J Clin Invest 32:44–51, 1953.
55. Bussolino F, Benedetto C, Massohrio M, Camussi G: Maternal vascular prostacyclin activity in pre-eclampsia. Lancet 2:702, 1980.
56. Fievet P, Fournier A, Agnes E, Herve MA, Carayon A, De Fremont JF, Miruran A, Dufour A, Verhoest P, Boulanger JC: Renin angiotensin aldosterone system urinary prostaglandins and kallikrein in pregnancy induced hypertension. Proc Eur Dial Transplant Assoc, 1984 (in press).
57. Remuzzi G, Zoja C, Marchesi D, Schieppati A, Mecca G, Misiani R, Donati MB, De Gaetano G: Plasmatic regulation of vascular prostacyclin in pregnancy. Br Med J 282:512–514, 1981.
58. Möhring J, Möhring B, Näumann HJ, Philippi A, Homsey E, Orth H, Dauda G, Kazda S, Gross F: Salt and water balance and renin activity in renal hypertension of rats. Am J Physiol 228:1847–1855, 1975.
59. Dal Canton A, Conte G, Fuiano G, Guasco R, Andreucci VE: Exaggerated natriuresis in the hypertensive man: clinical evidence for intrarenal hemodynamic heterogeneity. Nephron 27:-122–126, 1981.
60. Buckalew VM, Puschett JB, Kentzel JE, Goldberg M: Mechanism of exaggerated natriuresis in hypertensive man: impaired sodium transport in the loop of Henle. J Clin Invest 48:1007–1016, 1969.

2. PATHOGENESIS OF PREECLAMPSIA

GINA GREGORINI, NORBERTO PERICO, and GIUSEPPE REMUZZI

1. INTRODUCTION

Preeclampsia commonly occurs in primiparas [1], the usual clinical manifestations being hypertension, proteinuria, and edema. Even after a severe preeclampsia in the first pregnancy, however, these women may have no more trouble in subsequent pregnancies [2]. Preeclampsia, in fact, is rare in multiparas unless there are some predisposing factors, such as conditions associated with increased placental mass (hydatiform mole, Rh incompatibility, twin pregnancies) or previous maternal vascular diseases, such as essential hypertension, hypertensive nephropathies, or autoimmune disorders with vascular damage (scleroderma, systemic lupus erythematosus). Placental tissue, but not fetus, is required for development of preeclampsia, as in pregnancy complicated by hydatiform mole.

Preeclampsia appears typically in late pregnancy and dramatically resolves without residual damage within a short time after delivery, even in the severe forms [2]. Two main target organs are involved in this systemic disease: the kidney and the uterus. These organs share the same ability to produce renin and prostaglandins (PG), which seem to play a significant role in the pathogenesis of preeclampsia.

Although the etiology of preeclampsia remains unclear, our understanding of the pathophysiology of the disease has greatly increased in the last 30 years.

2. ANIMAL MODELS OF PREECLAMPSIA

Preeclampsia does not occur spontaneously in animals, and this lack of a natural model in laboratory animals has resulted in much effort to induce the disease experimentally. Several experimental models have been proposed, in which the disease may be induced by diet, uteroplacental ischemia, experimental hypertension, placental extract infusion, or immunologic damage to placenta.

2.1. Diet

For a long time, preeclampsia has been attributed to a deficiency of essential nutritional factors in relation to the increased needs of both mother and fetus. Consequently, changes in diet composition have been used to induce experimental toxemia.

In 1959, Stamler [3] studied the effects in pregnant rats of a low-vitamin-E (tocopherol) diet containing highly unsaturated fatty acids whose oxidative action was believed to annul the already low level of antioxidants. Rats 75 days old were fed this basic diet starting on day 13 of gestation. No evidence of illness occurred, however, until day 21 or 22 of gestation, when a majority of primigravidas died in rapid succession. Postmortem examination of the animals showed generalized venous engorgement, cardiac dilation, pulmonary congestion, and hemorrhagic edema. Microscopic examination revealed diffuse thrombosis of capillaries, arterioles, and venules in lungs, spleen, and kidneys, but rarely in adrenals, liver, and gastrointestinal tract. Unlike in human toxemia, fetuses were numerous, well developed, and usually alive and vigorous when examined immediately after maternal death. Clinical and pathologic signs of the disease were present only in pregnant rats, not in nonpregnant controls fed the same diet.

Subsequently the basic dietary regimen was greatly modified in many ways. Modifications in carbohydrate, mineral, and protein contents did not affect the toxicity of the diet, nor did supplementation with brewer's yeast or vitamins other than vitamin E. The toxicity of the diet increased only when the content of cod liver oil—rich in polyunsaturated fatty acids—was raised above 5% or when partial lipid peroxidation took place, suggesting that the lipid content was a critical component in the appearance of the disease. The addition to the diet of tocopherol preparations was the only completely successful means adequate to prevent the death of pregnant rats receiving the basic eclamptogenic diet; all of the other synthetic antioxidants could only partially replace tocopherol.

This model clearly indicates a relationship between the development of an acute fatal disease in pregnant rats and the intake of a substantial amount of partially oxidized polyunsaturated fatty acids in a diet with virtually no vitamin E as antioxidant. The protective action of α-tocopherol is presumably a function of its antioxidant nature, although a possible specific role in relation to an enzyme system is not excluded. In the context of this model, Spitz et al. [4] studied the production of prostacyclin (PGI_2)—an arachidonic acid (AA) metabolite with potent vasodilatory and antiaggregatory activity—by mesometrial triangles from pregnant rats.

These are vascular structures in the mesometrium associated with the developing placenta, comparable with the maternal part of human placenta. The authors observed that, in pregnant rats fed a diet containing very little tocopherol and highly unsaturated fatty acids (antivitamin-E stress diet), mesometrial triangles produced less PGI_2 than in rats fed a normal diet, and higher concentrations of free-radical oxidation products were found in the plasma. Furthermore, the group of rats fed the antivitamin-E stress diet developed toxemia-like symptoms. These findings have suggested that antivitamin-E stress diet induces an increase in free-radical oxidation products, which are known to inhibit PGI_2 synthetase and therefore vascular PGI_2 production, the major local defense mechanism in placental vessels during pregnancy.

Other authors investigated the role of selective depletion of divalent ions to induce a disease similar to human preeclampsia. A low-magnesium (Mg) diet was implicated in the etiology of preeclampsia. Early depletion of Mg in pregnant ewes induced hypertension, intrauterine growth retardation, and intrauterine death with placental infarcts. Renal involvement was indicated by significant proteinuria, and elevation of serum creatinine and blood urea, as well as by light- and electron-microscopic evidence of glomerular swelling and subendothelial fibrin deposition. Evidence for intravascular coagulation has been observed [5]. Similarly, zinc depletion and cadmium toxicity (which could potentiate the effects of zinc deficiency) have been shown to produce hypertension, vasospasm, proteinuria, sodium retention, edema, and convulsions in pregnant animals [6]. Since a possible association has been recently postulated between low calcium (Ca) intake and pregnancy-induced hypertension, the effect of a Ca-deficient diet before and during pregnancy has become the object of a more detailed analysis. Blood pressure in rats fed a Ca-free diet rose significantly after six weeks of treatment, compared with rats fed a normal diet. Thereafter, the animals were mated, but pregnant and nonpregnant animals on the Ca-free diet continued to present significantly higher blood pressure [7]. This supports the hypothesis that a low-Ca diet is associated with high blood pressure in pregnant and nonpregnant female rats.

Finally, several investigators have studied the effects of food restriction on cardiac output and blood flow to the uterus and placenta in pregnant rats. They observed that rats fed a 50% restricted diet from day 5 of gestation had lower body weight, and smaller fetuses and placentas; these rats also had a marked reduction in cardiac output and blood flow to placenta, but not to endometrium and myometrium [8, 9]. This suggests that food restriction reduces the expansion of uterine and placental blood flow by interfering with the increase in cardiac output that normally occurs in pregnancy.

2.2. Uteroplacental ischemia

Uteroplacental ischemia is assumed to increase blood pressure and induce fibrin deposition, releasing pressor substances and thromboplastic phospholipids into the systemic circulation [10]. Since reduced uterine blood flow is a characteristic of preeclampsia, different techniques have been used to induce a chronic reduction of uterine blood flow in pregnant animals.

Restricting the enlarging uterus in a cellophane wrapping failed to produce a model of preeclampsia in rats, but was effective in other species [11]. More satisfactory experimental models of preeclampsia in different species were obtained by severe constriction of the abdominal aorta to reduce uterine blood flow to 35%–40% [12]. This technique has been improved by reducing uterine blood flow in continuously controlled and monitored conditions to avoid fetal death and maintain an effective reduction of uterine blood flow. This experimental model, first applied to dogs, rabbits, cats, monkeys [12], and more recently to small animals like guinea pigs and rats [13], has also been used with primates (baboons) [14], whose reproductive physiology is very close to that of humans. It has been shown that severe interference in uterine blood flow in these animals produces placental ischemia with diffuse placental infarcts, suggesting that placental infarcts are directly related to induced ischemia [13]. It is important to note that placental infarcts rarely appear in pregnant animals [15], while they are a common occurrence in humans near term, especially in toxemia. Moreover, as in humans, the severity of experimental toxemia in the animals was related to the number of placental infarcts.

2.3. Preexisting experimental hypertension

In rats, and to some extent in other animals, the mere presence of hypertension before pregnancy is not always an adverse prognostic factor during pregnancy itself. It has been demonstrated, in fact, that spontaneously hypertensive rats do not develop preeclampsia, and their systemic blood pressure decreases in the last weeks of pregnancy [16]. Pregnant Goldblatt hypertensive rats—made hypertensive by removing one kidney and clamping the other one—behaved in the same way regarding blood pressure in late pregnancy, and no preeclampsia was observed [17]. Uninephrectomized DOCA–NaCl hypertensive rats, however, given 4 mg/kg day DOCA (desoxycorticosterone acetate) and drinking 0.9% NaCl rather than water, exhibited a worsening of hypertension, proteinuria, a rapid weight gain, and convulsions during pregnancy [17]. Fetal mortality increased to 34% while fetal weight and litter size decreased. Placentas showed frequent areas of hemorrhagic necrosis. Diffuse endothelial swelling and large deposits of dense fibrillar and granular material were found in the kidneys in comparison with nonpregnant hypertensive controls. In this model, however, the delivery did not effectively reduce blood pressure, which remained higher than in nonpregnant hypertensive controls with a progression of glomerular damage toward chronic renal failure [17].

2.4. Placental extract infusion

In order to test the hypothesis that a placental factor is responsible for at least some of the clinical signs of preeclampsia, extracts prepared from term placentas of preeclamptic and normotensive women were infused acutely and chronically in virgin female and pregnant rats [18]. In both groups, acute infusion of preeclamptic placental extracts produced a significant increase in blood pressure, proteinuria and, in the pregnant group, acute vasospasm. The angiotensin-II (AII) receptor blocker —salarasin—reversed these effects. Only pregnant rats, however, responded to chronic infusions of small doses of preeclamptic placental extracts with an increase in blood pressure. No differences in plasma renin activity (PRA), plasma angiotensin I (AI), or aldosterone levels between preeclamptic placental extracts, normal placental extracts, and saline-treated rats were found. This study suggests that the vascular effects of preeclamptic placental extracts are not the result of stimulation of the renin–angiotensin system, but that these extracts act upon AII receptors, either by binding to them or by increasing their number or affinity for circulating AII.

A toxemia-like syndrome was similarly induced in pregnant dogs by intraperitoneal injection of concentrates prepared from placentas of patients with preeclampsia or hydatiform mole [19]. Both of these concentrates progressively caused hypertension, proteinuria, disseminated intravascular coagulation, and hepatic dysfunction, in addition to intrauterine growth retardation or intrauterine death. This syndrome did not develop with concentrates prepared from placentas of normal term pregnancies. This experimental model of preeclampsia has been reproduced successfully by other authors, who found that oral administration of cyclosporin A intensified the changes induced by placental concentrates [20].

2.5. Immunologic damage to the placenta

Another experimental model was obtained by injuring the rat placenta by immunologic means. Pregnant and nonpregnant control rats were injected with placenta extracts in Freund adjuvant; this resulted in mild hypertension and proteinuria, but no definite histologic damage was observed in the placenta [21]. In order to injure the placenta more severely, pregnant and nonpregnant rats were injected with rabbit anti-rat placenta serum, rabbit anti-rat kidney serum, or normal rabbit serum; the antiplacenta serum produced hypertension in pregnant but not in nonpregnant rats, and the antikidney serum produced the same blood pressure elevation in pregnant and in nonpregnant animals [22].

By using immunofluorescent microscopy, Foidart et al. [23] found that 13 sera from 49 patients with severe preeclampsia contained antibodies reacting with placenta and kidney. These antibodies reacted with laminin (a large glycoprotein found in the lamina lucida of all basement membranes), but not with other basement membrane antigens, including collagen and proteoglycan. When injected intravenously into pregnant mice, antibodies to laminin induced a high incidence of fetal death, abortion, and proteinuria.

In conclusion, none of these experimental models is mimicking human preeclampsia. Animal models, however, are undoubtedly useful for studying some of the unsolved problems of preeclampsia.

3. PATHOGENESIS OF PREECLAMPSIA

3.1. Renin–angiotensin axis

3.1.1. Renin–angiotensin axis in normal pregnancy

During normal pregnancy, remarkable changes take place in the renin–angiotensin system. Their relationship with preeclampsia is obviously of great interest.

Renin is a proteolytic enzyme with a molecular weight of approximately 40,000 daltons. It acts upon a circulating renin substrate, an α-2-globulin, the angiotensinogen, to form AI, a 10-amino-acid peptide. AI is rapidly converted into the active vasoconstrictor AII during its circulation through capillary beds—particularly the pulmonary circulation—by an enzyme present in endothelial cells known as angiotensin-converting enzyme (ACE). Circulating AII is then inactivated by angiotensinases in tissues and blood. Therefore the level of plasma AII represents the net effect of renin release into the circulation, the concentration of the substrate angiotensinogen, the activity of ACE, and the activity of angiotensinases.

Over the last two decades it has been clearly established that PRA increases substantially early in normal pregnancy [24–33]. The renin substrate concentration in plasma also increases during pregnancy and influences the amount of angiotensin produced by renin in vivo [34]. It has been suggested that the rise in renin substrate during pregnancy is probably an effect of estrogens, since the same effect has been observed in women given estrogens or oral contraceptive agents containing estrogens [35]. Furthermore, plasma renin concentration (PRC) remains persistently high throughout pregnancy in all women. Thus, the combined increase in renin and in substrate concentration leads to a significant increase in PRA. New insights into the effects of renin–angiotensin system changes during pregnancy will be achieved by studying the tissue content of ACE and AII receptors. Although plasma ACE has been found to be consistently lower during pregnancy than in nonpregnant controls [36], the relevance of plasma ACE measurements to the actual conversion of AI to AII is open to question [37]. No correlation has been shown in pregnancy between plasma ACE and PRA or PRC or plasma AII. Direct studies of AII receptors have suggested that some changes in tissue responsiveness to AII are mediated by changes at the receptor level. Changes in AII receptor expression, in fact, were induced by steroids and dietary salt modifications [38]. Nevertheless, no data are available regarding the number and affinity of AII receptors in pregnancy.

Although plasma renin in pregnancy is primarly of renal origin, the high concentration of renin in uterus, placenta, and amniotic fluid makes these sites potential sources of plasma renin in pregnancy. Stakemann [39] and Gross [40] were the first authors to report that placental and uterine extracts of cats and rabbits had a pressor effect when injected intravenously, and produced a pressor substance similar to AII when incubated with serum. These studies were extended by Ferris et al. [41] and Gorden et al. [42], who demonstrated that neither stimuli reducing the concentration of renin in the kidney, such as variations in sodium intake, nor nephrectomy had any effect on the renin concentration in the uterus of pregnant rabbits. Cell cultures of human chorion and uterine muscle have been shown to synthesize renin [43]. As found in pregnant nephrectomized rabbits, reduction in uterine blood flow by either hemorrhagic hypotension or uterine artery ligation increased uterine renin secretion into the circulation [44]. It is not known whether uterine renin contributes to plasma renin in pregnancy. It seems unlikely, however, that uterine renin is responsible for the high PRA observed in pregnancy; in pregnant rabbits, in fact, uterine renin did not respond to changes either in salt intake (as mentioned) or in extracellular fluid volume, whereas plasma and kidney renin did [42]. On the other hand, renin activity was higher in uterine veins than in uterine arteries in women with toxemia at cesarean section [45, 46].

The role of uterine renin in the physiology of pregnancy remains unknown. A possible hypothesis suggests that uterine renin plays a role in the uterine blood flow regulation by increasing AII, as demonstrated in pregnant rabbits, dogs, and monkeys [44, 47, 48]. AII stimulates AA release from phospholipids of cell membranes and promotes PG synthesis [49, 50]. The increased uterine PGE_2 synthesis may be the cause of the fall in uterine vascular resistance and the consequent increase in uterine blood flow [48]. In favor of this hypothesis is the observation that the administration of captopril (a converting-enzyme inhibitor) to pregnant rabbits significantly reduced uterine blood flow without changing cardiac output or renal blood flow [51]; meanwhile, the PGE level in uterine vein was decreased. When captopril was given orally to pregnant rabbits from day 15 of gestation on, fetal mortality was almost 100% without changes in systemic blood pressure [51, 52]. These findings suggest that the reduction in uterine PGE synthesis induced by angiotensin blockade might be the cause of the high fetal mortality.

It has been shown that also human amniotic fluid contains a very high concentration of renin, mostly in an inactive form (prorenin), which is activated by incubation at acid pH [53, 54]. In the first trimester of pregnancy, inactive renin in plasma rapidly arises, then it declines slowly until midpregnancy and falls quickly to the normal range after delivery [55]. Therefore prorenin detectable in the plasma of pregnant women may be of amniotic origin. It has been recently suggested that whether or not activation of prorenin is involved in the normal regulation of active renin levels, this occurs more likely in the tissue of origin than in the circulation [56]. Thus, it is still unclear whether prorenin plays a physiologic role in normal pregnancy.

Even in normal pregnancy, renin release is under the control of several factors, such as renal perfusion pressure and sodium intake. Renin secretion in pregnancy, in fact, adequately responded to sodium restriction and volume expansion, although basal levels were persistently elevated [57–59]. Increased PG synthesis may also be involved in the high renin release in pregnancy. Intrarenal administration of AA in nonhypotensive doses in rats [60], rabbits [61], and dogs [62], in fact, has been shown to increase renin release. Similarly, in vitro incubation of AA, endoperoxides, or PGI_2 with renal cortical slices of rabbit caused release of renin, which was inhibited by indomethacin; these results demonstrate that prostaglandins directly stimulate renin release [63–66].

Patrono et al. [67] have demonstrated that PGI_2 infusion in healthy volunteers induced a substantial, dose-related rise in PRA and in circulating AII. On the other hand, AII has repeatedly been reported to release a PG-like material from several tissues and so it seems to be a specific releaser of PGI_2 from vascular tissue [50, 68, 69]. This is a receptor-mediated effect of AII, as the PGI_2 release is blocked by saralasin and captopril [50]. It has been recently postulated that PGI_2 release is triggered by AII through hypothetical receptors different from those used by AII to evoke the pressor response [70]. Thus, angiotensin appears to acquire the new, unsuspected function of promoting the biosynthesis of PGI_2 in vascular tissues. PGI_2, in turn, stimulates renin release in the kidney. This relationship between renin and PG synthesis might play a pivotal role in regulating not only the renal circulation, but also the circulation in other organs, the uteroplacental circulation in particular.

Finally, another determinant of renin secretion is vascular sensitivity to angiotensin. The level of angiotensin required to elicit a blood pressure response, in fact, varies with the sensitivity of the vasculature to angiotensin [38]. The factors controlling angiotensin sensitivity and receptor affinity, however, have not yet been identified. Changes of intracellular sodium and calcium concentration in the arterial wall or synthesis of angiotensin antagonists (such as PGs) in the blood vessel seem to be important in this respect [38].

3.1.2. Renin–angiotensin axis in preeclampsia

The balance between the production of vasodilator PGs in local vascular beds (chiefly uterus and kidney) and the renin–angiotensin system, in particular AII as a potent vasoconstrictor, may play a central role in the regulation of uterine blood flow and in the development of pregnancy-induced hypertension.

Broad variations in PRA during preeclampsia have been reported in the literature; almost all authors, however, have observed a PRA lower than in normal pregnancy, but still higher than in nonpregnant women [25, 28, 30, 32, 71, 72]. While there is evidence that, in preeclampsia, renin is not derived from the fetus or from the placenta, it might be uterine or decidual in origin. Since ischemia or anoxia of the pregnant uterus has been considered as a possible cause of preeclampsia, it has been postulated that uteroplacental ischemia increases the uteroplacental production of renin. As mentioned above, in fact, PRA was higher in uterine veins than in uterine arteries in women with toxemia [45] and, in a case of abdominal pregnancy with preeclampsia, PRA was high [73]. Moreover, in cases of hydatiform mole or with rhesus incompatibility, preeclampsia has been associated with much higher PRC, suggesting an increase in renin release because of an augmented placental mass [72]. This indicates a cause-and-effect relationship between uterine hypoperfusion with the resulting renin release and pregnancy-induced hypertension.

There is general agreement that preeclamptic women are more sensitive to the pressor effects of vasoconstrictor substances than are normal pregnant women. As early as 1937, Dieckmann and Michel [74] reported that vascular reactivity to the pressor effects of a vasoactive agent (crude vasopressin) was greater in preeclamptic than in normotensive pregnant women. Later studies have shown that, in normal human pregnancy, the vascular refractoriness to the pressor effects of AII was due to the decreased vascular smooth muscle response to AII more than to the altered blood volume or to the plasma concentration of AII [75–80]. It is important to note that, in nonpregnant subjects, plasma concentrations of renin and/or AII are inversely proportional to the vascular reactivity to AII. The concomitant synthesis of vasodilating PGs, either PGI_2 or PGE_2, might be involved in the regulation of vascular reactivity during human pregnancy. In this regard, it has been hypothesized that these PGs induce renal vasodilation and cause vascular refractoriness to AII in normal pregnancy, despite an increase in renin and AII concentrations [81, 82]. Gant et al. [83] suggested that a progestin mechanism may modulate the expression of PG-mediated vascular responsiveness to the pressor effects of AII. However, a direct effect of progestins upon vascular smooth muscle cannot be excluded at present. Disturbances in any of these components of the mechanism could lead to loss of refractoriness to AII, as shown in preeclampsia.

In conclusion, preeclampsia is characterized by an increased sensitivity to AII and other vasoactive agents, leading to generalized vasoconstriction with hypertension. The resulting ischemia of the pregnant uterus will increase renin production and consequently AII concentration, leading to a greater vasoconstrictor effect on the uteroplacental vasculature. Therefore the loss of vascular refractoriness to AII might play a central role in the pathogenesis of preeclampsia.

3.2. Vascular prostaglandin production

3.2.1. Vascular prostaglandin production in normal pregnancy

Striking changes occur in the cardiovascular system during pregnancy. Maternal and fetal circulation share some basic features, such as maximal generalized vasodilation, high blood volume, high cardiac output, and low systemic blood pressure [84–86]. In the fetus, low peripheral resistances allow very high cardiac output and lead to maximal exchanges with maternal blood as a compensatory mechanism for the low gradient in O_2 saturation at the fetoplacental unit [87]. The low blood pressure, despite high cardiac output, has been ascribed to low-resistance systems, such as umbilicoplacental circulation and vascular shunts [88]. However, the high blood flow found in several fetal organs points to systemic arterial vasodilation as an important factor in the low peripheral resistance [86, 87].

A possible role of PGs in hemodynamic changes in the fetal and maternal circulation was first suggested by Terragno et al. [89]. Investigating fetal, maternal, and nonpregnant bovine vascular tissues, they found a very high level of 6-keto-$PGF_{1\alpha}$—the stable breakdown product of PGI_2—in incubation medium from fetal blood vessels. This capacity, therefore, was not restricted to the ductus arteriosus, as commonly supposed [90, 91]. A significantly high PGI_2 production from fetal vessels has been observed in humans by Remuzzi et al. [92], who studied umbilical arteries and placental veins compared with vessels of healthy adults. It has been suggested that PGI_2 plays an important role in mediating maximal vasodilation and refractoriness to vasoconstrictor stimuli of fetal and placental circulation. The increased capacity to produce PGI_2 has been demonstrated also in maternal vasculature as a more general phenomenon of normal pregnancy. Goodman et al. [93] and Brash et al. [94] measured the urinary excretion of PGI_2 metabolites to estimate the maternal vessel biosynthesis of PGI_2 in pregnancy in comparison with nonpregnant controls. Although the absolute levels of these metabolites were much lower than the values obtained during infusion of effective doses of PGI_2, they were higher in pregnant than in nonpregnant women.

3.2.2. Vascular prostaglandin production in preeclampsia

Whichever mechanism operates in normal pregnancy, a fall in PGI_2 activity could be a link in the chain of events leading to preeclampsia [95]. Nowadays, measurements of circulating PGI_2 metabolites have given somewhat inconsistent results [96–98], but PGI_2 generation in fetal and maternal blood vessels seems to be reduced or inhibited in toxemia [99–102]. Remuzzi et al. [103] were the first to report that umbilical arteries from preeclamptic pregnancies synthesized less PGI_2-like substance than did normal umbilical arteries. This is consistent with the results obtained by other investigators using different experimental approaches [99, 101, 102, 104–107]. Thus, the pathologic features of preeclampsia, such as generalized vasoconstriction, increased maternal sensitivity to vasoconstrictors, blood volume contraction, and relative suppression of the renin–angiotensin system may all be accounted for by a deficiency in PGI_2 production.

Since PGI_2 level is related to factors affecting both its biosynthesis and its degradation, deficiency of PGI_2 in preeclampsia might be due to an unbalance between these factors [108]. An ability of a still undefined plasma component (plasmatic stimulating factor, PSF) to modulate PGI_2 synthesis was first reported by MacIntyre et al. [109], who demonstrated that normal cell-free plasma stimulates PGI_2 production by cultured endothelial cells from pig aorta. This finding was later confirmed in other experimental and clinical conditions, such as hemolytic uremic syndrome (HUS) [110] and uremia [111], in which PSF activity is reduced. PSF activity has been serially evaluated by Remuzzi et al. [112] and Gregorini et al. [113] in normal pregnancy and compared with nonpregnant controls: no difference was observed during early pregnancy, but PSF activity was significantly reduced during late pregnancy. The reduction in late pregnancy was not observed in patients with severe preeclampsia; in this case, PSF was normal but vascular production of PGI_2 was reduced. This result is difficult to reconcile with the good correlation observed between PSF and vascular production of PGI_2 in chronic uremic patients [111] and in patients with HUS [110].

A defective PG production by the vascular tissues in preeclampsia might depend on a reduced availability of AA, an unsaturated fatty acid derived from the linoleic acid, an essential fatty acid (EFA) [114]. It has been shown that dietary fat is necessary in pregnancy and that the active principle appears to be EFA [115]. In human pregnancy on a normal diet, deficiency of EFA has not been observed, as indicated by the blood levels of EFA that rise during the course of pregnancy until labor, when they peak [116]. Studies on pregnant rats fed a low EFA diet, however, showed prolonged dystocia and death of the fetuses, although the fetal growth was always satisfactory [117]. Prolonged dietary deprivation to produce EFA deficiency before pregnancy resulted in 30% smaller fetuses and in a reduction of placental weight [118]. The fatty acid composition of fetal and maternal tissues was markedly modified by accumulation of the eicosatrienoic 20:3w9, which cannot be converted to PG. Thus, maternal dietary deprivation was clearly responsible for fetal EFA deficiency, demonstrating the role of maternal diet in fetal plasma lipid composition. In order to establish whether the differences in PGI_2 synthesis between normal and preeclamptic pregnancies were related to AA availability, Ochard et al. [119] studied the free fatty acid composition of the umbilical artery tissue in normal pregnancies; free 5,8,11-eicosatrienoic acid (Mead acid) was identified in the umbilical artery tissue in a ratio with free AA ranging between 0.10 and 0.31. Unlike 8,11,14-eicosatrienoic acid, AA, and 5,8,11,14,17-eicosapentanoic acid, Mead acid is not a substrate for cyclooxygenase, but only for lipoxygenase, the enzyme-generating substances called leukotrienes of the three series (LT3) with vasoconstrictor activity [120]. If the substrate Mead acid is available at higher rates, one will expect LT3 to be increased. Thus, this phenomenon appears to be of importance in future approaches to the pathogenesis of preeclampsia.

AA metabolism can be modified by factors such as lipid peroxides, interfering with enzymatic activities involved in PG production [121, 122]. It has been shown that total serum lipids increase during pregnancy [123]. In preeclampsia, serum lipid concentration is significantly higher than in normal pregnancy, mainly because of increased triglycerides in the very low density lipoprotein (VLDL) and low-density lipoprotein (LDL) fractions [124, 125]. Serum lipid peroxides are particularly increased in normal pregnant women in comparison with nonpregnant subjects and their level is further elevated in preeclamptic women [124, 125]. In preeclampsia, the ratio between lipid peroxides and total lipids is higher than in normal pregnancy [125]. Serum high-density lipoproteins (HDL) are believed to be closely related to membrane lipids [126]. Thus, lipid peroxides produced in the cell membrane might be transferred to the HDL fraction together with lipids and circulate in the bloodstream, leading to various diseases. On the other hand, accumulation of peroxides is controlled by free-radical scavengers, namely, superoxide dismutase, catalase, glutathione peroxidase, and vitamin E [127]. A number of investigators have reported that circulating levels of tocopherol (vitamin E) are increased during the second and the third trimesters of pregnancy; compared with control plasma, however, vitamin-E levels are not altered in preeclampsia [128].

In conclusion, a steady increase in lipid-peroxide formation by activating the arachidonate cascade probably contributes to the physiologic modification of PG production in normal pregnancy; a sudden steep increase in lipid-peroxide formation that is not balanced by a corresponding increase in free-radical scavengers—as documented in preeclampsia—might promote accumulation of nonenzymatic derivatives that are biologically active and interfere with normal enzymatic activities (such as PGI_2 synthetase), thereby leading to a deficient PGI_2 production.

3.3. Uteroplacental ischemia

Preeclampsia is always associated with uteroplacental ischemia, various degrees of intrauterine fetal growth retardation and, in most severe cases, intrauterine death. Furthermore, this disease is also characterized by a low placental weight with areas of extensive infarction and ischemic necrosis on macro- or microscopic examination [129]. The remaining tissue presents ultrastructural abnormalities, such as cytotrophoblastic hyperplasia, focal syncitial necrosis, microvillous abnormalities, and thickening of trophoblastic basement membrane, which are very similar to those found in other conditions of placental ischemia, such as intrauterine fetal growth retardation and maternal smoking. Neither degenerative changes nor lesions related to accelerated aging have been demonstrated [130].

In order to understand the role of uteroplacental ischemia in the pathogenesis of preeclampsia, an adequate evaluation of uteroplacental blood flow and sequential events of normal placentation in human pregnancy is required. A substantial part of our knowledge on uteroplacental blood flow derives from animal experimental models, because of the complexity of uterine vascular supply and the difficulties associated with its measurement in humans. The clearance of dehydroepiandrosterone (DHEA), introduced by Gant et al. [131] as an indirect measurement of uterine blood flow (which depends upon the placental conversion of DHEA to estradiol), appeared to be reduced by approximately 50% in preeclampsia. Direct estimation of uteroplacental blood flow either by isotopic techniques [132, 133] or by Doppler ultrasound determination of blood flow velocity in the uterine vessels [134] indicated severe hypoperfusion. To ensure an adequate blood supply to the fetoplacental unit, complex adaptive changes are required during placentation in human pregnancy. Hemochorial placentation in humans and several mammals is characterized by trophoblastic cell invasion of the maternal vessel at the placental bed [135–137]. Starting at the opening into the intervillous space, trophoblastic cells retrogradely invade the lumen of spiral arteries. Subsequently, they cause endothelial disruption and penetrate the vascular wall by destroying the subendothelial layers. Thus, the smooth muscle cells of the media become unrecognizable and are replaced by fibrinoid material with "large cells" (trophoblastic cells). These vascular changes, referred to by Brosens [137] as "physiologic changes" to underline the essential role of normal placentation, occur in early pregnancy in the superficial decidual part of the spiral arteries. During the second half of pregnancy, these changes extend more deeply into the decidual and myometrial parts [136]. It has been shown that, in humans, trophoblastic invasion is particularly aggressive, reaching the myometrial end of the spiral arteries [137]. Spiral arteries become large (4–5 times the normal diameter) and unreactive because of loss of muscle-elastic structures. In spite of these major changes in the normal vascular wall, no thrombus formation has been seen. One possible explanation of this phenomenon is related to the observation that trophoblast specimens from early and late normal pregnancies and human trophoblastic cells in short-term culture produce a significant amount of PGI_2 [138, 139]. PGI_2 inhibits platelet aggregation, but also maintains blood vessel dilation [140]. This suggests that the ability of the invading trophoblast to colonize maternal blood vessels and avoid immobilization by platelet aggregates is PGI_2 dependent. These pregnancy-induced physiologic changes produce a significant reduction in peripheral vascular resistance in the placental bed, thereby allowing a much greater blood flow into and through the intervillous spaces of the placenta.

In preeclampsia, however, no trophoblastic cells have been found in myometrial segments of spiral arteries, the physiologic changes being restricted to the decidual segments [129, 136, 141]. Since, at this level, spiral arteries retain an essentially normal muscle-elastic structure, these segments are the most likely to develop stenosing hypertensive lesions, when pregnancy is complicated by severe preeclampsia [142, 143]. In their early stages, these lesions are characterized by endothelial damage, insudation of plasma constituents into the vessel wall, proliferation of myointimal cells with fat accumulation (foam cells), and medial necrosis. Gross endothelial damage, massive intramural fibrin deposition, luminal thrombosis, and vessel rupture with hemorrhage have been seen in later stages. Therefore a clear central role of occlusive lesions of maternal spiral arteries supplying the placenta appears in the pathogenesis of placental ischemia [144].

Recently, a new syndrome has been described that is characterized by repeated intrauterine death associated with the presence of a circulating "lupus-like" anticoagulant [145, 146]. This may be considered a model of uteroplacental ischemia and used to study the role of placental ischemia in the pathogenesis of preeclampsia. Like preeclampsia, this syndrome is characterized by fetal growth retardation and subsequent death in late pregnancy, due to the placental insufficiency [147]. The placenta, in fact, is small with extensive infarctions. The spiral arteries show the same lesions as in preeclamptic pregnancy: no or partial physiologic changes, intimal thickening, fibrinoid necrosis, acute atherosis, and intraluminal thrombosis. It is of interest that in both syndromes a defect of vascular PGI_2 has been reported, suggesting a common mechanism underlying the fetal growth retardation and death [148]. Despite the similarity of the uteroplacental lesions, however, the clinical feature of this new syndrome is quite different from that of classic preeclampsia. In particular, in the syndrome of recurrent abortion associated with the "lupus-like" anticoagulant, no evidence of hypertension or renal impairment has been reported [149]. Therefore pregnancies in patients with "lupus-like" anticoagulant and idiopathic intrauterine growth retardation do not support the hypothesis that uteroplacental ischemia is necessarily associated with preeclampsia.

3.4. Preeclampsia: a unifying hypothesis

A reduction in the synthesis of vasodilating PGs appears to play an important role in the pathogenesis of preeclampsia (figure 2-1) Several factors modulate AA metabolism, but our knowledge of their role in PG synthesis during pregnancy is still limited. It may be speculated, however, that an imbalance between lipoperox-

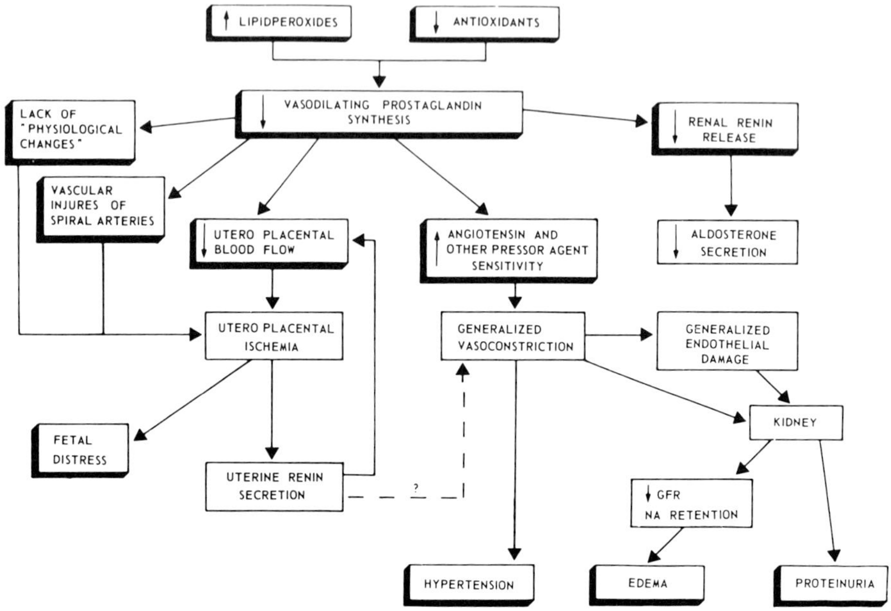

Figure 2-1. A unifying hypothesis for the pathophysiology of preeclampsia.

ides and the free-radical scavengers, which control their accumulation, interferes with normal enzymatic activities in the arachidonate cascade (such as that of PGI_2 synthetase), thereby reducing the synthesis of vasodilating PGs [150].

In the uterus, reduced PG synthesis may cause a reduction of uteroplacental blood flow, with consequent uteroplacental ischemia, intrauterine fetal growth retardation and, in severe cases, intrauterine death. Furthermore, lack of "physiologic changes," probably more frequent in the first pregnancy, and spiral artery lesions (that may be induced by the decrease in PGI_2 production) may account for uteroplacental ischemia and increased fetal distress. Since uteroplacental ischemia has been shown to increase uterine renin secretion, positive feedback may occur between uterine hypoperfusion, uterine renin release, and increase in uterine vascular resistance [45, 73].

These phenomena may contribute to the generalized vasoconstriction that is a characteristic feature of preeclampsia. Whether plasma renin in preeclampsia is of uteroplacental or rental origin, however, is still unknown. There is evidence that renal PG synthesis plays a role in renin secretion [67]. Consequently, in preeclampsia a reduction of vasodilating PG may cause a decrease in renal renin release, which in turn may cause a fall in aldosterone secretion. Moreover, in pregnancy-associated hypertension there is an increased sensitivity to the pressor effects of AII and other vasoconstrictor agents, in comparison with normal pregnancy. It has been shown that the refractoriness of normal pregnancy to AII may be abolished when women are treated with indomethacin, the inhibitor of PG synthesis [79]. Thus, in preeclampsia a decrease in PGI_2 synthesis in blood vessels might increase the vascular smooth muscle responsiveness to AII, thereby making the absolute level of renin or angiotensin less important than the sensitivity of arterioles to angiotensin. These changes of vascular sensitivity to pressor substances may cause a generalized vasoconstriction, which is responsible for hypertension and generalized endothelial damage. In the most severe case, proteinuria and sodium retention also occur.

In conclusion, this hypothesis suggests that PGI_2 deficiency plays a central role in the pathogenesis of preeclampsia and provides a pathophysiologic explanation for the clinical features of this disease.

REFERENCES

1. Chesley LC: False steps in the study of preeclampsia. In: Lindheimer M, Katz AI, Zuspan FP (eds) Hypertension in pregnancy. New York: John Wiley and Sons, 1976, pp 1–10.
2. Chesley LC: Remote prognosis after eclampsia. In: Lindheimer M, Katz AI, Zuspan FP (eds) Hypertension in pregnancy. New York: John Wiley and Sons, 1976, pp 31–40.
3. Stamler FW: Fatal eclamptic disease of pregnant rats fed anti-vitamin E stress diet. Am J Pathol 35:1207–1231, 1959.
4. Spitz B, Deckmyn H, Pijnenborg R, Van Assche FA, Vermylen J: Prostacyclin (PGI2) production by aortic rings and mesometrial triangles in pregnant rats, fed an anti-vitamin E stress diet [abstr]. In: Ninth international congress on thrombosis and hemostasis, Stockholm, July 1983, p 231.
5. Weaver K: Preeclampsia and eclampsia in magnesium depleted triplet bearing ewes [abstr]. In: Fourth world congress of the International Society for the Study of Hypertension in Pregnancy, Amsterdam, June 1984, p 251.
6. Chisolm JC: Role of zinc and cadmium in toxemia [abstr]. In: Fourth world congress of the International Society for the Study of Hypertension in Pregnancy, Amsterdam, June 1984, p 355.
7. Belizan JM, Pineda O, Sainz E, Menendez LA, Villar J: Rise of blood pressure in calcium-deprived pregnant rats. Am J Obstet Gynecol 141:163–169, 1981.
8. Ahokas RA, Anderson GD, Lipshitz J. Cardiac output and uteroplacental blood flow in diet-restricted and diet-repleted pregnant rats. Am J Obstet Gynecol 146:6–13, 1983.
9. Rosso P, Kava R: Effect of food restriction on cardiac output and blood flow to the uterus and placenta in the pregnant rat. J Nutr 110:2350–2354, 1980.
10. Ogden E, Hildebrand GJ, Page EW: Rise of blood pressure during ischemia of the gravid uterus. Proc Soc Exp Biol Med 43:49–54, 1945.
11. Douglas BH, Langford HG: Post-term blood pressure elevation produced by uterine wrapping. Am J Obstet Gynecol 97:231–238, 1967.
12. Abitbol MM: Experimental toxaemia in the pregnant dog and the aetiology of toxaemia. In: Bonnar J, MacGillivray I, Symonds M (eds) Pregnancy hypertension. Lancaster: MTP, 1980, pp 445–457.
13. Abitbol MM: Simplified technique to produce toxemia in the rat: consideration on cause of toxemia. Clin Exp Hypertens [B] 1:93–103, 1982.
14. Cavanagh D, Rao PS, Tsai CC, O'Connor TC: Experimental toxemia in the pregnant primate. Am J Obstet Gynecol 128:75–85, 1977.
15. Abitbol MM, Ober WB, Gallo GR: Experimental toxemia of pregnancy in the monkey. Am J Pathol 86:573–590, 1977.
16. Lindheimer MD, Katz AI, Koeppen B, Ordonez N, Oparil S: Renal function, the renin–angiotensin system, and volume homeostasis in pregnant and non pregnant spontaneous hypertensive rats [abstr]. In: Fourth world congress of the International Society for the Study of Hypertension in Pregnancy, Amsterdam, June 1984, p 326.
17. Douglas BH: The rat as a model for preeclampsia. Perspect Nephrol Hypertens 5:411–419, 1976.
18. Brianceschi SB, Papoutsis DV, Sloan HR, Curry JJ: Hypertensive actions of preeclamptic placental extracts in rats [abstr]. In: Fourth world congress of the International Society for the Study of Hypertension in Pregnancy, Amsterdam, June 1984, p 248.

19. Aladjem S, Lueck J, Brewer J: Experimental induction of toxemia-like syndrome in the pregnant beagle [abstr]. In: Fourth world congress of the International Society for the Study of Hypertension and Pregnancy, Amsterdam, June 1984, p 247.
20. Byrne TJ: Further work on a possible dog model of pre-eclampsia [abstr]. In: Fourth world Congress of the International Society for the Study of Hypertension in Pregnancy, Amsterdam, June 1984, p 306.
21. Langford HD, Douglas BH, Arhelger RB: A model of preeclampsia. I. Blood pressure changes produced by anti-placenta serum. Johns Hopkins Med J 120:213–219, 1967.
22. Smith SL, Douglas BH, Langford HG: A model of preeclampsia. II. Changes in renin content produced by anti-placenta serum. Johns Hopkins Med J 120:220–224, 1967.
23. Foidart JM, Hunt J, Mahieu P, Lapiere CM, Nusgens B, Derijcker C, Bruwier M, Risteli J, Lambotte C: A pathogenic role for antibodies to laminin in severe pre-eclampsia [abstr]. In: Ninth international congress of nephrology, Los Angeles, June 1984, p 279A.
24. Brown JJ, Davies DL, Doak PB, Lever AF, Robertson JIS: Plasma renin in normal pregnancy. Lancet 2:900–902, 1963.
25. Gordon RD, Parsons S, Symonds EM: A prospective study of plasma renin activity in normal and toxemic pregnancy. Lancet 1:347–349, 1969.
26. Weir RJ, Paintin DB, Robertson JIS, Tree M, Fraser R, Young J: Renin, angiotensin and aldosterone relationships in normal pregnancy. Proc R Soc Lond 63:1101–1102, 1970.
27. Skinner SL, Lumbers ER, Symonds EM: Analysis of changes in the renin–angiotensin system during pregnancy. Clin Sci 42:479–488, 1972.
28. Tapia HR, Johnson CE, Strong CE: Renin–angiotensin system in normal and in hypertensive disease of pregnancy. Lancet 2:847–850, 1972.
29. Weir R, Brown JJ, Fraser R, Lever AF, Logan RW, McIlwaine GM, Morton JJ, Robertson JIS, Tree MM: Relationship between plasma renin, renin–substrate, angiotensin II, aldosterone, and electrolytes in normal pregnancy. J Clin Endocrinol Metab 40:108–115, 1975.
30. Weinberg MH, Kramer NJ, Petersen LP, Cleary RE, Young PGM: Sequential changes in the renin–angiotensin–aldosterone systems and plasma progesterone concentration in normal and abnormal human pregnancy. In: Lindheimer M, Katz A, Zuspan F (eds) Hypertension in pregnancy. New York: John Wiley and Sons, 1976, pp 263–269.
31. Symonds EM: The renin–angiotensin system and sodium excretion during gestation. In: Lindheimer M, Katz A, Zuspan F (eds) Hypertension in pregnancy. New York: John Wiley and Sons, 1976, pp 271–279.
32. Weir RJ, Doig A, Fraser R, Morton JJ, Parboosingh J, Robertson JIS, Wilson A: Studies of the renin–angiotensin–aldosterone system, cortisol, DOC, and ADH in normal and hypertensive pregnancy. In: Lindheimer M, Katz A, Zuspan F (eds) Hypertension in pregnancy. New York: John Wiley and Sons, 1976, pp 251–258.
33. Wilson M, Morganti AA, Zervoudakis I, Letcher RL, Romney BM, Von Oeyon P, Papera S, Sealey JE, Laragh JH: Blood pressure, the renin–aldosterone system and sex steroids throughout normal pregnancy. Am J Med 68:97–104, 1980.
34. Tree M: Measurement of plasma renin substrate in man. J Endocrinol 56:159–171, 1973.
35. Weinberger MH, Collins RD, Dowdy AJ, Nokes GW, Luetscher JA: Hypertension induced by oral contraceptives containing estrogen and gestagen. Ann Intern Med 71:891–902, 1969.
36. Oats JN, Broughton Pipkin F, Symonds EM, Craven DJ: A prospective study of plasma angiotensin-converting enzyme in normotensive primigravidae and their infants. Br J Obstet Gynaecol 88:1204–1210, 1981.
37. Oparil S, Haber E: The renin–angiotensin system. N Engl J Med 291:389–401, 1974.
38. Brunner HR, Chang P, Wallach R, Sealey JE, Laragh JH: Angiotensin II vascular receptors: their affinity in relationship to sodium balance, the automatic nervous system and hypertension. J Clin Invest 51:58–67, 1972.
39. Stakemann G: A renin-like pressor substance found in the placenta of the cat. Acta Pathol Microbiol Immunol Scand 50:350–354, 1960.
40. Gross F, Schaechtelin G, Ziegler M, Berger M: A renin-like substance in the placenta and uterus of the rabbit. Lancet 1:914–916, 1964.
41. Ferris TF, Gorden P, Mulrow PJ: Rabbit uterus as a source of renin. Am J Physiol 212:698–702, 1967.
42. Gorden P, Ferris TF, Mulrow PJ: Rabbit uterus as a possible site of renin synthesis. Am J Physiol 212:703–706, 1967.

43. Symonds EM, Stanley MA, Skinner SL: Production of renin by in vitro cultures of human chorion and uterine muscle. Nature 217:1152–1153, 1968.
44. Ferris TF, Stein JH, Kauffman J: Uterine blood flow and uterine renin secretion. J Clin Invest 51:2827–2833, 1972.
45. Kokot F, Cekanski A: Plasma renin activity in peripheral and uterine vein blood in pregnant and non-pregnant women. J Obstet Gynecol 79:72–76, 1972.
46. Smith RW, Selinger HE, Stevenson SF: The uteroplacental complex. Am J Obstet Gynecol 105:1129–1131, 1969.
47. Assali NS, Holm LW, Segal N: Regional blood flow and vascular resistance of the fetus in uterine action of vasoactive drugs. Am J Obstet Gynecol 83:809–812, 1962.
48. Franklin GO, Dowd AJ, Caldwell BV, Speroff L: The effect of angiotensin II intravenous infusion on plasma renin activity and prostaglandin A, E, and F levels in the uterine vein of the pregnant monkey. Prostaglandins 6:261–280, 1974.
49. Dusting GJ, Mullins EM: Stimulation by angiotensin of prostacyclin biosynthesis in rats and dogs. Clin Exp Pharmacol Physiol 7:545–550, 1980.
50. Grodzinska L, Gryglewski RJ: Angiotensin-induced release of prostacyclin from perfused organs. Pharmacol Res Commun 12:339–347, 1980.
51. Ferris TF, Weir EK: Effect of captopril on uterine blood flow and prostaglandin E synthesis in the pregnant rabbit. J Clin Invest 71:809–815, 1983.
52. Broughton Pipkin F, Turner SR, Symonds EM: Possible risk with captopril in pregnancy: some animal data. Lancet 1:1256, 1980.
53. Sealey JE, Atlas SA, Laragh JH: Prorenin and other large molecular weight forms of renin. Endocr Rev 1:365–391, 1980.
54. Skinner SL, Cran EJ, Gibson R: Angiotensin I and II, active and inactive renin, renin substrate, renin activity, and angiotensinase in human liquor amnii and plasma. Am J Obstet Gynecol 121:626–630, 1975.
55. Hsueh WA, Luetscher JA, Carlson EJ, Grislis G, Fraze E, McHargue A: Changes in active and inactive renin throughout pregnancy. J Clin Endocrinol Metab 54:1010–1016, 1982.
56. Atias SA, Hesson TE, Sealey JE, Dharmgrongartama B, Laragh JH, Ruddy MC, Aurell M: Characterization of inactive renin ("prorenin") from renin-secreting tumors of non renal origin. J Clin Invest 73:437–447, 1984.
57. Bay WH, Ferris TF: Factors controlling plasma renin and aldosterone during pregnancy. Hypertension 1:410–415, 1979.
58. Weinberger MH, Kramer NJ, Grim GE, Petersen LP: The effect of posture and saline loading on plasma renin activity and aldosterone concentration in pregnant, non-pregnant, and estrogen-treated women. J Clin Endocrinol Metab 44:69–77, 1977.
59. Weinberger MH, Petersen LP, Herr MJ, Wade MB: The effects of supine and lateral recumbency on plasma renin activity during pregnancy. J Clin Endocrinol Metab 36:991–994, 1973.
60. Weber P, Holzgreve H, Stephan R, Herbst R: Plasma renin activity and renal sodium and water excretion following infusion of arachidonic acid in rats. Eur J Pharmacol 34:299–304, 1975.
61. Larsson C, Weber P, Anggard E: Arachidonic acid increases and indomethacin decreases plasma renin activity in the rabbit. Eur J Pharmacol 28:391–394, 1974.
62. Bolger PM, Eisner GH, Ramwell PW, Slotkoff LM: Effect of prostaglandin synthesis on renal function and renin in the dog. Nature 259:244–245, 1976.
63. Weber PC, Larsson E, Anggard E, Hamberg M, Corey EJ, Nicolaou KC, Samuelson B: Stimulation of renin release from rabbit renal cortex by arachidonic acid and prostaglandin endoperoxides. Circ Res 39:868–874, 1976.
64. Horton AR, Misono K, Hollifield J, Frölich JC, Inagami T, Oates JA: Prostaglandins and renin release. I. Stimulation of renin release from rabbit renal cortical slices by PGI2. Prostaglandins 14:1095–1104, 1977.
65. Gerber J, Olson RD, Nies AS: Interrelationship between prostaglandins and renin release. Kidney Int 19:816–821, 1981.
66. Henrich W: Role of prostaglandins in renin secretion. Kidney Int 19:822–830, 1981.
67. Patrono C, Pugliese F, Ciabattoni G, Patrignani P, Maseri A, Chierchia S, Peskar BA, Cinotti GA, Simonetti BM, Pierucci A: Evidence for a direct stimulatory effect of prostacyclin on renin release in man. J Clin Invest 69:231–239, 1982.
68. Gimbrone MA, Alexander RW: Angiotensin II stimulation of prostaglandin production in cultured human vascular endothelium. Science 189:219–220, 1975.

69. Danon A, Chang LCT, Sweetman BJ, Nies AS, Oates JA: Synthesis of prostaglandins by the rat renal papilla in vitro: mechanism of stimulation by angiotensin II. Biochim Biophys Acta 388:71–83, 1975.
70. Swies J, Radomski M, Gryglewsky RJ: On the mechanism of angiotensin II induced release of prostacyclin. Pharmacol Res Commun 13:37–40, 1981.
71. Brown JJ, Davies DL, Doak PB, Lever AF, Robertson JIS, Trust P: Plasma renin concentration in hypertensive disease of pregnancy. Lancet 2:1219, 1965.
72. Brown JJ, Davies DL, Doak PB, Lever AF, Robertson JIS, Trust P: Plasma renin concentration in the hypertensive diseases of pregnancy. J Obstet Gynaecol Br Commonw 73:410–417, 1966.
73. Baeler RW, Copeland WE, Stein JH, Ferris TF: Plasma renin and aldosterone in an abdominal pregnancy with toxemia. Am J Obstet Gynecol 122:545–548, 1975.
74. Dieckmann WJ, Michel HL: Vascular–renal effect of posterior pituitary extracts in pregnant women. Am J Obstet Gynecol 33:131–137, 1937.
75. Abdul-Karim R, Assali NS: Pressor response to angiotensin in pregnant and non-pregnant women. Am J Obstet Gynecol 82:246–251, 1961.
76. Gant NF, Daley GL, Chand S, Walley PJ, MacDonald PC: A study of angiotensin II pressor response throughout primigravid pregnancy. J Clin Invest 52:2682–2689, 1973.
77. Gant NF, Chand S, Whalley PJ, MacDonald PC: The nature of pressor responsiveness to angiotensin II in human pregnancy. Obstet Gynecol 43:854–860, 1974.
78. Cunningam FG, Cox K, Gant NF: Further observation on the nature of pressor responsivity to angiotensin II in human pregnancy. Obstet Gynecol 46:581–583, 1975.
79. Everett RB, Worley RJ, MacDonald PC, Gant NF: Effect of prostaglandin synthetase inhibitors on pressor response to angiotensin II in human pregnancy. J Clin Endocrinol Metab 46:-1007–1010, 1978.
80. Everett RB, Worley RJ, MacDonald PC, Gant NF: Modification of vascular responsiveness to angiotensin II in pregnant women by intravenously infused 5 α-dihydroprogesterone. Am J Obstet Gynecol 131:352–357, 1978.
81. Gant NF, Worley RJ, Everett RB, MacDonald PC: Control of vascular responsiveness during human pregnancy. Kidney Int 18:253–258, 1980.
82. Paller MS: Mechanism of decreased pressor responsiveness to ANGII, NE, and vasopressin in pregnant rats. Am J Physiol 247:H100–H108, 1984.
83. Gant NF, Whalley PJ, Everett RB, Worley RJ, MacDonald PC: Evidence for a vasodepressor prostaglandin deficiency in pregnancy-induced hypertension. In: Lewis PJ, Moncada, S, O'-Grady J (eds) Prostacyclin in pregnancy. New York: Raven, 1983, pp 99–107.
84. Hytten FE, Paintin DB: Increase in plasma volume during normal pregnancy. J Obstet Gynaecol Br Commonw 70:402–407, 1963.
85. MacGillivray I, Rose GA, Rowe B: Blood pressure survey in pregnancy. Clin Sci 37:395–407, 1969.
86. Rudolph AM, Heymann MA: Circulatory changes during growth in the fetal lamb. Circ Res 26:289–299, 1970.
87. Rudolph AM, Heymann MA: Fetal and neonatal circulation and respiration. Annu Rev Physiol 36:187–207, 1974.
88. Nuwayhid B, Vaughn D, Brinkman CR, Assali NS: Circulatory shock in pregnant sheep. IV. Fetal and neonatal circulatory responses to hypovolaemia: influence of anaesthesia. Am J Obstet Gynecol 132:658–666, 1978.
89. Terragno NA, McGiff JC, Murray S, Terragno A: Patterns of prostaglandin production in the bovine fetal and maternal vasculature. Prostaglandins 16:847–855, 1978.
90. Pace-Asciak CR, Rangaraj G: The 6-keto-prostaglandin Flα pathway in the lamb ductus arteriosus. Biochim Biophys Acta 486:583–585, 1977.
91. Terragno NA, Terragno A, McGiff JC, Rodriguez DJ: Synthesis of prostaglandins by the ductus arterious of the bovine fetus. Prostaglandins 14:721–727, 1977.
92. Remuzzi G, Misiani R, Muratore D, Marchesi D, Livio M, Schieppati A, Mecca G, de Gaetano G, Donati MB: Prostacyclin and human foetal circulation. Prostaglandins 18:341–348, 1979.
93. Goodman RP, Killam AR, Brash AR, Branch RA: Prostacyclin production during pregnancy: comparison of production during normal pregnancy and pregnancy complicated by hypertension. Am J Obstet Gynecol 142:817–822, 1982.
94. Brash AR, Goodman RP, Fitzgerald GA: Endogenous prostacyclin production in human

pregnancy. In: Lewis JP, Moncada S, O'Grady J (eds) Prostacyclin in pregnancy. New York: Raven, 1983, pp 71–77.
95. Ferris TF: Post partum renal insufficiency. Kidney Int 14:383–391, 1978.
96. Lewis PJ, Shepherd GL, Ritter J, Chan SMT, Bolton PJ, Jogee M, Myatt L, Elder MG: Prostacyclin and pre-eclampsia. Lancet 1:559, 1981.
97. Mitchell MD: Prostacyclin during human pregnancy and parturition. In: Lewis PJ, O'Grady J (eds) Clinical pharmacology of prostacyclin. New York: Raven, 1981, pp 121–129.
98. Ylikorkala O, Viinikka L: Maternal plasma levels of 6-keto-prostaglandin F during pregnancy and puerperium. Prostaglandins 7:95–99, 1981.
99. Carreras LO, Defreyn G, Van Houtte E, Vermylen J, Van Assche A: Prostacyclin and pre-eclampsia. Lancet 1:422, 1981.
100. Remuzzi G, Marchesi D, Zoja C, Muratore D, Mecca G, Misiani R, Rossi E, Barbato M, Capetta P, Donati MB, de Gaetano G: Reduced umbilical and placental vascular prostacyclin in severe pre-eclampsia. Prostaglandins 20:105–110, 1980.
101. Downing I, Shepherd GL, Lewis PJ: Reduced prostacyclin production in pre-eclampsia. Lancet 2:1374, 1980.
102. Stuart MJ, Clark DA, Sunderji SG, Allen JB, Yambo T, Elrad H, Slott JH: Decreased prostacyclin production: a characteristic of chronic placental insufficiency syndromes. Lancet 1:1126–1128, 1981.
103. Remuzzi G, Marchesi D, Mecca G: Reduction of fetal vascular prostacyclin activity in pre-eclampsia. Lancet 2:310, 1980.
104. Bussolino F, Benedetto C, Massobrio M, Camussi G: Maternal vascular prostacyclin activity in pre-eclampsia. Lancet 2:702, 1980.
105. Dadak C, Kefalides A, Sinzinger H, Weber G: Reduced umbilical artery prostacyclin formation in complicated pregnancies. Am J Obstet Gynecol 144:792–795, 1982.
106. Hamberg M, Tuoemo T, Svenson J, Ionsson CF: Formation and action of prostacyclin in isolated human umbilical artery. Acta Physiol Scand 106:289–292, 1979.
107. Ritter JM, Ongari M, Gordon-Wright AP, Blair IA, Orchard MA, Lewis PJ: Prostacyclin synthesis by human umbilical artery rings: stimulation of arteries from women with normal pregnancies and preeclampsia by a factor in human serum. In: Lewis PJ, Moncada S, O'Grady J (eds) Prostacyclin in pregnancy. New York: Raven, 1983, pp 159–163.
108. Pearson JD: Plasma factors regulating prostaglandin biosynthesis and catabolism. In: Herman AG, Van Houtte PM, Goosens A, Denolin H (eds) Cardiovascular pharmacology of the prostaglandin. New York: Raven, 1982, pp 23–33.
109. MacIntyre DE, Pearson JD, Gordon JL: Localisation and stimulation of prostacyclin production in vascular cells. Nature 271:549–551, 1978.
110. Remuzzi G, Misiani R, Marchesi D, Livio M, Mecca G, De Gaetano G, Donati MB: Haemolytic–uraemic syndrome: deficiency of plasma factor(s) regulating prostacyclin activity? Lancet 2:871–872, 1978.
111. Remuzzi G, Livio M, Cavenaghi AE, Marchesi D, Mecca G, Donati MB, De Gaetano G: Unbalanced prostaglandin synthesis and plasma factors in uremic bleeding: a hypothesis. Thromb Res 13:531–536, 1978.
112. Remuzzi G, Zoja C, Marchesi D, Schieppati A, Mecca G, Misiani R, Donati MB, De Gaetano G: Plasmatic regulation of vascular prostacyclin in pregnancy. Br Med J 282:512–514, 1981.
113. Gregorini G, Ongari M, Imberti L, Mecca G, Remuzzi G: Plasmatic regulation of prostacyclin production in pregnancy. In: Lewis PJ, Moncada S, O'Grady J (eds) Prostacyclin in pregnancy. New York: Raven, 1983, pp 153–158.
114. Crawford MA: Background to essential fatty acids and their prostanoid derivatives. Br Med Bull 39:210–213, 1983.
115. Lunven P: Nutrition in pregnancy. Lancet 2:400, 1983.
116. Ogburn PL, Johnson SB, Williams PP, Holman RT: Levels of free fatty acids and arachidonic acid in pregnancy and labor. J Lab Clin Med 95:943–949, 1980.
117. Leat WMF, Northrop CA: Effect of dietary linoleic and linolenic acids on gestation and parturition in the rat. Q J Exp Physiol 66:99–103, 1981.
118. Menon NK, More C, Dhopeshwarkar GA: Effect of essential fatty acid deficiency on maternal, placental and fetal rat tissues. J Nutr 111:1602–1610, 1981.
119. Orchard MA, Lewis PJ, Ongari MA, Waddell KA, Blair IA: Free 5,8,11-eicosatrienoic acid in

human umbilical artery. In: Lewis PJ, Moncada S, O'Grady J (eds) Prostacyclin in pregnancy. New York: Raven, 1983, pp 59–63.
120. Hammarstrom S: Conversion of 5,8,11 eicosatrienoic acid to leukotrienes C_3 and D_3. J Biol Chem 256:2275–2279, 1981.
121. Salmon JA, Smith DR, Flower RJ, Moncada S, Vane JR: Further studies on the enzymatic conversion of prostaglandin endoperoxide into prostacyclin by porcine aorta microsomes. Biochim Biophys Acta 523:250–262, 1978.
122. Okuma M, Takayama H, Uchino H: Generation of prostacyclin-like substance and lipid peroxidation in vitamin E-deficient rats. Prostaglandins 19:527–536, 1980.
123. Mullick S, Bagga OP, Duhmullick V: Serum lipids studies in pregnancy. Am J Obstet Gynecol 89:766–770, 1964.
124. Ishihara M: Studies on lipoperoxide of normal pregnant women and of patients with toxemia of pregnancy. Clin Chim Acta 84:1–9, 1978.
125. Maseki M, Nishigaki I, Hagihara M, Tomoda Y, Yagi K: Lipid peroxide levels and lipid content of serum lipoprotein fractions of pregnant subjects with or without pre-eclampsia. Clin Chim Acta 115:155–161, 1981.
126. Stein Y, Stein O, Goren R: Metabolism and metabolic role of serum high density lipoproteins. In: Gotto AM, Miller NE, Dliver MF (eds) High density lipoprotein and atherosclerosis. Amsterdam: Elsevier, 1978, pp 37–49.
127. Dormandy TL: Free-radical oxidation and antioxidants. Lancet 1:647–650, 1978.
128. Jagadeesan V, Prema K: Plasma tocopherol and lipid levels in pregnancy and oral contraceptive users. Br J Obstet Gynaecol 87:903–907, 1980.
129. Jones CJP, Fox H: An ultrastructural and ultrahistochemical study of the human placenta in maternal pre-eclampsia. Placenta 1:61–76, 1980.
130. Van der Veen F, Fox H: The human placenta in idiopathic intrauterine growth retardation: a light and electron microscopic study. Placenta 4:65–78, 1983.
131. Gant NF, Hutchinson HT, Siiteri PK, MacDonald PC: Study of the metabolic clearance rate of dehydroepiandrosterone-sulfate in pregnancy. Am J Obstet Gynecol 111:555–562, 1971.
132. Olkkonen HS, Suonio S, Haring P: Determination of placental blood flow by external monitoring of ^{113}In. Nuklearmedizin 15:168–172, 1976.
133. Lunell NO, Nylund LE, Lewander R, Sarby B: Uteroplacental blood flow in preeclampsia measurements with indium-113 m and a computer-linked gamma camera. Clin Exp Hypertens [B] 1:105–117, 1982.
134. Khong TY, Pearce JMF, Robertson WB, Campbell S: Pathological correlation of changes in blood flow in preeclampsia [abstr]. In: Fourth world congress of the International Society for the Study of Hypertension in Pregnancy, Amsterdam, June 1984, p 69.
135. Marais WD: Human decidual spiral artery studies. IV. Human atherosis of a few weeks duration: histopathogenesis. J Obstet Gynaecol Br Commonw 69:234–238, 1962.
136. Dixon HG, Robertson WB: Vascular changes in the placental bed. Pathol Microbiol 24:-622–629, 1961.
137. Brosens I: A study of the spiral arteries of the decidua basalis in normotensive and hypertensive pregnancies. J Obstet Gynaecol Br Commonw 71:222–230, 1964.
138. Rakoczi I, Tihanyi K, Falkay G, Rozsa I, Demeter J, Gati I: Prostacyclin production in trophoblast. In: Lewis PJ, Moncada S, O'Grady J (eds) Prostacyclin in pregnancy. New York: Raven, 1983, pp 15–23.
139. Jogee M, Myatt K, Moore P, Elder MG: Prostacyclin production by human placental cells in short-term culture. Placenta 4:219–230, 1983.
140. Moncada S, Higgs EA, Vane JR: Human arterial and venous tissues generate prostacyclin (prostaglandin x), a potent inhibitor of platelet aggregation. Lancet 1:18–21, 1977.
141. Robertson WB, Bronsens I, Dixon HG: The pathological response of the vessels of the placental bed to hypertensive pregnancy. J Pathol Bacteriol 93:581–592, 1967.
142. Zeek PM, Assali NS: Vascular changes in the decidua associated with eclamptogenic toxemia of pregnancy. Am J Clin Pathol 20:1099–1106, 1950.
143. De Wolf F, Robertson WB, Brosens I: The ultrastructure of acute atherosis of the spiral arteries in hypertensive pregnancy. Am J Obstet Gynecol 123:164–174, 1975.
144. Brosens I, Renaer N: On the pathogenesis of placental infarcts in preeclampsia. J Obstet Gynaecol Br Commonw 79:794–799, 1972.

145. Perico N, Pusineri F, Remuzzi G: The lupus anticoagulant. Proc Soc Exp Biol Med 176:-337–341, 1984.
146. Nilsson JM, Astedt B, Hedner U, Berezin D: Intrauterine death and circulating anticoagulant. Acta Med Scand 197:153–159, 1975.
147. De Wolf F, Carreras LO, Moerman P, Vermylen J, Van Assche A, Renaer M: Decidual vasculopathy and extensive placental infarction in a patient with repeated thromboembolic accidents, recurrent fetal loss, and a lupus anticoagulant. Am J Obstet Gynecol 142:829–834, 1982.
148. Vermylen J, Carreras LO, Deckmyn H, Van Assche A, De Wolf F, Spitz B: Abnormal prostacyclin release in pregnancy. In: Lewis PJ, Moncada S, O'Grady J (eds) Prostacyclin in pregnancy. New York: Raven, 1983, pp 171–174.
149. Soulier JP, Boffa MC: Avortéments à répétition, thromboses et anticoagulant circulant antithromboplastine. Nouv Presse Med 9:859–864, 1980.
150. Editorial: Pregnancy and the arachidonic acid cascade. Lancet 1:997–998, 1982.

3. COAGULATION AND PREGNANCY

EDOARDO ROSSI, MARIA MATILDE COSSU, and PIERO CAPETTA

1. INTRODUCTION

During the course of normal pregnancy the hemostatic system undergoes major changes resulting in fibrin deposition in the uteroplacental vasculature that is very important for the normal development of pregnancy. Such changes are interpreted as a physiologic adaptation to prepare the hemostatic system for its role during placental separation; in late pregnancy, in fact, the uterine blood flow to the placenta reaches 600–800 ml/min and at parturition it must be arrested within a few seconds. The effectiveness of such modifications is such that childbirth in pregnant women with congenital hemorrhagic disorders (e.g., von Willebrand disease) involves very slight hemorrhagic risk (and need of treatment) and less risk than in events other than pregnancy such as surgical interventions.

Knowledge of the physiology of hemostasis during pregnancy is thus necessary in order to have a rational basis for treating any hemorrhagic or thromboembolic complications; furthermore, monitoring the pattern of the hemostatic changes may provide indications on the evolution of any disorders occurring during pregnancy and consequently on fetal outcome.

2. CHANGES IN THE HEMOSTATIC SYSTEM

2.1. Coagulation system

The plasma levels and activity of most of the clotting factors are increased during normal pregnancy, except for factors XI and XIII (decreased activity) and factor

V (unchanged activity) [1]. This increase is progressive during the course of pregnancy; it is already evident in the second month and reaches the maximum in the third trimester. In table 3-1, the values of the clotting factors at the end of pregnancy are reported. The most significant increase is observed in fibrinogen and in factors VII, VIII, and X. All the components of factor VIII are increased, although the increase of F VIII R:AG–F VIII vWF (synthesized in the endothelium) is greater than that of F VIII:C [2]. The increase in clotting factors is even more marked when taking into account the effect of hemodilution due to the expansion of plasma volume that is typical of pregnancy. This means that by the end of pregnancy the fibrinogen concentration, for example, has almost doubled. Changes in concentration of clotting factors reflect the balance between synthesis (increased in pregnancy) and consumption. During pregnancy the concentrations and activity of the most important natural inhibitors of coagulation (i.e., antithrombin III, anti-Xa, and protein C) are maintained at the same or slightly lower levels than in the nonpregnant state. All the changes induced by pregnancy normalize after childbirth, at a rate proportional to the half-life of each factor.

2.2. Platelets

During normal pregnancy there is a slight reduction in the count of circulating platelets, attributable to the plasma volume expansion; platelet life span, determined with nonradioisotopic methods, in fact, is within the normal range [3].

No significant alterations are observed in platelet function when investigated with the usual aggregation and adhesiveness tests. Also the plasma platelet-specific proteins β-thromboglobulin and PF_4) and the platelet concentration of β-thromboglobulin and 5-hydroxytryptamine are not significantly different from nonpregnancy values [4]. There is no significant change in the production of platelet thromboxane A_2 [5].

2.3. Fibrinolytic enzyme system

A significant progressive reduction of fibrinolytic activity of the plasma (as measured by euglobulin lysis time) [1] and of fibrinolytic response to venous occlusion

Table 3-1. Clotting factors in late pregnancy

Fibrinogen	4.0–6.5 g/liter
Factor II	100%–125%[a]
Factor V	100%–150%
Factor VII	150%–250%
Factor VIII	200%–500%
Factor IX	100%–150%
Factor X	150%–250%
Factor XI	50%–100%
Factor XII	100%–150%
Factor XIII	40%–70%
Antithrombin III	80%–110%
Protein C	80%–100%

[a]%, percent of normal values.

[6] is characteristic of pregnancy, and normalizes rapidly after separation of the placenta [1].

The placenta produces an inhibitor of urokinase-induced fibrinolysis [7]. A fall in the levels of plasminogen activator, responsible for reduced fibrinolytic activity of plasma in vitro, could be the consequence of its absorption to fibrin, and thus not necessarily be an in vivo expression of fibrinolysis impairment during normal pregnancy.

Furthermore, in pregnancy there is a 50% decrease in the plasma concentration of histidine-rich glycoprotein (HRG) [8]. This protein has an affinity for the lysine binding sites of plasminogen and thus plays a role in the regulation of fibrinolysis. The decrease in its levels in pregnancy results in more free plasminogen being available for binding to fibrin. It is interesting that there is a similar decrease in HRG levels during contraceptive treatment with estrogen–progesterone combinations [9].

As a result of these modifications, the fibrinolytic enzyme system may be rapidly and efficiently activated in pregnancy.

3. CLOTTING ACTIVATION DURING NORMAL PREGNANCY

3.1. Signs of clotting activation

When considered together, the hemostatic changes that occur in normal pregnancy are compatible with the development of clotting activation, that is, with the presence in the circulation of intermediate activated coagulation factors that are the expression of thrombin formation in excess of the capacities of antithrombin control mechanisms. At least in the third trimester of pregnancy, in fact, there are always signs of increased thrombin formation such as those shown in table 3-2 [2, 10–13]. It is still controversial, however, whether the increase in the F VIII R:AG–F VIII:C ratio in pregnancy is due to a thrombin-induced loss of coagulant activity of factor VIII as a result of activation of the coagulation system. The increased endothelial synthesis of F VIII R:AG, in fact, might have a different pattern than the nonendothelial synthesis of F VIII:C. However, the presence of other signs that certainly indicate increased thrombin formation, such as fibrinopeptide A (FPA) and high molecular weight fibrin(ogen) complexes (HMWFC), and the fact that the one-stage assay (influenced by the presence of thrombin and Xa) gives higher values of F VIII:C than the two-stage assay (not influenced by circulating thrombin), suggests that the increase of the F VIII R:AG–F VIII:C ratio

Table 3-2. Signs of clotting activation usually observed in pregnancy

High molecular weight fibrin(ogen) complexes (HMWFC) [10]
Fibrinopeptide A (FPA) [11]
Increased F VIII R:AG–F VIII:C ratio [2]
Cold promoted activation of thrombotest (occasionally) [12]
Thrombin-like influence on factor-V activity [13]

is due at least in part to the thrombin-induced loss of factor-VIII coagulant activity.

A characteristic aspect of clotting activation in normal pregnancy that is not observed in other prothrombotic states is the absence of signs of platelet activation, despite the evident signs of enhanced thrombin production in the plasma.

3.2. Cause of clotting activation

Clotting activation in normal pregnancy is attributable to the endothelial damage caused by migration of the trophoblast in the maternal vessels. In human hemochorial placentation, in fact, the trophoblast causes fragmentation and discontinuation of the endothelium of the spiral arteries and penetrates the arterial walls up to the myometrium; thus, elastic lamina and smooth muscle cells are replaced by a matrix containing fibrin and by trophoblastic cells. These structural changes of the spiral arteries ("physiologic changes") cause an expansion of the lumina, thereby allowing the increase in blood flow normally occurring as pregnancy advances; furthermore, these physiologic changes make the uteroplacental vessels less responsive to maternal vasomotory stimuli and favor the institution of low peripheral resistances in the uteroplacental vasculature. The endothelial damage induced by trophoblast migration causes local activation of the coagulation system, which results in a compensatory increase of clotting factors that exceeds the rate of consumption. Furthermore, the placenta and decidua are rich in tissue thromboplastin, the release of which may activate the coagulation system.

3.3. Results of clotting activation

The enhanced thrombin production results in an increase in fibrin formation and deposition. Fletcher et al. [10] have evaluated the plasma HMWFC concentration in normal pregnancy and calculated a threefold increase in fibrin formation in the second month of pregnancy, compared with the nonpregnant state, and a fivefold or more increase in late pregnancy. This indicates that daily formation of fibrin in the third trimester is 150–250 mg.

The progressive reduction in the plasma levels of factor XIII is also consistent with the progressive increase in fibrin formation [14]. Fibrin deposition may be demonstrated in the media of the spiral arteries supplying the placenta; a fibrin deposit in the intervillous space is normally present in pregnancy and is probably important in its development since it serves to regulate the maternal–fetal exchanges. Furthermore, numerous mural thrombi in various stages of organization can be observed in late pregnancy.

3.4. Control mechanisms of clotting activation

The nonparticipation of platelets in clotting activation in pregnancy and the control of fibrin deposits are both due to the increased availability of antiaggregant prostaglandins and the efficacy of the fibrinolytic system despite the fall in plasma levels of plasminogen activator.

Systemic and uterine maternal vessels, umbilical vessels, placenta [15], myometrium [16], and other components of the fetoplacental unit synthesize notable quantities of prostacyclin (PGI_2), the most important prostaglandin produced by the vessel walls, which inhibits platelet aggregation and causes the vascular smooth muscle tissue to relax. The increased availability of PGI_2 may explain why there is normally no vascular thrombosis in the spiral arteries despite the presence of major endothelial lesions caused by trophoblast penetration of the arterial wall. The trophoblast secretes PGI_2 [17], and there is reason to believe that the interaction of the migrating trophoblast with the uterine arterial wall, which is the crucial event of normal placentation, is a prostacyclin-dependent phenomenon; that is, the capacity of the invading tissue to colonize maternal vessels is related to its capacity to produce PGI_2, thereby preventing immobilization by platelet aggregates. The efficacy of this antiaggregant mechanism in normal pregnancy is demonstrated not only by the nonparticipation of platelets in clotting activation, but also by the absence of arterial thrombosis in the spiral arteries despite major disendothelization.

The reduced plasma concentration of plasminogen activator, which causes the decrease of plasma fibrinolytic activity in vitro, could be due to adsorption of the activator on the fibrin fibers. Such a mechanism might effectively limit fibrin deposits and might also account for the usual difficulty in histologic demonstration of fibrin deposits [18]. Furthermore, the reduced plasma levels of HRG increase the availability of free plasminogen for binding to fibrin.

4. ACUTE COAGULATION DEFECTS IN PREGNANCY: THE DISSEMINATED INTRAVASCULAR COAGULATION (DIC)

4.1. Pathogenesis

Acute coagulation defects arise in several complications of pregnancy and labor. These hemostatic defects are the consequence of acute disseminated intravascular coagulation (DIC). DIC is more frequent in pregnancy pathologies than in other diseases because of the changes in the hemostatic system occurring during normal pregnancy

Acute DIC is a complex multifactorial syndrome caused by the generalized formation of thrombin in amounts far beyond the capacity of the antithrombin mechanisms to control. In patients with acute DIC, the factors consumed during normal coagulation (fibrinogen, factors V and VIII, platelets, antithrombin III, protein C) are greatly reduced or even disappear from circulation. Secondary hyperfibrinolysis also occurs, due to simultaneous activation of the fibrinolytic enzyme system, which promotes the clearance of intravascular fibrin deposits especially by the kidney; this hyperfibrinolysis acts also on the plasma clotting factors, thereby aggravating the hemostatic defect due to excessive consumption of these factors. This serious condition of decompensated DIC is preceded by a phase of compensated DIC in which the signs of clotting factors consumption are slight or even absent (because synthesis of clotting factors is increased) and there are only a few signs of hyperfibrinolysis.

4.2. Clinical picture

The clinical consequences of acute DIC are mainly hemorrhage and/or ischemic organ damage, anemia and shock. Hemorrhage is the most important and the greatest threat to life. It is caused by excess consumption of clotting factors and may manifest in any district although the genital district is most commonly involved. The lost blood has a characteristic aspect of incoagulability and fluidity that is mainly due to the reduced levels of circulating fibrinogen. The visible hemorrhage, however, is not a good indication of the amount of blood lost or of the severity of the hemostatic defect. This may be demonstrated by prolonged bleeding from the sites of venipuncture, by spontaneous cutaneous and mucosal hemorrhages, by hematomas at the sites of injections or sutures, or by hemorrhage during surgery. The first diagnostic indication of the hemostatic defect is often the failure to clot of the blood sample sent for testing to the laboratory.

The site and extent of ischemic organ damage depend on the relationship between thrombin–fibrinogen and plasmin–fibrin interactions. Micro- and macro-thrombosis occur in the late stages of DIC, especially in the forms with a chronic course. The organs most frequently affected by ischemic damage are kidneys, brain, lungs, skin, and liver.

Anemia is fundamentally posthemorrhagic; a hemolytic–microangiopathic component may be present that, however, is more typical of the forms of DIC with a chronic course (preeclampsia) or of the later phases of acute DIC associated with thrombotic microangiopathy.

Posthemorrhagic hypovolemic shock is the most dangerous consequence of DIC since it increases this coagulation defect. In the pregnant woman, in fact, shock may trigger intravascular clotting. The severity of shock generally depends on severity of the hemorrhage, but it may be enhanced following the activation of the vasoactive kinins usually present in DIC.

The pathologies of pregnancy that are most frequently complicated by acute DIC are listed in table 3-3. Acute DIC may exhibit different clinical pictures. When it occurs in the presence of an efficient fetoplacental unit (e.g., abruptio placentae) it is characterized by a major hemorrhagic symptomatology and a hypovolemic shock, while ischemic organ damage develops much later either as the consequence of no or inadequate treatment of the acute phase or as the result of prolonged shock.

Table 3-3. Pathologies of pregnancy most frequently complicated by disseminated intravascular coagulation (DIC)

Abruptio placentae
Amniotic fluid embolism
Prolonged retention of dead fetus
Intrauterine infection
Eclampsia and preeclampsia
Shock of any etiology
Severe fetomaternal bleeding

The symptomatology related to ischemic organ damage is typical of the acute DIC that manifests itself some time after the loss of function of the fetoplacental unit (e.g., prolonged retention of the dead fetus). This difference may be due to the presence or absence of the factors that normally control clotting activation in pregnancy. Thus, the increased availability of antiaggregant and vasodilatory prostaglandins and the efficacy of fibrinolysis do not protect against hemorrhagic risk, but do prevent thrombotic microangiopathy by means of reduced platelet participation and effective clearance of fibrin.

4.3. Diagnosis

The diagnosis of acute coagulation defects is based on signs of excessive consumption of clotting factors and secondary hyperfibrinolysis. Prothrombin time (PT), partial thromboplastin time (PTT), fibrinogen concentration, platelet count, and rapid assays measuring the levels of fibrin(ogen) degradation products (FDP) provide information on the patient's coagulation status; more sophisticated tests are too time-consuming, and do not provide more useful information. In Table 3-4 the tests are reported that are commonly used to diagnose both the compensated and decompensated phases of DIC. Obviously, precise knowledge of modifications of the clotting factors in pregnancy is essential; furthermore, serial checks at short intervals may give early information on the evolution from normality to compensated DIC or from the compensated to the decompensated stage of DIC.

Early diagnosis of DIC is clearly important to avoid the catastrophic consequences of the overt clinical phase. Diagnosis must be made immediately after the appearance of any pathology of pregnancy that may be complicated by DIC. In DIC that develops when the fetoplacental unit is functioning efficiently, consumption of the clotting factors varies greatly and is sometimes severe, whereas the reduction of the platelet count is more modest; signs of secondary hyperfibrinolysis are always evident. DIC that develops some time after the fetoplacental unit has ceased to function as an efficient unit is characterized by a modest consumption of the clotting factors, severe thrombocytopenia, and slight signs of

Table 3-4. Laboratory tests in pathologies of pregnancy complicated by disseminated intravascular coagulation (DIC) and defective hemostasis

	Acute or decompensated phase	Compensated phase
Platelet count	Reduced (< 100,000/ml)	Normal or reduced
Thrombin clotting time	Prolonged ++	Prolonged +
Fibrinogen	Reduced	Normal
Fibrin(ogen) degradation products (FDP)	Raised ++	Raised +
One-stage prothrombin time	Prolonged	Normal
Activated partial thromboplastin time	Prolonged	Normal
Factor-VIII level	Reduced	Normal

hyperfibrinolysis. This different pattern is explained, at least in part, by the presence or absence of the mechanisms that regulate the physiologic clotting activation in pregnancy.

4.4. Treatment

The treatment proposed for acute coagulation defects in obstetric patients is largely based on the observation of a few cases, since no adequate trials of the therapeutic measures have been performed. There are three main steps in treatment: removal of the cause of DIC, replacement therapy, and anticoagulant therapy.

The cause of DIC should be removed whenever possible, regardless of the hemostatic situation; this is the most important therapeutic approach since it is practically impossible to obtain normalization of the coagulation defect without eliminating the cause of DIC. Removal of the cause is often followed by spontaneous regression of DIC.

Replacement therapy has the aim of correcting the hemostatic defect, anemia, and shock. Fresh frozen plasma is the most useful blood component to correct the hemostatic defect, since it is generally difficult to procure sufficient amounts of fresh whole blood (no older than 6 h). Fresh frozen plasma provides adequate amounts of the labile factors V and VIII in addition to fibrinogen, antithrombin III, and protein C. Platelet concentrates may be used in cases of severe thrombocytopenia; concentrates of antithrombin III have also been used successfully. The use of stored whole blood, which is deprived of factors V and VIII and platelets, is contraindicated, since it would further dilute these factors in the recipient. Furthermore, stored whole blood is rich in microaggregates that will be entrapped in the lung, thereby contributing to the respiratory distress syndrome that not infrequently complicates DIC in pregnancy. Treatment with fibrinogen concentrates is not recommended, since it may aggravate intravascular coagulation.

Anemia may be effectively controlled with transfusions of packed red cells.

It is vitally important to correct shock since shock per se in pregnant women promotes intravascular coagulation.

Prompt replacement of the blood volume is fundamental in preventing acute renal failure. Blood volume replacement should be guided by monitoring central venous pressure and urinary output until complete normalization of the hemostatic function. The latter must thus be carefully and frequently checked.

The efficacy of anticoagulant therapy with heparin in DIC is still controversial. It may serve to block consumption of the clotting factors and prevent microthrombosis, but, if the vascular compartment is not intact, such treatment may increase hemorrhage, especially when there is severe thrombocytopenia with reduced availability of PF_4.

In our experience, removal of the cause of DIC and adequate treatment of hypovolemic shock are sufficient to induce spontaneous regression of DIC, without anticoagulant therapy. The use of antifibrinolytic agents is contraindicated since they may interfere with fibrin clearance in the microcirculation.

5. HEMOSTATIC SYSTEM IN PREECLAMPSIA

The modifications of the hemostatic system in preeclampsia are the result of failure in the mechanisms that control clotting activation in pregnancy. In preeclamptic pregnancy, there are evident signs of increased thrombin production. In particular, FPA and HMWFC are increased, demonstrating increased formation and deposition of fibrin. Moreover, there is reduced availability of PGI_2 [15] and inefficient fibrinolytic activity.

The platelets, which are not involved in clotting activation of normal pregnancy, play an important role in preeclampsia: there is an early fall in platelet count coinciding with increase in uric acid levels and increased sensitivity to angiotensin [18]; platelet life span is reduced [3]; circulating platelets respond less to aggregating agents, and there is a decrease in their serotonin content [19]; and plasma levels of the platelet-specific proteins are increased [4]. There is, therefore, evidence of platelet activation. It is still not established whether these platelet abnormalities in preeclampsia are due to actual consumption connected with phenomena of vascular microthrombosis with reduced platelet survival [3], or to a temporary and reversible sequestration in some districts of platelets with normal survival [19].

Concerning fibrinolysis, in preeclampsia there is a greater increase in euglobulin lysis time than in normal pregnancy, and a slower normalization after parturition. This indicates a greater absorption of the activator on the fibrin fibers and consequently a greater fibrinolytic activation that is evidenced by the increase in serum FDP that is characteristic of preeclampsia. Despite this increased activation, the insufficiency of fibrinolytic control is shown by the pathologic deposition of fibrin at the placenta, with occlusions of the spiral arteries, and consequent placental infarcts and fetal underdevelopment. Thrombotic microangiopathy may involve also other microcirculatory districts (particularly that of the kidney) and may generalize during eclamptic crises.

In preeclamptic pregnancy, there is also an early pathologic increase of the F VIII R:AG–F VIII:C ratio, which correlates with fetal growth retardation and perinatal mortality [20]. The increase of this ratio is connected both with increased endothelial synthesis of F VIII R:AG (and this confirms the existence of endothelial activation or damage) and with a more marked thrombin-induced loss of factor-VIII coagulation activity. Our sequential studies in preeclamptic women have demonstrated that the F VIII R:AG–F VIII:C ratio increased progressively up to a maximum, after which it decreased progressively until normalization: in this second phase the signs of deterioration of placental function and increased fetal risk became more marked [21]. An increase of the F VIII R:AG–F VIII:C ratio indicates abnormal endothelial stimulation and activation of the clotting system originating in the uteroplacental circulation with abnormal thrombin generation: its progressive decrease suggests that the factor triggering the clotting activation gradually disappears so that thrombotic lesions occur and are followed by irreversible cessation of the deciduoplacental function.

The early major involvement of the platelets and factor-VIII complex in preeclampsia indicates that abnormalities of the relation between the platelets and endothelium play an important role in the genesis and course of this disease; moreover, recent data attribute an initial and fundamental role to abnormalities of vessel walls in preeclampsia (see chapter 2).

6. CONCLUSION

The hemostatic system undergoes major adaptation to the state of pregnancy. This consists of physiologic signs of clotting activation that originate in the uteroplacental circulation as a consequence of changes in the uteroplacental vasculature necessary to allow an adequate flow of blood to the placenta as pregnancy advances. The result of such clotting activation is fibrin deposition at the uteroplacental level. These changes of the hemostatic system well account for the frequency and importance of the acute coagulation defects with DIC in pregnancy.

Careful monitoring of hemostasis in pregnancy may provide useful indications regarding the functioning of the deciduoplacental microcirculation, especially in pathologies of pregnancy characterized by fetal growth retardation.

REFERENCES

1. Bonnar J, McNicol GP, Douglas AS: The coagulation and fibrinolytic mechanism during and after normal childbirth. Br Med J 2:200–203, 1970.
2. Van Royen EA, Ten Cate JW: Antigen–biological activity ratio for factor VIII in late pregnancy. Lancet 2:449–450, 1973.
3. Rakoczi I, Tallian F, Bagdany S, Gati I: Platelet life-span in normal pregnancy and pre-eclampsia as determined by a non-radioisotope technique. Thromb Res 15:553–556, 1979.
4. Airoldi ML, Capetta P, Cattaneo S, Paracchini ML, Rossi E, Tantalo V: Livelli plasmatici di β-TG e PF_4 nella gravidanza normale e pre-eclampsia. In: Doni A, Gasparri F (eds) Haemostasis and pregnancy. Florence: Giuntina, 1983, pp 193–199.
5. Wallenburg HCS, Rotmans N: Enhanced reactivity of the platelet thromboxane pathway in normotensive and hypertensive pregnancies with insufficient fetal growth. Am J Obstet Gynecol 144:523–528, 1982.
6. Astedt B, Isacson S, Nilsson IH: Fibrinolytic activity of veins during pregnancy. Acta Obstet Gynecol Scand 49:171–173, 1970.
7. Uszynski M, Abildgaard U: Separation and characterisation of two fibrinolytic inhibitors from human placenta. Thromb Diathes Haemorrh 25:580–589, 1971.
8. Morgan WT, Koskelo P, Koenig H, Conway TP: Human histidine-rich glycoprotein. II. Serum levels in adults, pregnant women and neonates. Proc Soc Exp Biol Med 158:647–651, 1978.
9. Jespersen J, Kluft C: Decreased levels of histidine-rich glycoprotein (RHG) and increased levels of free plasminogen in women on oral contraceptives low in estrogen. Thromb Haemost 48:283–285, 1982.
10. Fletcher AP, Alkjaersig NK, Burstein R: The influence of pregnancy upon blood coagulation and plasma fibrinolytic enzyme function. Am J Obstet Gynecol 134:743–751, 1979.
11. Weiner CP, Kwaan H, Hauck WW, Duboe FJ, Paul M, Wallemark CB: Fibrin generation in normal pregnancy. Obstet Gynecol 64:46–48, 1964.
12. Gjonnaess H: Cold promoted activation of factor VII. Gynecol Invest 4:61–721, 1973.
13. Van Royen EA: Haemostasis in human pregnancy and delivery. Thesis, University of Amsterdam, 1974.
14. Coopland A, Alkjaersig N, Fletcher AP: Reduction in plasma factor XIII (fibrin stabilizing factor) concentration during pregnancy. J Lab Clin Med 73:144–153, 1969.
15. Remuzzi G, Marchesi D, Zoia C, Muratore D, Mecca G, Misiani R, Rossi E, Barbato M, Capetta P, Donati MB, De Gaetano G: Reduced umbilical and placental vascular prostacyclin in severe pre-eclampsia. Prostaglandins 20:105–110, 1980.
16. Omini C, Folco GC, Pasargiklian R, Fono M, Berti F: Prostacyclin (PGI_2) in the pregnant human uterus. Prostaglandins 17:113–120, 1979.

17. Rakoczi I, Tihanyi K, Falkay G, Rósza I, Demeier J, Gáti I: Prostacyclin production in trophoblast. In: Lewis PJ, Moncada S, O'Grady J (eds) Prostacyclin and pregnancy. New York: Raven, 1983, pp 15–23.
18. Redman CWG, Bonnar J, Beilin CJ: Early platelet consumption in pre-eclampsia. Br Med J 1:467–469, 1978.
19. Whigham KAE, Howie PW, Drummond AH, Prentice CRM: Abnormal platelet function in pre-eclampsia. Br J Obstet Gynaecol 85:28–32, 1978.
20. Thornton CA, Bonnar J: Factor VIII related antigen and factor VIII coagulant activity in normal and pre-eclamptic pregnancy. J Obstet Gynaecol Br Commonw 84:919–923, 1977.
21. Capetta P, Rossi E, Mondonico P, Gianotti GA, Polvani F: Factor VIII related antigen/factor VIII ratio and pre-kallikrein activity in monitoring the hypertensive diseases of pregnancy. In: Bonnar J, MacGillivray I, Symonds M (eds) Pregnancy hypertension. Lancaster UK: MTP, 1979, pp 383–391.

4. PATHOLOGY OF THE KIDNEY IN PREECLAMPSIA

JAMES R. TAYLOR and BENJAMIN H. SPARGO

1. INTRODUCTION

The inability to identify properly the underlying condition resulting in gestational hypertension and other renal dysfunctions during pregnancy using clinical criteria alone has led to a great deal of confusion in the literature [1–3]. An evolution in the pathologic nomenclature and the now widespread use of electron and immunofluorescent microscopy in addition to light microscopy has allowed for a more precise distinction of lesions of true preeclampsia from others that mimic preeclampsia clinically. In the 1950s, one of the authors (B.H.S.) recalls the frustration of Dieckmann not only in the inability to clinically distinguish preeclampsia from other causes of hypertension in pregnancy, but also by the discrepancy between his clinical impression and the pathologist's report and the irreproducibility of the pathologic interpretation [4]. The scope of this problem of clinical variability has been more recently revealed in several studies in which postpartum renal biopsy in women, diagnosed to have preeclampsia clinically, revealed renal lesions other than those ascribed to preeclampsia in as many as 45% of the patients [2, 5]. These other renal lesions include primary renal diseases such as glomerulonephritis, membranous nephropathy, "minimal change" nephropathy, tubulointerstitial lesions, and nephrosclerosis, in addition to lesions associated with systemic disease such as sickle cell and diabetic nephropathies [5]. These conditions were not infrequently found superimposed on the renal changes felt to be characteristic of preeclamptic toxemia (PET).

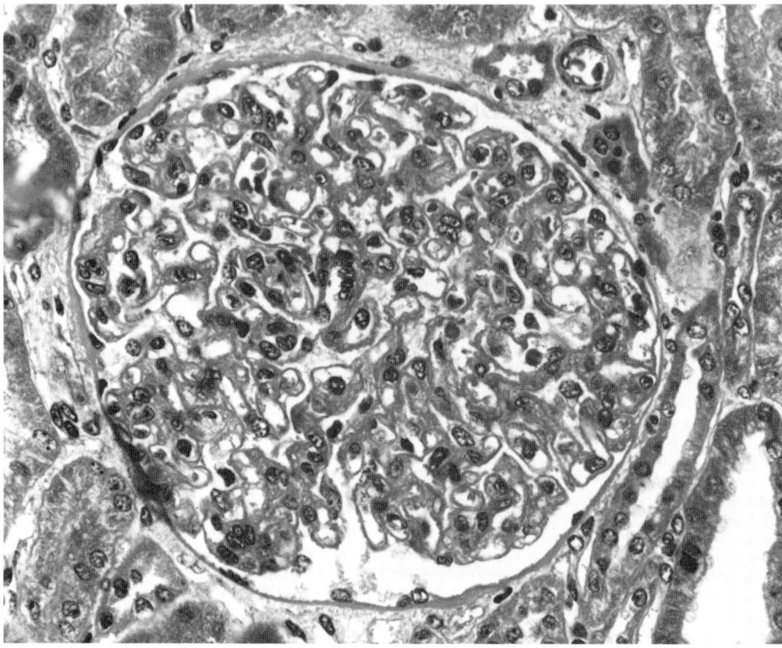

Figure 4-1. Preeclamptic nephropathy. The glomerulus is swollen and fills Bowman's space. There is a decrease in the vascularity, resulting in a bloodless appearance. The glomerulus is normocellular. H & E, × 400.

Since 1958, postpartum renal biopsy of patients with gestational hypertension has been intensively studied at the University of Chicago, resulting in the collection of more than 200 cases. Not only severely preeclamptic and eclamptic patients, but also patients with only mild hypertension, were biopsied. This has resulted not only in a variety of lesions, but also a wide spectrum of severity. All of these have been studied by both light and electron microscopy and the majority have also been subjected to immunohistologic analysis. We feel that only by the utilization of all three of these complementary modalities can the various lesions associated with gestational hypertension be accurately distinguished. This can be exemplified in the situation when the pathologist is faced with the differential diagnosis of a renal lesion in which frequent double contours of the basement membrane and interpositioning of mesangial cytoplasm are seen by light microscopy and electron microscopy, respectively. These features are seen not only in preeclampsia, but also membranoproliferative glomerulonephritis. The demonstration of a granular reaction for both immunoglobulin and complement by immunofluorescence would indicate that the lesion was a complex trapping glomerulonephritis. Similarly, in a recent study, it was shown that IgA nephropathy (the diagnosis of which requires immunohistology for demonstration of the specific nature of the deposits) was not associated with progression of the renal disease during pregnancy whereas membranoproliferative lesions did progress [6]. This again underscores the importance

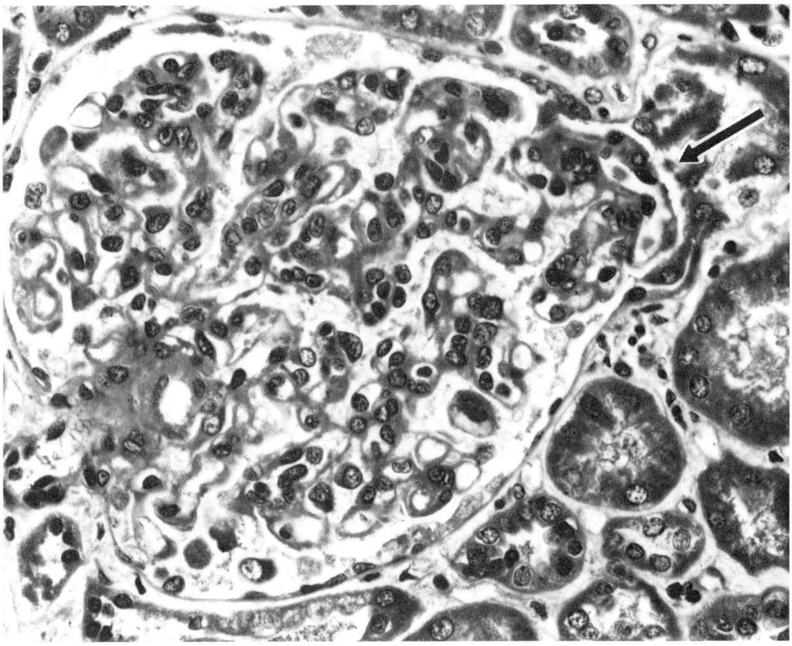

Figure 4-2. The swelling of the mesangial and endothelial cells has resulted in partial occlusion of the capillary lumina and herniation of the tuft into the proximal tubule *(arrow).* H & E, × 400.

of the pathologist using all the tools available to him. This chapter summarizes the morphologic criteria we use to distinguish the lesion of PET from other conditions. The importance of this distinction can be appreciated in follow-up studies that have confirmed the complete reversibility and and excellent long-term prognosis of pure preeclampsia [1, 5, 7].

2. LIGHT AND ELECTRON MICROSCOPY

There are no substantive differences in the renal lesions between preeclampsia and eclampsia [2], and in general the severity of the clinical signs and symptoms is matched in a proportionate degree by the severity of the morphologic alteration [8]. The most consistent and biologically important renal changes occur in the glomeruli that are diffusely enlarged and swollen [2, 8, 9]. A focal variation in the intensity of the changes is often observed, particularly as they resolve [10] (figure 4-1). Measurements on postmortem material by Sheehan and Lynch [11] have shown that the toxemic glomerulus is about 10% larger than that of the normal. Occasional giant glomeruli (two times the mean normal glomerular size) are seen, particularly in eclamptics [12]. The enlarged glomerular tuft fills the Bowman space and, in more severe cases, herniation of the tuft into the proximal tubule in a process dubbed "pouting" by Sheehan and Lynch is occasionally seen [2, 5, 8, 11, 12] (figure 4-2).

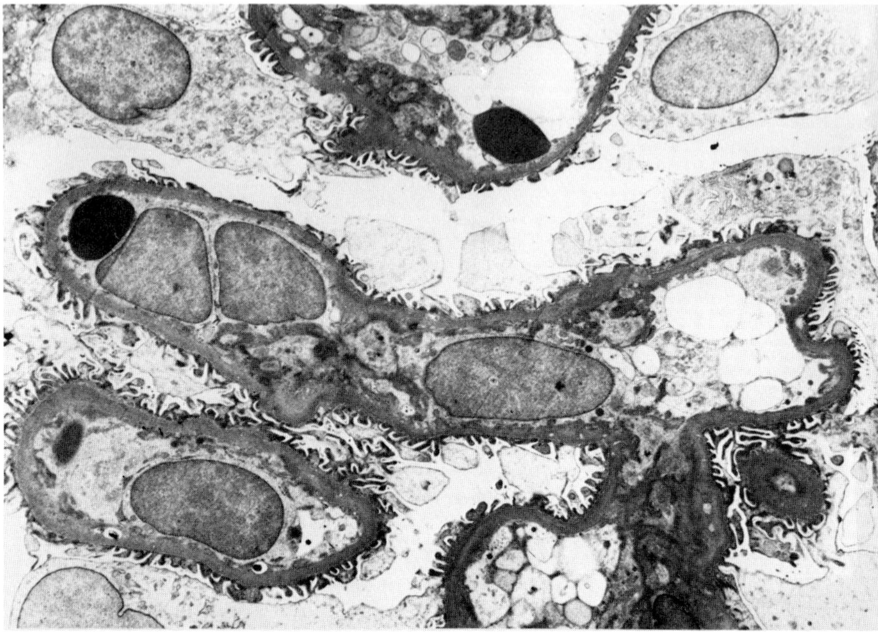

Figure 4-3. An electron micrograph showing the characteristic cigar-shaped distortion of the lobule seen in preeclampsia. × 7500.

Significant hypercellularity, such as that which is seen in inflammatory lesions such as glomerulonephritis, is not a feature of PET [2, 8, 13]. Postinflammatory changes such as segmental adhesions are also not seen [2, 10, 14]. Apposition and bridging of the glomerular capillary loops to the capsular epithelium can be demonstrated ultrastructurally at the peak of severity in some cases, but this change is reversible. The hyalinization and adherence noted by several authors may represent cases of mild glomerulonephritis that were erroneously included in the PET group [8, 12, 15].

Characteristically the glomeruli in PET have an obstructed, bloodless appearance with a marked decrease in vascularity and a characteristic pattern of longitudinal capillary collapse producing cigar-shaped lobules [16] (figure 4-3). The degree of obstruction can be so marked in the most severe cases as to result in infarction of glomeruli and renal cortical necrosis (figure 4-4). This encroachment on the lumen is due to a marked mesangial and endothelial cell cytoplasmic hypertrophy, a feature that is more easily appreciated ultrastructurally [16] (figure 4-5). This cytoplasmic swelling extends from the stalk area out to the peripheral capillary loops and is responsible for the dilatation and beading of the stem and ballooning of the capillary loops, particularly in severe cases [8, 12]. The cytoplasmic hypertrophy results in the ultrastructural impression of an increased number of cytoplasmic organelles [15]. Vacuolation of the mesangial and endothelial cells due to the accumulation of fluid and lipid is a prominent feature that is best appreciated at the light-microscopic level

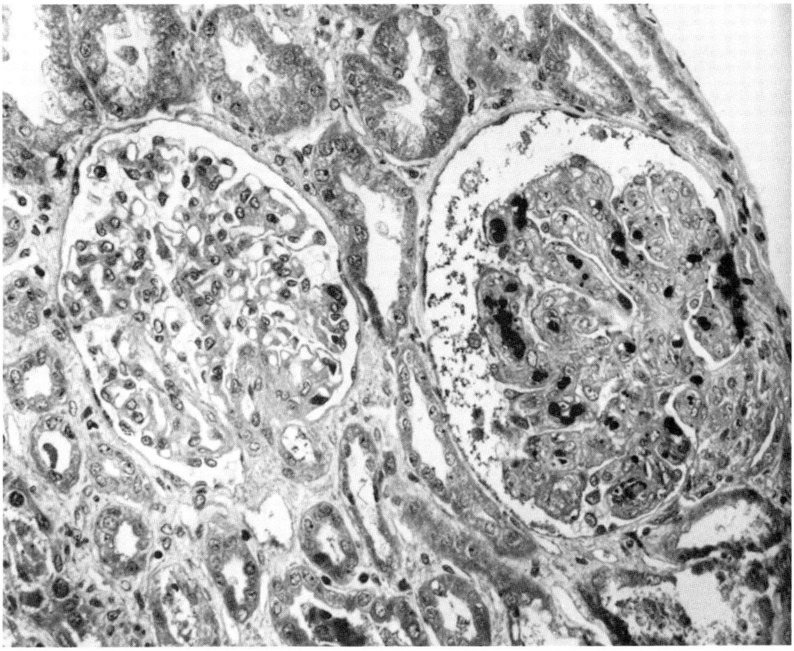

Figure 4-4. There is marked variation in the degree of obstruction. The glomerulus on the right is preinfarcted. H & E, × 300.

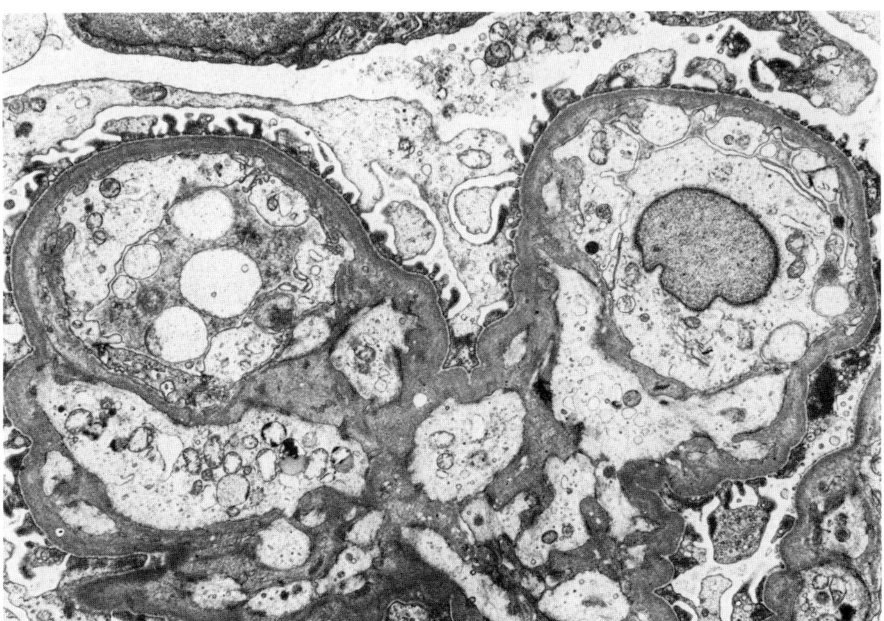

Figure 4-5. An electron micrograph showing prominence of endothelial cytoplasm with no residual lumen. The epithelial cell foot processes are intact. × 11,250.

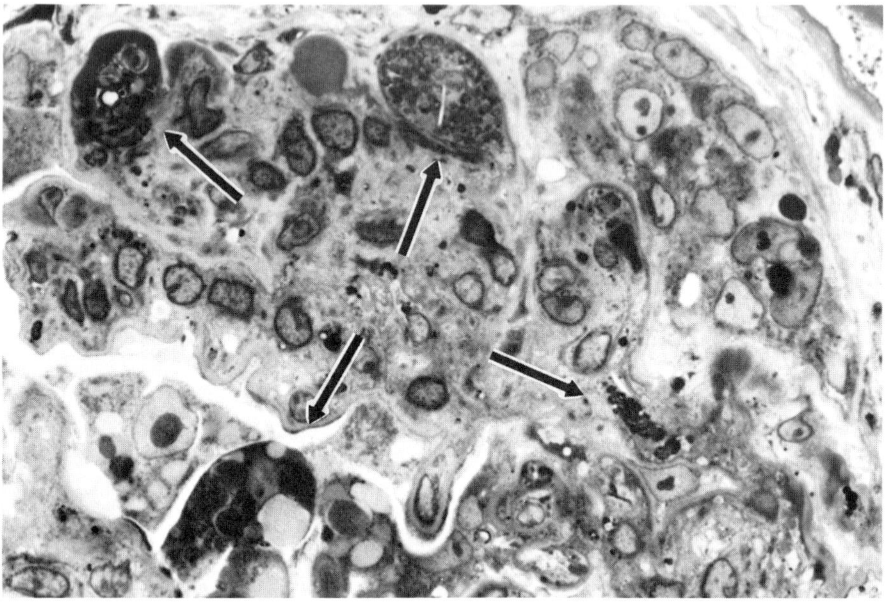

Figure 4-6. Prominent lipid accumulation seen in endothelial and mesangial cells *(arrows)*. Plastic embedded, toluidine blue stain, × 1000.

in the osmium-fixed–toluidine-blue-stained "thick" sections, presumably due to the superior lipid fixation of osmium over aldehyde fixatives (figures 4-6 and 4-7). Also nicely demonstrated in the thick section is the occasional presence of foam cells [8, 12, 15] in the mesangium. Electron microscopy reveals the mesangial and endothelial vacuolization to be due to a heterogeneous array of fluid and lipid resulting in an impressive cytoplasmic lysosomal change with numerous myelin-like figures and fine droplets of neutral fats [5, 8, 10, 12] (figure 4-8). Occasionally, cholesterol clefts can be seen in cases biopsied after a long postpartum interval [17] (figure 4-9). It was this finding of numerous vacuoles, along with the marked cytoplasmic swelling in the endothelial cells, that led to the use of the term *endotheliosis* in one of the early electron-microscopic descriptions of this lesion by one of the authors (B.H.S.) [18]. This very characteristic finding is not often seen throughout the entire glomerulus and frequently step sectioning of the epon-embedded material is required before the extent of the lesion is revealed. There appears to be a correlation between the clinical severity of the patient's signs and symptoms and the amount of endotheliosis. The change is occasionally superimposed on other lesions, but has never been seen in nonpregnant women.

In some cases of PET, electron microscopy reveals deposits of a finely granular, electron-dense material. This is found most frequently distributed subendothelially, but is also seen interposed between the endothelial and mesangial cells [3, 19–21] (figure 4-10). Although this material has been interpreted as immune complexes

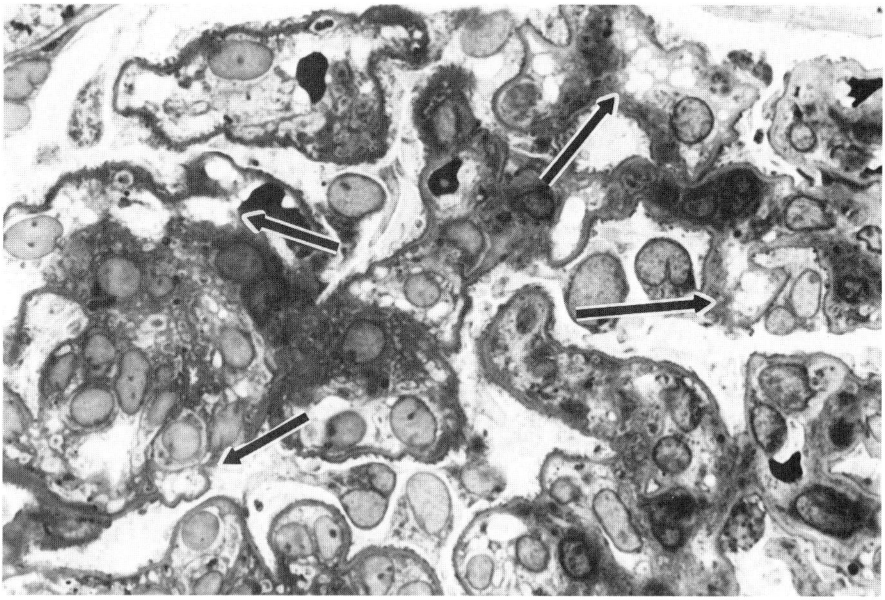

Figure 4-7. There is an accumulation of fluid vacuoles in the opposite pole of same glomerulus as in figure 4-6 *(arrows)*. Plastic embedded, toluidine blue stain, × 1000.

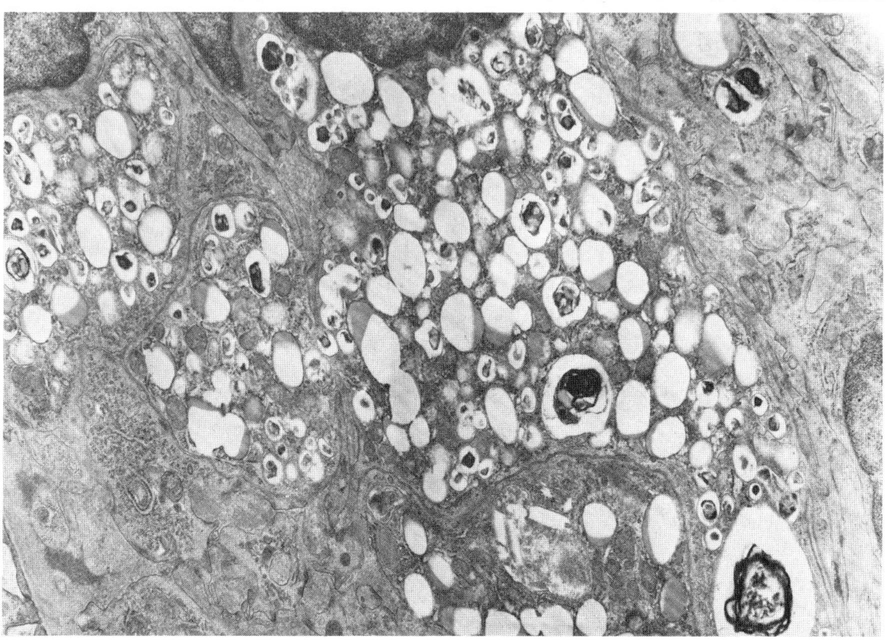

Figure 4-8. An electron micrograph showing many vacuoles that have a fluid–lipid interface. Myelin-like figures are also present. × 15,000.

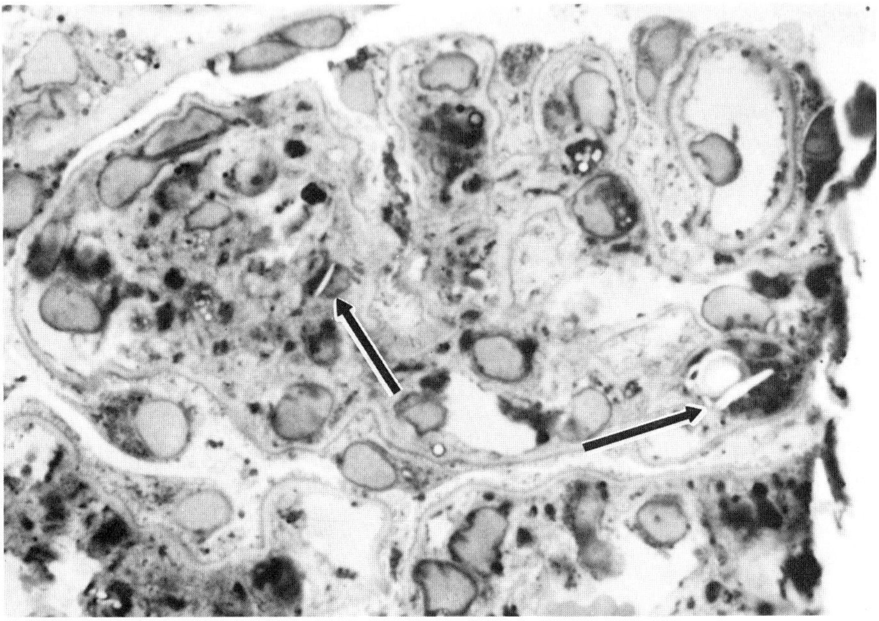

Figure 4-9. A glomerulus with vacuolization and cholesterol clefts *(arrows)*. Plastic embedded, toluidine blue stain, × 1000.

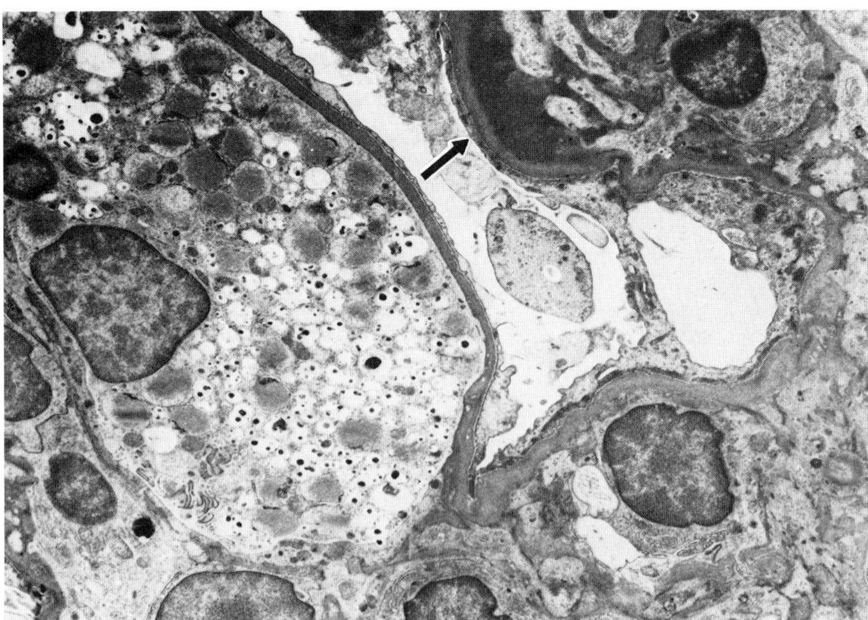

Figure 4-10. Electron-dense, subendothelial material is present *(arrow)*. Numerous lipid-containing vacuoles are seen in an adjacent endothelial cell. × 10,000.

by some authors [15, 22, 23], because of our immunofluorescent data that will be summarized later and because this material lacks the electron-dense, granular appearance characteristic of immune complexes, we feel that it frequently represents fibrin and fibrin precursors. In fact, in the most florid cases of PET, fibrin tactoids showing their characteristic periodicity are seen sporadically in the mesangium [3, 24], subendothelium [3, 5, 13, 25], and exceptionally in the urinary space [15]. This electron-dense material may also be due in part to the accumulation of several basement membrane proteins such as laminin, type-IV collagen, fibronectin, and a proteoglycan, all of which have been demonstrated recently in the mesangium and the thickened glomerular capillary walls of patients with PET [24]. An accumulation of a similar, finely granular material is seen in hemolytic uremic syndrome and postpartum renal failure. These conditions, however, are distinguished from PET by their lack of endothelial reactive changes and the frequent fibrin thrombi in the afferent arterioles. Fibrin thrombi are seen in only the most severe cases of PET. Furthermore, the prompt and complete resolution so characteristic of PET also distinguishes it from these other lesions.

Early observers noted what they felt to be a thickened basement membrane by light microscopy in this condition and likened PET to a membranous glomerulonephritis [26]. More recently, statements attesting to [2, 20, 27] and refuting [8, 10, 13] light-microscopic thickening have been made. It has been repeatedly shown ultrastructurally that in fact the basement membrane is not thickened [12, 18, 19, 28]. A double contour of the basement membrane or "splitting" of the basement membrane has also been noted, particularly with the use of silver stains [15, 24, 25, 27, 29]. Electron microscopy shows that this appearance is a consequence of the tremendous mesangial cell hypertrophy that results in interpositioning of the mesangial cell cytoplasm and mesangial matrix between the peripheral capillary endothelial cell and the basement membrane [24, 25, 27].

Epithelial cell proliferation in the form of crescents is only occasionally seen in the most severe cases of preeclampsia and eclampsia [8, 12] (figure 4-11). Much more frequently, one sees protein transport droplets (a manifestation of the proteinuria characteristic of this condition) and vacuolation and swelling of the epithelial cells [2, 3, 13, 30]. Vacuoles as well as phagolysosomes are also seen with electron microscopy [14, 15]. The proteinuria does not seem to depend on epithelial cell foot process obliteration, as this is only seen focally [2, 5, 18, 28] and does not appear to be more frequent in our preeclamptics with nephrotic levels of proteinuria [31]. Other authors, also studying patients with nephrotic levels of proteinuria in PET, have found an average of only 5%–10% obliteration of the epithelial cell foot processes [14]. The massive protein losses seen in many of these patients with morphologically normal epithelial cells and swollen, reactive endothelial cells supports the conclusion by Kanwar [32] in his recent summary on the biophysiology of glomerular filtration and proteinuria where he states, "Any disturbance that alters the 'integrated' functions of the cellular and extracellular elements [of the glomerular capillary wall], regardless of how minor, can result in the abnormal loss of plasma proteins into the urinary space."

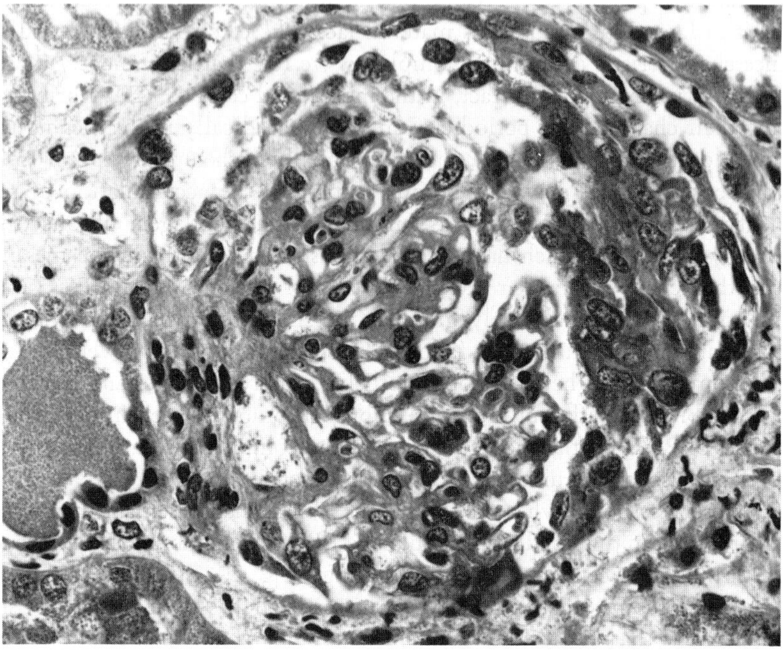

Figure 4-11. A cellular crescent is formed by proliferation of epithelial cells. The preeclamptic glomerulus is not inflamed or hypercellular. H & E, × 450.

The presence of a fibrillar proteinaceous debris in the Bowman space noted by several authors [2, 9] probably is the result of cytolysis of the frequently poorly preserved parietal epithelial cells.

Once one leaves the glomerulus, the renal changes associated with PET become less frequent and much less specific. We feel that there are no specific arterial or arteriolar alterations in PET in accordance with the experience of others [8, 10]. The arteriosclerosis, arteriolosclerosis, and insudative changes noted in the "preeclamptic" patients of several studies [3, 12, 14] that were similarly noted and felt to persist postpartum by others [20, 33] would be grounds for placement of such patients into a nephrosclerosis or a nephrosclerosis with superimposed preeclampsia category depending on whether the aforementioned characteristic glomerular changes of PET were present or not. Similarly, the findings by Aber [34], who demonstrated residual structural abnormalities in lobular, interlobular, and arcuate arteries in patients with a previous history of gestational hypertension using serial renal angiography, would suggest to us that these patients must have underlying renovascular pathology. It has been suggested that underlying renal vascular lesions can result in a condition of latent hypertension that is unmasked by the pregnancy [1].

Similarly, no significant changes in the tubulointerstitium are noted aside from the hyaline protein reabsorption droplets [8, 9, 18] that are a manifestation of the proteinuria.

3. IMMUNOHISTOLOGY

The development of immunofluorescent-labeling techniques in the early 1960s provided a powerful tool for the specific glomerular localization of fibrin and its precursors, immunoglobulin-complement complexes, and a variety of other serum proteins. No other single area has generated as much controversy with regard to the pathogenesis of the renal lesion in PET.

Originally the descriptions by Vassalli et al. [35] and Fiaschi and Naccarato [20], who demonstrated primarily fibrinogen/fibrin and lesser degrees of immunoglobulin in the glomerular basement membrane, resulted in suggestions that an intravascular coagulation disturbance was the underlying disorder in toxemia. More recently, with the refinement in specific antiimmunoglobulin antisera, a number of authors have described finding immunoglobulins, most frequently IgM [3, 15, 22, 27], in addition to fibrin/fibrinogen in the subendothelial position, within capillary lumina, and sometimes in the mesangium. Also, complement staining has been noted in a significant number of biopsies by some investigators [14, 15], leading to proposals that the renal lesions of PET were immunologically mediated much as a glomerulonephritis. Much lower frequencies of positivity with all reagents have been recorded in our data as well as that by other groups [5, 12, 36]. We interpret the low-intensity staining of fibrin and immunoglobulin to be due to nonspecific trapping secondary to narrowing of the glomerular capillary lumina by the swollen mesangial and endothelial cells similar to that described in other conditions with pronounced glomerular ischemia such as amyloidosis and diabetic glomerulosclerosis. Indeed, through the use of the freeze-substitution technique, the demonstration of soluble proteins such as albumin and transferrin colocalizing with fibrinogen, IgM, and β_1C-globulin [13] would seem to suggest that the positivity of the latter three is insudative consequent to the increased permeability of the capillary wall.

The discrepancy between our findings and those who claim frequent intense positivity is not easily explained, but does not appear to be a function of the postpartum interval [13]. More likely it is a manifestation of patient selection, with our series containing many more patients with only mild cases of PET.

4. CLINICAL PATHOLOGIC CORRELATION: PROGNOSTIC IMPLICATIONS

The importance of the renal biopsy in the setting of gestational hypertension is realized when discrete diagnostic groups that are not clinically distinct can be separated by pathologic criteria and when the long-term morbidity of these distinct groups is found to differ. Table 4-1 lists the pathologic diagnoses in the renal biopsies of 104 primigravidas and 72 multiparas in a recently published biopsy series from the University of Chicago [5]. Note that, despite the clinical diagnosis of preeclampsia in the vast majority of patients, only 55% showed the reversible changes of PET that we have just described. In addition, it can be seen that more

Table 4-1. Renal pathology in 176 hypertensive pregnant patients

Diagnosis	No.	Primigravidas	Multiparas
Preeclampsia	96	79	17
with nephrosclerosis	13	6	7
with renal disease	3	1	2
with both	2	1	1
Nephrosclerosis	19	3	16
with renal disease	4	2	2
Renal disease	31	12	19
Normal histology	8	0	8
Total	176	104	72

From Fisher et al. [5], by copyright permission of the Williams and Wilkins Company.

than 80% of the patients with PET are primigravidas, confirming the notion that this is a disease of the first pregnancy.

As mentioned previously, we feel that there are no specific arterial or arteriolar changes in PET. By definition then, those patients who had kidney biopsies showing interlobular artery alterations such as fibroelastic arterial thickening, reduplication of the internal elastic lamina, medial hypertrophy, and insudative hyaline trapping in the afferent arterioles were placed in the nephrosclerosis category (figure 4-12). Disagreement exists in the literature between those who have felt that these changes, which are designated as arteriolosclerosis, are the cause of hypertension and that they are only rarely found in nonhypertensives [37, 38], and those who consider them as part of an aging process that may be exacerbated and accelerated by hypertension and metabolic diseases such as diabetes [39, 40]. Our finding these vascular changes in a group of young pregnant hypertensive patients does not allow us to distinguish between these two notions and emphasis is placed on the vascular lesions primarily to select out those patients who may not have the excellent long-term prognosis as those with the completely reversible glomerular lesions of PET. Of the patients in our series, 15 showed both the glomerular lesion of PET and nephrosclerosis. One might postulate that the elevation in blood pressure produced by the glomerular swelling resulted in secondary arteriolosclerosis in these patients. We feel, however, that the duration of hypertension in PET is insufficient to produce the arteriolar changes seen in nephrosclerosis. In follow-up analysis, these patients with both lesions were felt to behave like the group with nephrosclerosis alone.

Table 4-2 lists follow-up clinical information in 86 patients from our series [5]. Note that in the 53 women who had PET alone the prevalence of hypertension was 9.4%. This is not significantly different from the prevalence of hypertension in an age-, sex-, and race-adjusted control population from a large epidemiologic survey used for comparison [41]. These findings concur with those of other investigators [7, 29]. Chesley et al. [29], who recognized the difficulty in clinically separating true preeclampsia from latent essential hypertension unmasked by preg-

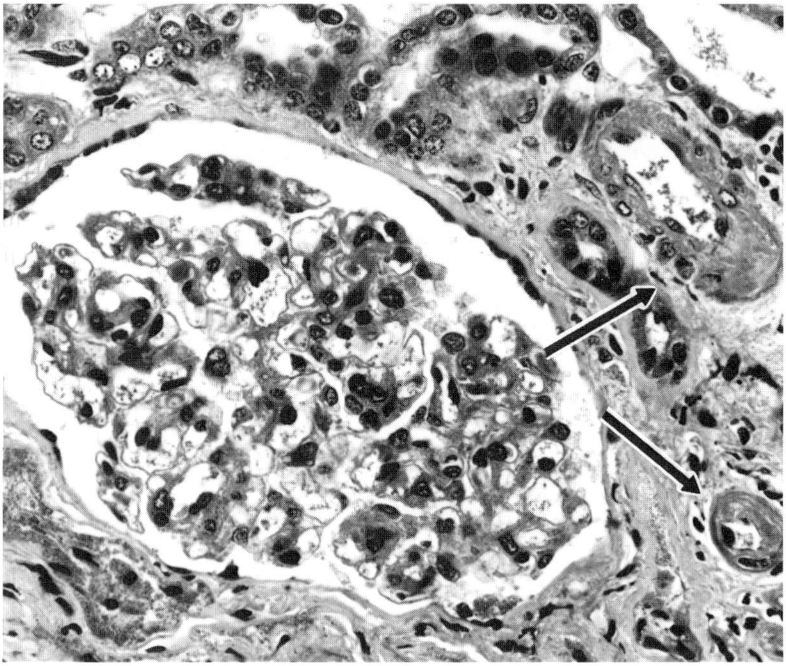

Figure 4-12. Two arterioles show moderately severe hyaline arteriolosclerosis *(arrows)* in a patient with hypertensive nephrosclerosis. H & E, × 400.

nancy, limited their observations to patients with eclampsia, the diagnosis of which is clinically much more secure. In their most recent follow-up, published in 1976, they have compiled one of the most thorough epidemiologic surveys, spanning over 40 years. They found no significant difference in follow-up in the prevalence of hypertension between primiparous eclamptic women and women matched for age and race. In contrast, multiparous eclamptics, many of whom had had antecedent hypertension, showed a significantly greater prevalence of hypertension in follow-up, associated with a mortality rate 2–5 times greater than that for the primiparous eclamptics. Furthermore, they found that, although there was no

Table 4-2. Follow-up observations

Biopsy diagnosis	No. examined	Average no. of months after delivery	Hypertension (%)	Increased urinary protein (%)
Preeclampsia	53	68.1	9.4	7.5
Nephrosclerosis	19	74.0	74.0	32.0
Renal disease	14	83.8	7.2	29.0

Modified from Fisher et al. [5], by copyright permission of the Williams and Wilkins Company.

significant difference in the prevalence of hypertension between those eclamptic women who had had subsequent pregnancies and those who had not, those who had at least one subsequent hypertensive pregnancy showed a greater prevalence of essential hypertension than those whose subsequent pregnancies were all normotensive. In addition, their data suggested that subsequent hypertensive pregnancies might accelerate the development of permanent hypertension in those destined to develop it. They concluded that eclampsia and true preeclampsia were neither a predictive sign nor a cause of hypertension.

Others [42–44] have claimed to show an association between clinically "toxemic" patients and the eventual development of hypertension. The discrepancies between their data and the studies that have just been summarized [5, 29] probably result in part from their inclusion of preeclamptic patients. As mentioned earlier, we feel that it is clinically difficult to distinguish reliably between true preeclampsia and patients with essential, gestationally induced hypertension. Furthermore, the former studies [42–44] compared the patients with clinical preeclampsia to a control group of normotensive gravidas. Although this might appear a logical choice, actually this group of normotensive "controls" seriously underrepresents the remote incidence of hypertension because gestation frequently induces transient increases in the blood pressure of women who will ultimately develop permanent hypertension later in life [29].

Our data suggest that many of those women who are destined to develop permanent essential hypertension can be identified by postpartum renal biopsy. Of the patients in our nephrosclerosis category, 74% were found on follow-up examination to have developed hypertension (table 4-2) [5]. The dramatic difference in the prevalence of hypertension between this group and the PET group underscores the importance of separating these two groups morphologically.

Our findings corroborate those reported by Peyser et al. [45], who reevaluated 13 patients who had had postpartum biopsies interpreted as nephrosclerosis. Although only three of 13 had been hypertensive at six months postpartum, when the follow-up was extended to between two and seven years, ten of the 13 had developed hypertension. Similarly, the irreversibility of the arteriolar lesion was demonstrated by Smyth et al. [46], who found that, in seven patients who had a postpartum biopsy that showed nephrosclerosis, all seven who had a follow-up biopsy some time later had persistent arteriolar changes. Subsequently, four patients who had later pregnancies all redeveloped gestational hypertension.

The other major group separated morphologically from PET in our biopsy series of gestational hypertensives is a heterogeneous collection of renal diseases. Chronic glomerulonephritis was the single most common lesion demonstrated, followed in order of decreasing frequency by tubulointerstitial lesions, membranous nephropathy, sickle cell nephropathy, poststreptococcal glomerulonephritis, minimal change nephropathy, and diabetic nephropathy. PET occasionally was seen superimposed on these lesions (table 4-1) [5].

In the setting of gestational hypertension where the clinical impression is usually preeclampsia, the pathologist must keep in mind the possibility of finding these other lesions. It is interesting to note that more than one-half of these patients did not have symptoms of their renal diseases until they became pregnant [47]. Similarly, in a recent series reported by Surian et al. [6], 40% of the patients with a variety of renal disease had been asymptomatic before pregnancy.

As mentioned previously, we feel that the use of electron microscopy and immunofluorescence in addition to light microscopy maximizes the ability of the pathologist to distinguish PET from other glomerular lesions that may produce symptoms in pregnancy. We cannot concur with the suggestion that, in the setting of gestational proteinuria, the presence of even one hyalinized, sclerosed, or fibrosed glomerulus indicates that the patient is probably suffering from some underlying glomerulonephritis [36]. The study by Kaplan et al. [48] showed that as many as 10% of glomeruli may be sclerotic in normal individuals under the age of 40 years and this would certainly seem to make such a conclusion hazardous.

Again the importance of separating this group of renal diseases from PET is dramatized by examination of follow-up clinical studies that show an increased prevalence of significant proteinuria among those patients with an underlying renal disease (table 4-2) [5, 47]. These lesions obviously do not demonstrate the reversibility of PET. Fortunately, however, recent studies have shown that, at least in women with preserved kidney function at conception, the pregnancy does not appear to worsen the course of the renal disease [6, 49].

5. CONCLUSION

In writing this chapter, we have attempted to show that, by renal biopsy, patients with true preeclampsia can be distinguished from those patients with latent essential hypertension or underlying renal disease that have come to clinical attention in the last months of pregnancy due to the increased demands placed on the kidney at that time. The morphologic alterations of true preeclampsia are distinctive, and the differential diagnosis between these lesions is usually not difficult, particularly when light and electron microscopy and immunofluorescence are used in conjunction.

It has been shown that, in this setting, renal biopsy affords the clinician the most accurate prognostic information regarding the development of permanent hypertension or worsening of renal function. True preeclamptic toxemia is a completely reversible lesion that has no correlation with the development of permanent hypertension. Eventual permanent hypertension, however, is associated with those patients who have biopsies that show arterial nephrosclerosis. Recent studies have shown that, in general, patients with preserved renal function do not experience deterioration as a result of pregnancy in short-term follow-up studies [49], although lesions with a poor prognosis outside of pregnancy also tend to progress in gravid patients [6, 49]. In individuals with inflammatory glomerular lesions, a peripartum assessment of glomerular scarring may provide the best available information as to the long-term prognosis of renal function in much the same way as a chronicity index is now used to predict which patients with lupus glomerulonephritis will probably progress to renal failure [50].

REFERENCES

1. Chesley LC: Hypertension in pregnancy: definitions, familial factor, and remote prognosis. Kidney Int 18:234–240, 1980.
2. Pollak VE, Nettles JB: The kidney in toxemia of pregnancy: a clinical and pathologic study based on renal biopsies. Medicine (Baltimore) 39:469–525, 1960.
3. Nochy D, Birembant P, Hinglais N, Freund M, Idatte JM, Jacquot C, Chartier M, Gariety J: Renal lesions in the hypertensive syndromes of pregnancy: immunomorphological and ultrastructural studies in 114 cases. Clin Nephrol 13:155–162, 1980.
4. Dieckmann WJ: Seminar. Sharp & Dohme 16:19, 1954.
5. Fisher KA, Luger A, Spargo BH, Lindheimer MD: Hypertension in pregnancy: clinical–pathological correlations and remote prognosis. Medicine (Baltimore) 60:267–276, 1981.
6. Surian M, Imbasciati E, Cosci P, Banfi G, Barbiano di Belgiojoso G, Brancoccio D, Minetti L, Ponticelli C: Glomerular disease and pregnancy: a study of 123 pregnancies in patients with primary and secondary glomerular diseases. Nephron 36:101–105, 1984.
7. Bryans CI: The remote prognosis in toxemia of pregnancy. Clin Obstet Gynecol 9:973–990, 1966.
8. Sheehan HL: Renal morphology in preeclampsia. Kidney Int 18:241–252, 1980.
9. Altchek A, Albright NL, Sommers SC: The renal pathology of toxemia of pregnancy. Obstet Gynecol 31:595–607, 1968.
10. Thomson D, Paterson WG, Smart GE, MacDonald MK, Robson JS: The renal lesions of toxemia and abruptio placentae studied by light and electron microscopy. J Obstet Gynaecol Br Commonw 79:311–320, 1972.
11. Sheehan HL, Lynch JB: Pathology of toxemia of pregnancy. Edinburgh: Churchill Livingstone, 1973.
12. Crocker DW: The pathology of renal diseases in pregnancy. In: De Alvarez RR (ed) The kidney in pregnancy. New York: John Wiley and Sons, 1976, pp 167–214.
13. Pollak VE: The role of intravascular coagulation in toxemia of pregnancy. In: McIntosh RM, Guggenheim SJ, Schrier RW (eds) Kidney disease: hematologic and vascular problems. New York: John Wiley and Sons, 1977, pp 107–124.
14. First MR, Ooi BS, Jao W, Pollak VE: Pre-eclampsia with the nephrotic syndrome. Kidney Int 13:166–177, 1978.
15. Seymore AE, Petrucco OM, Clarkson AR, Haynes WDG, Lawrence JR, Jackson B, Thompson AJ, Thomson NM: Morphological and immunological evidence of coagulopathy in renal complications of pregnancy. In: Lindheimer MD, Katz AI, Zuspan FP (eds) Hypertension in pregnancy. New York: John Wiley and Sons, 1976, pp 139–153.
16. Spargo BH, Seymore AE, Ordonez NG: Renal biopsy pathology with diagnostic and therapeutic implications. New York: John Wiley and Sons, 1980.
17. Spargo BH, Lichtig C, Luger AM, Katy AI, Lindheimer MD: The renal lesion in pre-eclampsia. In: Lindheimer MD, Katz AI, Zuspan FP (eds) Hypertension in pregnancy. New York: John Wiley and Sons, 1976, pp 129–137.
18. Spargo BH, McCartney CP, Winemiller R: Glomerular capillary endotheliosis in toxemia of pregnancy. Arch Pathol 68:593–599, 1959.
19. Farquhar MF: Review of normal and pathologic glomerular ultrastructure. In: Metcoff J (ed) Proceedings of the 10th annual conference on the nephrotic syndrome. New York: National Kidney Disease Foundation, 1959, pp 2–29.
20. Fiaschi E, Naccarato R: The histopathology of the kidney in toxemia: serial renal biopsies during pregnancy, peurperium and several years postpartum. Virchows Arch [Pathol Anat] 345:299–309, 1968.
21. McKay DG: Chronic intravascular coagulation in normal pregnancy and pre-eclampsia. Contrib Nephrol 25:108–119, 1981.
22. Petrucco OM, Thompson NM, Lawrence JR, Weldon MW: Immunofluorescent studies in renal biopsies in pre-eclampsia. Br Med J 1:473–476, 1974.
23. Gallery EDM, Gyory AZ: Immunoglobulin deposition in the kidney in pre-eclampsia: its significance. Aust NZ J Med 8:408–12, 1978.
24. Foidart JM, Noeby D, Nusgens B, Foidart JB, Mahieu PR, Lapiere CM, Lambotte R, Bariety J: Accumulation of several basement membrane proteins in glomeruli of patients with pre-eclampsia and other hypertensive syndromes of pregnancy: possible roles of renal prostaglandins and fibronectin. Lab Invest 49:250–259, 1983.
25. Robson JS: Proteinuria and the renal lesion in preeclampsia and abruptio placentae. In: Lind-

heimer MD, Katz AI, Zuspan FP (eds) Hypertension in pregnancy. New York: John Wiley and Sons, 1976, pp 61–73.
26. Rhinehart JF, Farquhar MG, Jung HC, Abul-Haj SK: The normal glomerulus and its basic reactions in disease. Am J Pathol 29:21–31, 1953.
27. Tribe CR, Smart GE, Davies DR, Mackenzie JC: A renal biopsy study in toxemia of pregnancy. J Clin Pathol 32:681–692, 1979.
28. McKay DG: Blood coagulation and toxemia of pregnancy. In: Kincaid-Smith P (ed) Glomerulonephritis: morphology, natural history, and treatment. New York: John Wiley and Sons, 1972, pp 963–995.
29. Chesley LC, Annitto JE, Cosgrove RA: The remote prognosis of eclamptic women. Am J Obstet Gynecol 124:446–459, 1976.
30. Dieckmann WJ, Potter EL, McCartney CP: Renal biopsies from patients with toxemia of pregnancy. Am J Obstet Gynecol 73:1–16, 1957.
31. Fisher KA, Ahuja S, Luger A, Spargo BH, Lindheimer MD: Nephrotic proteinuria with pre-eclampsia. Am J Obstet Gynecol 129:643–646, 1977.
32. Kanwar YS: Biology of disease: biophysiology of glomerular filtration and proteinuria. Lab Invest 51:7–21, 1984.
33. Kincaid-Smith P: The similarity of lesions and underlying mechanism in preeclamptic toxemia and postpartum renal failure. In: Kincaid-Smith P (ed) Glomerulonephritis: morphology, natural history, and treatment. New York: John Wiley and Sons, 1972, pp 1013–1025.
34. Aber GM: Intrarenal vascular lesions associated with pre-eclampsia. Nephron 21:297–309, 1978.
35. Vassalli P, Morris RH, McCluskey RT: The pathogenic role of fibrin deposition in the glomerular lesions of toxemia of pregnancy. J Exp Med 118:467–476, 1963.
36. Kincaid-Smith P, Fairley KF: The differential diagnosis between toxemia and glomerulonephritis in patients with proteinuria during pregnancy. In: Lindheimer MD, Katz AI, Zuspan FP (eds) Hypertension in pregnancy. New York: John Wiley and Sons, 1976, pp 157–167.
37. Allen AC: The kidney: medical and surgical diseases. New York: Grune and Stratton, 1962, p 564.
38. Moritz AR, Oldt MR: Arteriolar sclerosis in hypertensive and non-hypertensive individuals. Am J Pathol 13:679–728, 1937.
39. Smith JP: Hyaline arteriosclerosis in the kidney. J Pathol Bacteriol 69:147–168, 1955.
40. Heptinstall RH: Renal biopsies in hypertension. Br Heart J 16:133–141, 1954.
41. Hypertension and hypertensive heart disease in adults. US Public Health Service publ 1000, ser 11, N13, Washington DC, 1966.
42. Reid DE, Teel HM: Non-convulsive pregnancy toxemias: their relationships to chronic vascular and renal disease. Am J Obstet Gynecol 37:886–896, 1939.
43. Epstein FH: Late vascular effects of toxemia of pregnancy. N Engl J Med 271:391–395, 1964.
44. Singh MM, Macgillivary I, Mahaffy RG: A study of the long term effects of pre-eclampsia on blood pressure and renal function. J Obstet Gynaecol Br Commonw 81:903–906, 1974.
45. Peyser MR, Toaff R, Leiserowitz DM, Aviram A, Griffel B: Late follow up in women with nephrosclerosis diagnosed at pregnancy. Am J Obstet Gynecol 132:480–484, 1978.
46. Smythe CM, Bradham WS, Dennis EJ, McIver FA, Howe HG: Renal arteriolar disease in young primiparas. J Lab Clin Med 63:562–573, 1964.
47. Katz AI, Davison JM, Hayslett JP, Singson E, Lindheimer MD: Pregnancy in women with kidney disease. Kidney Int 18:192–206, 1980.
48. Kaplan C, Pasternack B, Shah H, Gallo G: Age-related incidence of sclerotic glomeruli in human kidneys. Am J Pathol 80:227–234, 1975.
49. Katz AI, Lindheimer MD: Effect of pregnancy on the natural course of kidney disease. Semin Nephrol 4:252–259, 1984.
50. Austin HA, Muenz LR, Joyce KM, Antonovych TA, Kullick ME, Klippel JH, Decker JL, Balow JE: Prognostic factors in lupus nephritis: contribution of renal histologic data. Am J Med 75:382–391, 1983.

5. RENAL FUNCTION DURING NORMAL PREGNANCY AND THE EFFECT OF RENAL DISEASE AND PREECLAMPSIA

JOHN M. DAVISON

1. INTRODUCTION

Alterations in the mother's appearance are obvious as pregnancy advances. Less obvious, but just as significant, are the alterations in the mother's internal environment, whereby the fetus somehow overrides and resets maternal homeostatic mechanisms in the interests of the pregnancy. The changes in the physiology of the renal tract are particularly prominent aspects of the adaptive process. This chapter focuses on changes in renal hemodynamics, tubular function, and volume homeostasis and discusses their clinical relevance in normal pregnancy as well as in the presence of renal disease and preeclampsia.

2. RENAL BLOOD FLOW

Changes in renal hemodynamics [renal blood flow (RBF) and glomerular filtration rate (GFR)] have been discussed in detail in chapter 1. What follows therefore deals only with the main contribution to our understanding of alterations in RBF and GFR.

As an index of RBF, the renal clearance of para-amino hippurate (PAH) is used, which is a measure of effective renal plasma flow (ERPF). The increment in ERPF in pregnancy has probably been substantially underestimated because of inappropriate correction of data to a standard body surface area, the mixing of cross-sectional with serial data, and inaccuracies due to small sample size in a measurement with considerable individual variation [1]. The problems have been compounded by the fact that not all of the measurements were performed at identical gestational ages and some subjects were not investigated at all in the nonpregnant state or in the first trimester.

It can be seen from figure 5-1 that the many different patterns of change in mean ERPF described by various investigators [2–5] can be almost entirely encompassed within a range equal to 1 standard deviation of either side of the mean of the most recent and reliable serial study [6]. It is now generally accepted that ERPF increases significantly during pregnancy with midpregnancy increments attaining 60%–80% followed by a significant decrement in the third trimester, which is not related to the effects of posture.

3. GLOMERULAR FILTRATION RATE

There is close agreement for mean values of GFR, measured by inulin clearance, in the studies of earlier workers [2–5, 8] (figure 5-1). When results are not adjusted to a standard surface area, GFR is increased by approximately 50% throughout pregnancy. None of these studies suggests a significant decrease during the third trimester of pregnancy, but relatively little information is available after gestational week 37.

4. FILTRATION FRACTION

Bearing in mind the changes in ERPF and GFR just described, it might be anticipated that filtration fraction (FF), the ratio of GFR to ERPF, should decrease from nonpregnant values during early pregnancy, but should increase again during

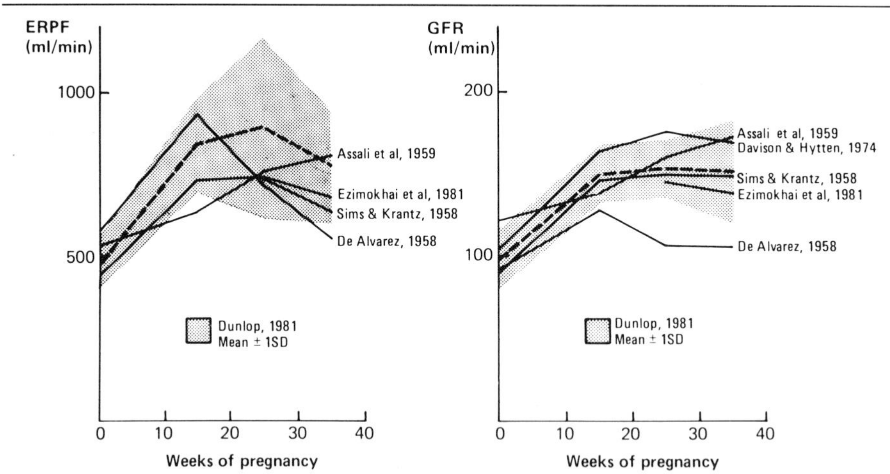

Figure 5-1. Changes in mean effective renal plasma flow *(ERPF)* and glomerular filtration rate *(GFR)* in pregnancy. Data not corrected for standard body surface area. Results taken from references 2–6 and 8. Modified from Davison and Dunlop [7], with permission by Grune and Stratton Inc.

the third trimester. This pattern of change is indeed confirmed by a more intensive search of the available literature [1]. Interestingly, mean arterial pressure alters in a pattern that is a mirror image of that suggested for ERPF (compatible with the opposing effects of variation in peripheral resistance), but which is parallel with that of FF (implying either hemodynamic changes within the glomerulus or possibly transient loss of filtration pressure equilibrium).

5. CHANGES IN THE RENAL HANDLING OF CREATININE AND UREA

5.1. Creatinine clearance

Creatinine, unlike inulin, is not renally inert. Consequently some of the creatinine appearing in the urine is derived from tubular secretion. In the nonpregnant situation the resultant error is sufficiently small to be of no significance in clinical practice and therefore 24-h creatinine clearance can be used as an index of GFR [9]. Throughout gestation, creatinine and inulin clearances do not differ significantly under infusion conditions, although the results of both are slightly greater than those obtained for creatinine clearance calculated over the preceding 24 h [8]. Since 24-h creatinine clearance is a noninvasive investigation, it has been found to be particularly valuable in circumstances where infusion would be undesirable or difficult to implement, especially when serial measurements are needed.

By week 8 of pregnancy (six weeks after conception), a mean increment of 45% has occurred in 24-h creatinine clearance, a change well beyond the limits of laboratory error and biologic variability [10]. Throughout the second trimester, creatinine clearance remains elevated, but during the weeks preceding delivery there is a consistent decrease to nonpregnant values [11].

Immediately after delivery, 24-h creatinine clearance increases compared with results obtained in the same subjects before labor. Values obtained on postnatal day 6 do not differ significantly from nonpregnant values. It is not clear whether this pattern reflects alteration in GFR itself, in creatine and/or creatinine metabolism, or in the renal handling of creatinine. At this time there is a very substantial diuresis that occurs on day 4 after delivery, but the peak value for creatinine clearance does not always occur on this day. Figure 5-2 demonstrates the overall extent of the changes in 24-h creatinine clearance during and after normal pregnancy.

5.2. Urea clearance

Much of the initial work on urea clearance during pregnancy was confusing because of arguments about the optimal conditions for the determination of this parameter [12]. It was known that, under certain conditions, the rate of urea excretion was related to the rate of urine flow but that above an "augmentation limit" of about 2 ml/min, the renal handling of urea was independent of flow. Another factor that had to be taken into account was the progressive decline during late pregnancy in the kidney's ability to handle a water load that, when linked with an inadequate diuresis, would have the effect of reducing urea clearance as pregnancy progressed [13]. Overall, it appears that the studies where diuresis was

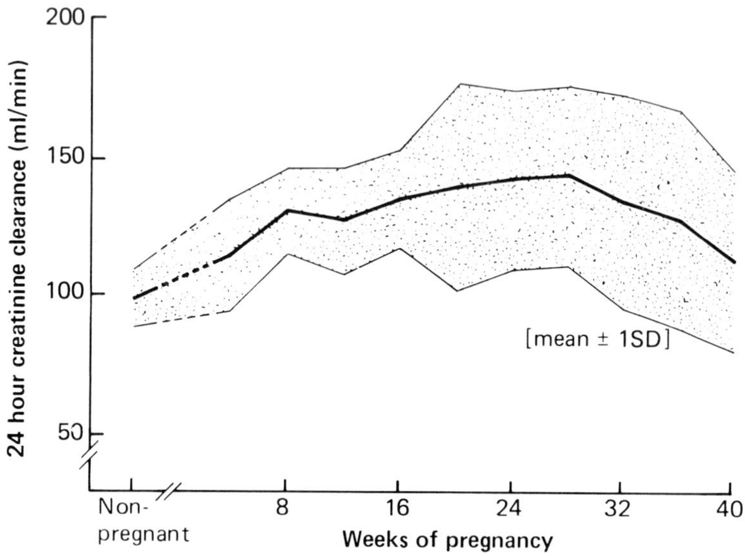

Figure 5-2. Changes in 24-h creatinine clearance during normal pregnancy. Data derived from study of 15 healthy women from before conception and at regular intervals throughout pregnancy.

inadequate were those in which the now well-documented increment in urea clearance was unrecognized.

Particularly significant is the study by Nice [14] because, not only did she publish the results of a control group of nonpregnant women (most other workers compared their results during pregnancy with those of men), but she studied her subjects serially, thus enabling each to act as her own control. Unfortunately, the increases in urea clearance that she described (and that we now accept as physiologic) were considered excessive and were disbelieved by the succeeding generation of research workers.

5.3. Clinical relevance

5.3.1. Plasma creatinine and urea concentration

The plasma levels of creatinine and urea decrease [12]. Creatinine levels decrease from a nonpregnant value of 73 μmol/liter (0.82 mg/dl) to 65, 51, and 47 μ mol/liter (0.73, 0.58, and 0.53 mg/dl, respectively) in successive trimesters. Similarly, urea levels fall from nonpregnancy values of 4.3 mmol/liter (25.8 mg/dl) to pregnancy values of 3.5, 3.3, and 3.1 mmol/liter (21.0, 19.8, and 18.6 mg/dl, respectively). Familiarity with these changes is vital because values considered normal in nonpregnant women may signify decreased renal function in pregnancy. Values of plasma creatinine of 75 μmol/liter (0.85 mg/dl) and urea of 4.5 mmol/liter (27 mg/dl) should alert the clinician to further assess renal function [15]. (Plasma creatinine can be converted from μmol/liter to mg/dl by multiplying by

0.0113, and plasma urea can be converted from mmol/liter to mg/dl by multiplying by 6.0.)

5.3.2. Assessment of renal function

Caution is necessary when serially assessing renal function just on the basis of plasma creatinine levels. An individual may lose up to 50% of renal function yet still maintain a plasma creatinine level of less than 130 μmol/liter (1.47 mg/dl) (Fig. 5-3). If renal function is more severely compromised, however, a small decrement in GFR causes a marked rise in plasma creatinine and, under these conditions, creatinine excretion is diminished [15]. This may be related to muscle mass, but there is evidence of extrarenal clearance with recycling of creatinine to creatine and irreversible degradation to products other than creatinine, such as sarcosine, hydantoin, and methylamine [16].

Plasma creatinine, its reciprocal, or its logarithm are often used to gauge GFR. Indeed, formulas have been devised to calculate a value for GFR from plasma

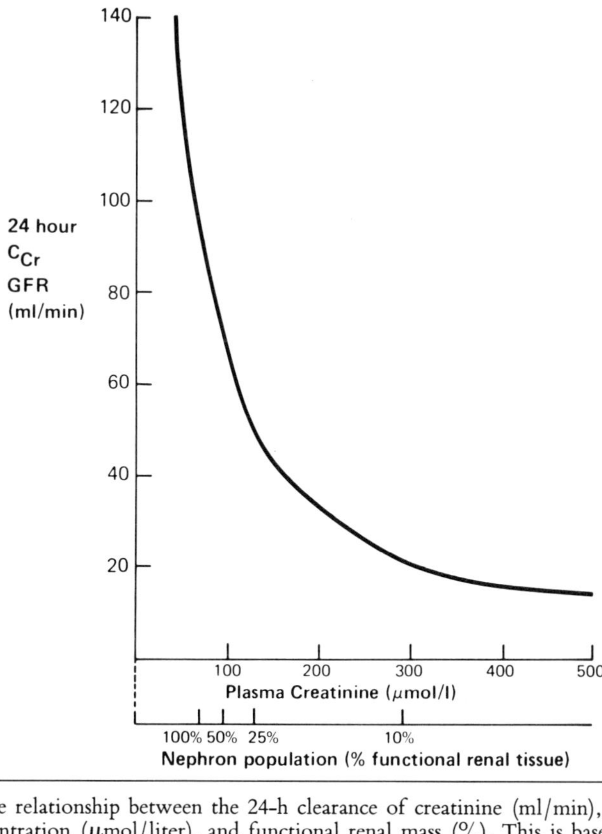

Figure 5-3. The relationship between the 24-h clearance of creatinine (ml/min), plasma creatinine concentration (μmol/liter), and functional renal mass (%). This is based on the assumption that 24-h creatinine excretion is constant at approximately 11.5 mmol.

creatinine level, provided there is information available on the patient's age, height, weight, and sex. It is erroneous, however, to use this approach in pregnancy where body size or weight does not reflect renal size [12]. In pregnancy, at least, evaluation of renal function must be based on the clearance of creatinine and not on a plasma determination alone. Toward the end of the third trimester, for example, there can be a 15%–20% decrease in function that affects plasma creatinine minimally [11].

5.3.3. Attention to detail during clearance measurements

To overcome such problems as "washout" from changes in urine flow, 24-h urine samples are used for clearances and this also avoids difficulties caused by diurnal variations. Dilation of the urinary tract in pregnancy can lead to collection errors, but these can be minimized if the woman is sufficiently hydrated to ensure a high urine flow rate and if she is positioned in lateral recumbency for an hour before the start and at the end of the collection, so as to standardize the procedure and minimize dead-space errors.

Many methods of determining creatinine in plasma also measure noncreatinine chromogens, thus leading to overestimates. This obviously has an effect on the calculation of clearance that must be taken into account. In addition, recent intake of cooked meat can increase plasma creatinine levels by up to 16 μmol/liter (0.18 mg/dl) (because cooking converts preformed creatine into creatinine) and awareness of this is necessary when timing a blood sample during a clearance period [17].

5.3.4. Urea clearance measurements as an index of renal function

Urea clearance must never be used because it is dependent on urine flow rate as well as GFR [7]. There have been attempts to reintroduce the test with modifications or to combine it with creatinine clearance in the hope that the errors of both would cancel each other out, but these have not gained acceptance.

6. CHANGES IN THE RENAL HANDLING OF URIC ACID

Normal pregnancy induces relative hypouricemia. Plasma uric acid concentrations decrease by over 25% as early as week 8 of pregnancy, but increase again during the third trimester to attain levels close to the nonpregnant mean [18]. The main reason for this pattern of events is alteration in the renal handling of uric acid, which, although freely filtered, is subsequently so actively reabsorbed that effectively only about 10% of the original filtered load appears in the urine. The physiology is more complex than simple tubular reabsorption because, while a large proportion of filtered uric acid is reabsorbed proximally, any final excretion depends on balance distally between active secretion and further reabsorption.

The hypouricemia of early and midpregnancy reflects an alteration in the fractional clearance of uric acid (uric acid clearance ÷ GFR), with a decrease in net tubular reabsorption [19]. Later in pregnancy the kidney appears to excrete a smaller proportion of the filtered uric acid load and it is this increase in net reabsorption that is associated with an increase in plasma uric acid concentration.

From the clinical viewpoint it is of interest that uric acid concentration and renal absorption are significantly higher in pregnancies complicated by preeclampsia or intrauterine growth retardation (see section 12.2.2). Above a critical blood level of 350 μmol/liter (5.9 mg/dl) there is significant perinatal mortality in hypertensive patients [20], and serial measurements can be used in monitoring progress in preeclampsia. It must be remembered, however, that physiologic variability can be such that some healthy women have high blood levels without problems [18] and that single random measurements are of no use clinically.

7. CHANGES IN THE RENAL HANDLING OF GLUCOSE

7.1. Glucose excretion during pregnancy

Clinically detectable glycosuria is more common during pregnancy [1]. The excretion of glucose increases very early in pregnancy and may exceed nonpregnancy values (20–100 mg in 24 h) by a factor of 10. The glycosuria can vary dramatically during a 24-h period and from day to day, with the intermittency being unrelated to either blood sugar levels or to the stage of pregnancy. By one week after delivery, nonpregnant glucose excretion patterns are reestablished.

7.2. Physiologic basis of glycosuria in pregnancy

7.2.1. Physiology of renal reabsorption of glucose

The kinetics of renal glucose reabsorption are complex. The original description of the renal handling of glucose was, in retrospect, an oversimplification and the concept of a maximal reabsorptive capacity for glucose, the Tm glucose or Tm_G, has had to be modified [1, 21]. It is now well established (a) that glucose is always present in normal urine; (b) that Tm_G is not constant, but varies with changes in extracellular fluid volume and GFR, which is itself altered by hyperglycemia; (c) that glucose is absorbed at sites other than the proximal tubule; and (d) that increased glucose excretion is probably due to deficient reabsorption from the 5% of filtered glucose that normally escapes proximal tubular reabsorption.

Serial studies of the renal handling of glucose under infusion conditions in women with varying degrees of glycosuria revealed that glucose reabsorption was less complete during pregnancy than it was 8–12 weeks after delivery [22]. Reabsorption was always less complete in pregnant women with obvious glycosuria and these women, although no longer clinically glycosuric after pregnancy, still showed less complete reabsorption under infusion conditions when nonpregnant.

It is not known why the renal handling of glucose is altered in pregnancy [1]. Two significant physiologic adaptations in pregnancy have the potential to affect glucose reabsorption in opposite ways: volume expansion may inhibit the reabsorption of sodium and hence glucose, whereas increased GFR may stimulate glucose reabsorption. Obviously, the hormones of pregnancy, particularly the sex steroids, suggest themselves as etiologic factors and, because their concentrations in the body decline rapidly after delivery in much the same way as glucose excretion, this supports such an idea. Whatever the explanation, however, there must also be moment-by-moment intrarenal change(s) of some sort to account for the classic intermittency of glucose excretion.

7.3. Clinical relevance

Glycosuria of pregnancy reflects an alteration in renal function rather than one in carbohydrate metabolism. Consequently, the testing of random urine samples during pregnancy is both unhelpful in the diagnosis and control of diabetes mellitus and also unrepresentative of the degree of glycosuria present.

A recent investigation has suggested that women with more than usual glycosuria in pregnancy may have sustained renal tubular damage from earlier untreated urinary tract infections, although no longer bacteriuric when pregnant [23]. Infection can impair distal tubular function as evidenced by reduced urine-concentrating ability, a manifestation of tubular dysfunction that is reversed once infection is eradicated. With the renal handling of glucose, however, if distal tubular sites are affected by infection, full recovery may not occur.

8. OTHER CHANGES IN RENAL TUBULAR FUNCTION

Excretion of most amino acids and several water-soluble vitamins increases during pregnancy. Renal bicarbonate reabsorption and proton excretion appear unchanged by pregnancy [15]. Urinary protein excretion is increased so that proteinuria should not be considered abnormal until it exceeds 300 mg in 24 h [24]. Furthermore, increasing protein excretion (in the absence of hypertension) in women with known renal disease does not necessarily indicate progression of the disease.

9. SODIUM HOMEOSTASIS

Total body water increases by 6–8 liters, 4–6 of which are extracellular. There is also a cumulative retention of about 950 mmol of sodium distributed between the maternal extracellular compartment and the products of conception. The physiologic significance of the plasma volume expansion and the attendant "hemodilution" remains ill-defined. In essence, it constitutes a "physiologic hypervolemia" that is sensed and accepted as "normal." Whether or not the increment is "necessary" remains to be elucidated, but there is evidence that smaller increments are associated with poor pregnancy outcome and/or low birth weight [25]. Furthermore, it has been suggested that the alterations in extracellular fluid volume may affect renal hemodynamics. The establishment of increments in ERPF and GFR occur well before the increases in extracellular volume, however, and subsequently there is no further augmentation of renal hemodynamics as plasma volume continues to increase.

Renal sodium is the prime determinant of volume homeostasis. Even allowing for the 4–5-mmol/liter decrease in plasma sodium that occurs in early pregnancy, the filtered load of sodium will still increase from nonpregnant levels of approximately 20,000 mmol/day to as much as 30,000 mmol/day. This change must be accompanied by parallel increments in tubular reabsorption of sodium or massive sodium depletion would ensue. This adaptive increase in tubular reabsorption not only equals the large increase in filtered load, but additionally 2–6 mmol of sodium are reabsorbed daily for fetal and maternal stores. This change represents the largest renal adjustment during pregnancy. Amid all of this, a pregnant woman is probably not prone to excessive sodium retention and handles ingested salt similarly to nonpregnant women or is even a subtle sodium waster [15, 26].

The influence of humoral changes during normal pregnancy on renal sodium handling and volume regulation is incompletely understood. Aldosterone secretion and excretion and levels of plasma desoxycorticosterone, cortisol estrogen, prolactin, and prostaglandins all increase during normal gestation. These and other factors that may influence renal sodium handling during gestation have been mentioned elsewhere [15, 26, 27–30] and are discussed in chapter 6.

10. CHANGES IN THE RENAL HANDLING OF WATER

Early in pregnancy, plasma osmolality decreases to a level about 10 mOsm/kg below the nonpregnant norm and this can be accounted for by the concomitant fall in plasma sodium and associated anions [31]. It might therefore be anticipated that a pregnant woman would stop secreting antidiuretic hormone, arginine vasopressin (AVP), and be in a state of continuous water diuresis. This does not happen because the osmotic thresholds for both AVP secretion and thirst decrease by approximately 10 mOsm/kg each during pregnancy [32].

There is a paucity of data regarding the nonosmotic factors that control AVP secretion in pregnancy [15]. Decreases in mean arterial pressure stimulate AVP secretion, but in the pregnant woman the decrease in plasma osmolality antedates the fall in blood pressure and the lower body tonicity is sustained until term, when pressures return to nonpregnant levels. Plasma volume is an important determinant of AVP release: hypovolemia stimulates, while hypervolemia may blunt, AVP secretion. In pregnancy, absolute blood volume increases markedly, but presumably the volume-sensing AVP secretion mechanism is reset so that the increased volume is sensed as normal [33].

11. PREGNANCY AND CHRONIC RENAL DISEASE

11.1. Renal dysfunction and its repercussions

In women with renal disease, pathology may be both clinically and chemically silent. Most will remain symptom free until GFR has decreased to less than 25% of its original level and many plasma constituents can be normal until a late stage of the disease (see section 5.3.2). Conceiving and sustaining a viable pregnancy is related to the degree of functional impairment rather than to the underlying renal lesion. Nature adds a helping hand by blunting fertility as renal function falls, and when plasma creatinine and urea levels before conception exceed 275 μmol/liter (3.10 mg/dl) and 10 mmol/liter (60 mg/dl) respectively, normal pregnancy is rare. There are exceptions, however, and cases have been reported where women with moderate to severe disease (including patients requiring maintenance hemodialysis) have conceived and successfully completed their pregnancies (see chapter 11).

Nevertheless, it is preferable to restrict pregnancy to women whose plasma creatinine levels are 150–200 mmol/liter (1.70–2.25 mg/dl) or less and who have a diastolic blood pressure of 90 mm Hg or lower [34]. Some are more strict and recommend that pregnancy should not be undertaken when plasma creatinine concentrations exceed 135 μmol/liter (1.53 mg/dl) [35]. Whatever level is decided upon, it should take cognizance of the fact that degrees of impairment that do not cause symptoms or appear to disrupt homeostasis in nonpregnant individuals can certainly jeopardize pregnancy. If a woman with chronic renal disease wishes to have children, the sooner she sets about it the better, as renal function will in any case diminish with age.

11.2. Effects of disease on pregnancy and of pregnancy on disease

Clinicians do not always have the chance to counsel patients before conception. Often pregnancy in a patient with known chronic renal disease or suspected of having renal disease presents as a fait accompli. In view of the radically different outlook in women with different degrees of renal insufficiency, it is useful to consider the impact of pregnancy by categories of renal functional status prior to pregnancy.

11.2.1. Preserved renal function and minimal hypertension

Women with chronic renal disease but normal or only mildly decreased renal function at conception usually have a successful obstetric outcome and pregnancy does not adversely affect the course of their disease [34, 36, 37]. While generally true for most patients, this statement has to be tempered somewhat in lupus nephropathy and perhaps IgA nephropathy, which appear more sensitive to intercurrent pregnancy [38–40] (see chapter 9).

Most pregnant women show increments in GFR although there are less than those of normal women. Increased proteinuria is the most common renal effect of pregnancy, occurring in almost 50% of pregnancies [34]. Increments occur in nearly all types of renal disease, although rarely in women with chronic pyelonephritis. Protein excretion can be massive, often exceeding 3 g/24 h and frequently leading to nephrotic edema.

A common diagnostic problem during pregnancy is the distinction between superimposed preeclampsia and an exacerbation or worsening of the underlying renal condition. Whereas it is widely accepted that pregnant women with preexistent renal disease are more susceptible than control populations to develop preeclampsia, the true incidence in women with renal disease not accompanied by hypertension is not known. This is in part because the diagnosis of preeclampsia cannot be made with certainty on clinical grounds alone, because hypertension and proteinuria may be manifestations of the underlying renal disease.

11.2.2. Moderate renal insufficiency

Prognosis is more guarded where renal function is moderately impaired before pregnancy (plasma creatinine 160μmol/liter, 1.80 mg/dl). It is difficult to draw firm conclusions about pregnancy in these women, chiefly because the number of cases reported is still small. It seems that the chance for a successful pregnancy is good, but the optimistic fetal prognosis must be tempered by the fact that some will experience significant renal functional deterioration during pregnancy that may not improve after delivery, thus accelerating the downhill course of the underlying disease [35, 41]. More prospective studies of the impact of pregnancy on underlying renal disease are needed in this group of women.

11.2.3. Severe renal insufficiency

As most women with severe renal insufficiency have amenorrhea and/or anovulatory menstrual cycles, they have difficulty conceiving and therefore the likelihood of a normal pregnancy and delivery is low. Information about such patients is very limited so it is difficult to evaluate whether pregnancy has an adverse effect on their disease; since renal function is already severely compromised, however, this issue is largely irrelevant. Nonetheless, pregnancy in patients with advanced renal failure can have a serious impact on their health.

Mistakenly generalizing, clinicians assume that all uremic women cannot conceive and often neglect contraceptive counseling for patients on maintenance dialysis. While conception is not common—an incidence of one in 200 patients has been quoted recently—its true frequency is unknown, because most pregnancies in dialyzed patients probably end in early abortion [42]. The incidence of conception may increase in the future with the expanding use of continuous ambulatory peritoneal dialysis (CAPD), a therapeutic modality apparently associated with maintenance (or resumption) of reproductive function in a higher proportion of uremic women. Indeed, there have been isolated case reports of women on CAPD who carried the pregnancy to the stage of potential viability or to successful delivery [43].

Despite the occasional delivery of a viable infant, most authorities do not recommend attempts at pregnancy or its continuation after it has occurred in women with severe renal insufficiency [44]. First, the unsuccessful cases, and those that might have ended in disaster, are probably not reported, so that the true incidence of successful pregnancy is even smaller than would be suggested by the handful of reports in the literature. Second, these women are prone to volume overload, severe exacerbations of their hypertension, and/or superimposed preeclampsia, besides heavy fetal wastage at all stages of pregnancy. In such women, pregnancy represents an excessive risk for the mother, with an uncertain (but very low) chance of producing a healthy infant, and therefore should be discouraged. This discussion is taken further in chapters 9 and 11, and pregnancy in renal allograft recipients is considered in chapter 12.

12. THE KIDNEY IN PREECLAMPSIA

This topic is discussed in chapters 7 and 9. It is clear that the literature is confusing and controversial, largely because it is often difficult to distinguish clinically among preeclampsia, essential hypertension, chronic renal disease, and combinations of these separate entities [15, 34]. For instance, some women with undiagnosed essential hypertension show a decrement in blood pressure in early pregnancy and normal levels if first examined in midpregnancy so that, when significantly raised pressures are recorded near term, they are then erroneously labeled as preeclamptic. Furthermore, an accelerated phase of essential hypertension (albeit a rare event during pregnancy), certain forms of renal disease (glomerulonephritis and systemic lupus erythematosus), and pheochromocytoma may all mimic preeclampsia.

These diagnostic dilemmas are clearly emphasized in studies where renal biopsy was performed immediately after pregnancies complicated by hypertension [45]. Table 4–1 (chapter 4) shows the pathologic diagnosis on postpartum renal biopsy in 176 patients biopsied because pregnancy was complicated by hypertension, proteinuria, and edema, and where in most instances the clinical diagnosis was preeclampsia. This diagnosis was wrong in 25% of primiparas and was wrong more often than not in multiparas. In addition, a surprisingly large number of patients had unsuspected parenchymal renal disease. Such information emphasizes the pitfalls inherent in interpreting reports where the diagnosis is based on clinical criteria alone.

12.1. Alterations in renal morphology (see also chapter 4)

In preeclampsia the characteristic morphologic lesion is glomeruloendotheliosis [15, 45], which is completely reversible. The glomeruli are large and swollen, but not hypercellular, due to swelling of the intracapillary cells (mainly endothelial but also mesangial) that encroach on the capillary lumina, giving the appearance of a bloodless glomerulus. The lesion is considered by most, but not all, investigators to be virtually pathognomic of the disease.

12.2. Alterations in renal function (see also chapter 1)

12.2.1. Renal hemodynamics

Both ERPF and GFR decrease in preeclampsia. The decrement in GFR is approximately 25%–35% in mild cases whereas the normal increase in pregnancy ranges 40%–50% above values postpartum. Thus, despite morphologic evidence of glomerular cell swelling, ischemia, and obliteration of the urinary space, GFR in preeclamptic women often remains above prepregnancy values. The decrement may not be appreciated unless serial monitoring is undertaken and if there is not familiarity with norms for pregnancy (see Sections 2, 3, and 5). It should be emphasized that, while functional decrements in preeclampsia are usually mild or moderate and reverse rapidly after delivery, occasionally a patient may progress to acute tubular necrosis, especially when treatment or intervention is neglected [15].

12.2.2. Uric acid clearance

In preeclampsia, uric acid clearance decreases and renal reabsorption increases. These changes can occur earlier (sometimes weeks prior to any other signs or symptoms of the disease) and be more profound than the change in GFR. The increase in renal uric acid reabsorption is accompanied by increased plasma levels of this solute and the level of hyperuricemia correlates directly with the decrement in plasma volume that occurs in preeclampsia and indirectly with the plasma renin activity. High uric acid levels (> 350 μmol/liter, > 5.9 mg/dl) correlate with the severity of the preeclamptic lesion as well as with poor fetal outcome [20].

12.2.3. Protein excretion

Abnormal proteinuria almost always accompanies preeclampsia and the diagnosis is suspect without this sign, even though glomerular endotheliosis has sometimes been described in the absence of increased protein excretion. Proteinuria may be minimal, moderate, or severe (i.e., in the nephrotic range). The occurrence of the nephrotic syndrome deserves emphasis for, in the past, heavy proteinuria was believed to be uncommon in preeclampsia and, when it occurred, it was considered indicative of a severe form of the disease. It is now apparent that preeclampsia is the most common cause of the nephrotic syndrome in pregnancy [45]. The severity of maternal disease is similar in preeclamptic women with heavy proteinuria and those excreting less than 3.5 g/day, although small but significant increases in fetal loss occur in the women with severe proteinuria.

The proteinuria is nonselective. It has been attributed to vasopressin as well as to the actual glomerular lesion itself. There is evidence that the magnitude of the proteinuria correlates with the severity of the morphologic lesion [46].

12.2.4. Volume homeostasis

Edema and rapid weight gain are characteristic findings in preeclampsia, yet these signs may be observed frequently in healthy pregnant women [12]. Nevertheless, when compared with normal individuals, preeclamptic patients can have significant plasma volume contraction, increased to a body exchangeable sodium and a markedly expanded interstitial space. The enigma of volume homeostasis in preeclampsia is compounded by the observation that the disease can occur without fluid retention, in which case it actually may be more severe.

The cause of sodium retention in certain women with preeclampsia is obscure [27]. The decrease in GFR (often to levels that are comparable to or still above those in nonpregnant women) seems an insufficient explanation. Aldosterone levels are normal in early and midpregnancy in women destined to develop third-trimester hypertension while production, plasma concentrations, and urinary excretion of the hormone actually decrease when preeclampsia occurs [47]. Plasma levels of desoxycorticosterone (DOC), another potent mineralocorticoid, have been reported to be both decreased and unchanged in preeclampsia [27]. Prolactin, another hormone that may cause sodium retention, might play a role in the pathophysiology of this disease, but reports on circulating levels have yielded contradictory results [48].

Decrements in the levels of hormones with natriuretic activity could conceivably lead to pathologic sodium retention in preeclampsia [15]. While several investigators have found plasma levels of progesterone unaltered in preeclamptic women, it has recently been suggested that extraadrenal conversion of this natriuretic hormone to the potent sodium-retaining steroid DOC may be accelerated in these patients [49]. Also, production and urinary levels of prostaglandins with potent vasodilating and natriuretic effects may be decreased during preeclampsia [30, 50].

There is controversy regarding the occurrence and clinical significance of plasma volume depletion in preeclampsia and whether it is a cause or an effect of the disease process [51, 52]. It has been suggested that reduced plasma volume in primigravid patients might serve as an early indicator of the possible development of hypertension and may contribute significantly to the reduced uteroplacental blood flow in preeclamptic pregnancies, resulting in infants of smaller birth weight when compared with infants of nonhypertensive control patients [25]. On the other hand, it has been reported that plasma volume in mild preeclampsia is related to infant birth weight rather than to the development of preeclampsia [53]. Furthermore, recent studies indicate that plasma volume is not reduced in most patients with mild preeclampsia, but it is reduced in those pregnancies resulting in small-for-gestational-age infants [54].

13. CONCLUSION

Changes in the renal physiology of the renal tract during normal pregnancy are so marked that nonpregnant norms cannot be used for the management of pregnant women. Furthermore, it must also be remembered that, as pregnancy advances, the normal baseline undergoes further change and cognizance of all these alterations is essential if kidney problems in pregnancy are to be suspected, detected, and managed correctly.

ACKNOWLEDGMENTS

This work was supported by the Medical Research Council (England). I am indebted to Mrs. A. Gaffney for excellent secretarial assistance.

REFERENCES

1. Davison JM, Dunlop W: Renal hemodynamics and tubular function in normal human pregnancy. Kidney Int 18:152–161, 1980.
2. Sims EAH, Krantz KE: Serial studies of renal function during pregnancy and the puerperium in normal women. J Clin Invest 37:1764–1774, 1958.
3. De Alvarez RR: Renal glomerulotubular mechanisms during normal pregnancy. I. Glomerular filtration rate, renal plasma flow and creatinine clearance. Am J Obstet Gynecol 75:931–944,1958.
4. Assali NS, Dignam WJ, Dasgupta K: Renal function in human pregnancy. II. Effects of venous pooling on renal hemodynamics and water, electrolyte and aldosterone excretion during normal gestation. J Lab Clin Med 54:394–408, 1959.
5. Ezimokhai M, Davison JM, Philips PR, Dunlop W: Non-postural serial changes in renal function during the third trimester of normal human pregnancy. Br J Obstet Gynaecol 88:465–471, 1981.
6. Dunlop W: Serial changes in renal hemodynamics during normal human pregnancy. Br J Obstet Gynaecol 88:1–9, 1981.
7. Davison JM, Dunlop W: Changes in renal hemodynamics and tubular function induced by normal human pregnancy. Semin Nephrol 4:198–207, 1984.
8. Davison JM, Hytten FE: Glomerular filtration during and after pregnancy. J Obstet Gynaecol Br Commonw 81:588–595, 1974.

9. Brod J, Sirota JH: The renal clearance of endogenous "creatinine" in man. J Clin Invest 27:645–654, 1948.
10. Davison JM, Noble MCB: Serial changes in 24 hour creatinine clearance during normal menstrual cycles and the first trimesters of pregnancy. Br J Obstet Gynaecol 88:10–17, 1981.
11. Davison JM, Dunlop W, Ezimokhai M: 24 hour creatinine clearance during the third trimester of normal pregnancy. Br J Obstet Gynaecol 87:106–109, 1980.
12. Hytten FE, Leitch I: Physiology of human pregnancy, 2nd edn. Oxford: Blackwell, 1971.
13. Janney JC, Walker EW: Kidney function in pregnancy. I. Water diuresis in normal pregnancy. JAMA 99:2078–2083, 1932.
14. Nice M: Kidney function during normal pregnancy. I. The increased urea clearance of normal pregnancy. J Clin Invest 14:575–578, 1935.
15. Lindheimer MD, Katz AI: The renal response to pregnancy. In: Brenner BM, Rector RC Jr (eds) The kidney, 2nd edn). Philadelphia: WB Saunders, 1981.
16. Mitch WE, Collier VU, Walser M: Creatinine metabolism in chronic renal failure. Clin Sci 58:327–335, 1980.
17. Jacobsen FK, Christensen CK, Mogensen CE, Heilskow HSC: Evaluation of kidney function after meals. Lancet 1:319, 1980.
18. Lind T, Godfrey KA, Otun H, Philips PR: Changes in serum uric acid concentration during normal pregnancy. Br J Obstet Gynaecol 91:128–132, 1984.
19. Dunlop W, Davison JM: The effect of normal pregnancy upon the renal handling of uric acid. Br J Obstet Gynaecol 84:13–21, 1977.
20. Redman CWG, Beilin LJ, Bonnar J, Wilkinson R: Plasma urate measurements in predicting fetal death in hypertensive pregnancy. Lancet 1:1370–1373, 1976.
21. Atherton JC, Green R: Renal function in pregnancy. Clin Sci 65:449–456, 1983.
22. Davison JM, Hytten FE: The effect of pregnancy on the renal handling of glucose. J Obstet Gynaecol Br Commonw 82:374–381, 1975.
23. Davison JM, Sprott MS, Selkon JB: The effect of covert bacteriuria in schoolgirls on renal function at 18 years and during pregnancy. Lancet 2:651–655, 1984.
24. Davison JM: The effect of pregnancy on kidney function in renal allograft recipients. Kidney Int 27:74–79, 1984.
25. Arias F: Expansion of intravascular volume and fetal outcome in patients with chronic hypertension in pregnancy. Am J Obstet Gynaecol 123:610–616, 1975.
26. Bay WH, Ferris TF: Factors controlling plasma renin and aldosterone during pregnancy. Hypertension 1:410–19, 1979.
27. Nolten WE, Ehrlich EN: Sodium and mineralocorticoids in normal pregnancy. Kidney Int 18:162–172, 1980.
28. Wilson M, Morganti AA, Zervoudakis I, Letcher RL, Romney BM, Oevon PV, Papera S, Sealy JE, Laragh JH: Blood pressure, the renin–aldosterone system and sex steroids throughout normal pregnancy. Am J Med 68:97–102, 1980.
29. Barron WM, Lindheimer MD: Renal sodium and water handling in pregnancy. Obstet Gynecol Annu 13, 1984.
30. Goodman RP, Killam AP, Brash AR, Branch RA: Prostacyclin production during pregnancy: comparison of production during normal pregnancy and pregnancy complicated by hypertension. Am J Obstet Gynecol 142:817–820, 1982.
31. Davison JM, Vallotton MB, Lindheimer MD: Plasma osmolality and urinary concentration and dilution during and after pregnancy: evidence that lateral recumbency inhibits maximal urinary concentrating ability. Br J Obstet Gynaecol 88:472–479, 1981.
32. Davison JM, Gilmore EA, Durr J, Robertson GL, Lindheimer MD: Altered osmotic thresholds for vasopressin secretion and thirst in human pregnancy. Am J Physiol 246:F105–F109, 1984.
33. Davison JM: Renal haemodynamics and volume homeostasis in pregnancy. Scand J Clin Lab Invest 44:15–27, 1984.
34. Katz AI, Davison JM, Hayslett JP, Singson E, Lindheimer MD: Pregnancy in women with kidney disease. Kidney Int 18:192–206, 1980.
35. Bear RA: Pregnancy in patients with chronic renal disease. Can Med Assoc J 18:663–665, 1978.
36. Surian M, Imbasciati E, Cosci P: Glomerular disease and pregnancy: a study of 123 pregnancies in patients with primary and secondary glomerular disease. Nephron 36:101–105, 1984.
37. Davison JM, Lindheimer MD: Chronic renal disease. Clin Obstet Gynecol 27:891–901, 1984.

38. Kincaid-Smith P, Whitworth JA, Fairley KF: Mesangial IgA nephropathy in pregnancy. Clin Exp Hypertens 2:821–838, 1980.
39. Gimovsky ML, Moutoro M, Paul RH: Pregnancy outcome in women with systemic lupus erythematosus. Obstet Gynecol 63:686–692, 1984.
40. Mor-Josef S, Navot D, Rabinowitz R, Schenker JG: Collagen diseases and pregnancy. Obstet Gynecol Surv 39:67–84, 1984.
41. Hou SH, Grossman SD, Madias NE: Pregnancy in women with renal disease and moderate renal insufficiency. Am J Med 78:185–194, 1985.
42. Editorial: Pregnancy after renal transplantation. Br Med J 1:733–734, 1976.
43. Cattran DC, Benzie RJ: Pregnancy in continuous ambulatory peritoneal dialysis patient. Peritoneal Dial Bull 3:13–14, 1983.
44. Davison JM, Katz AI, Lindheimer MD: Management of renal complications of pregnancy and pregnancy in the renal disease, dialysis and transplant patient. In: Suki WN, Massry SG (eds) Therapy of renal disease and related disorders. The Hague: Martinus Nijhoff 1984, pp 347–376.
45. Fisher KA, Luger A, Spargo BH, Lindheimer MD: Hypertension in pregnancy: clinical–pathological correlations and remote prognosis. Medicine (Baltimore) 60:167–174, 1981.
46. Pollak VE, Nettles JB: The kidney in toxemia of pregnancy: a clinical and pathological study based on renal biopsies. Medicine (Baltimore) 39:469–477, 1960.
47. Weinberger MH, Kramer MJ, Petersen LP, Cleary RE, Young PCM: Sequential changes in the renin–angiotensin–aldosterone systems and plasma progesterone concentration in normal and abnormal pregnancy. In: Lindheimer MD, Katz AI, Zuspan FP (eds) Hypertension in pregnancy. New York: John Wiley and Sons, 1976, pp 263–269.
48. Yuen BH, Cannon W, Woolley S, Charles E: Maternal plasma and amniotic fluid prolactin levels in normal and hypertensive pregnancy. Br J Obstet Gynaecol 85:293–298, 1978.
49. Winkel CA, Casey ML, Guerami A, Rawlins SC, Cox K, MacDonald SC, Parker RC: Ratio of plasma deoxycorticosterone (DOC) levels to plasma progesterone (P) levels in pregnant women who did or did not develop pregnancy-induced hypertension [abstr 341]. Society for Gynecologic Investigation, 30th annual meeting, Washington DC, March 1983.
50. Editorial: Pregnancy and the arachidonic acid cascade. Lancet 1:997–998, 1982.
51. Gallery EDM, Hunyor SN, Gyory AZ: Plasma volume contraction: a significant factor in both pregnancy-associated hypertension (pre-eclampsia) and chronic hypertension in pregnancy. Q J Med [New Ser] 48:593–602, 1979.
52. Goodlin RC, Dobry CA, Anderson JC, Woods RE, Quaife M: Clinical signs of normal plasma volume expansion during pregnancy. Am J Obstet Gynecol 145:1001–1009, 1983.
53. Campbell DM, MacGillivray I: Evans blue disappearance rate in normal pregnancy and pre-eclampsia. In: Bonnar J, MacGillivray I, Symonds EM (eds) Pregnancy hypertension. Lancaster UK: MTP, 1980, pp 191–195.
54. Sibai BM, Anderson GD, Spinnato JA, Shaver DC: Plasma volume findings in patients with mild pregnancy-induced hypertension. Am J Obstet Gynecol 147:16–19, 1983.

6. SODIUM METABOLISM IN NORMAL PREGNANCY AND IN PREECLAMPSIA

WOLFRAM E. NOLTEN and EDWARD N. EHRLICH

1. INTRODUCTION

During the course of normal gestation, major changes in volume, distribution, and concentration of body fluids occur in the maternal organism, in order to meet the requirements of the developing conceptus. In pregnant as in nonpregnant subjects, sodium and water balance are governed by hypothalamic centers that control the release of antidiuretic hormone and influence thirst sensation, by renal adjustments of sodium and fluid excretion, and by secretion of gluco- and mineralocorticoids by the adrenal cortex. These homeostatic mechanisms in pregnant women must accommodate increasing levels of salt-retaining, natriuretic, and vasodepressor factors associated with advancing pregnancy if sodium and water balance are to be maintained.

It is commonly accepted that abnormal sodium retention and associated volume hyperexpansion can result in hypertension, as exemplified by the occurrence of elevated blood pressure in Conn's syndrome. A failure of any of the many regulatory mechanisms to respond appropriately to the changing requirements of pregnancy could disrupt salt and/or volume homeostasis and lead to hypertension.

It is therefore appropriate to review the alterations in body fluids that take place in normal pregnancy, and the factors that regulate them, so that we can gain some insight into the pathophysiology of hypertensive complications of gestation.

2. WEIGHT GAIN AND CHANGES IN FLUID VOLUMES IN PREGNANCY

2.1. Weight gain in pregnancy

Healthy primigravidas, who ingest an unrestricted diet and do not develop generalized edema, gain during the course of gestation an average of 12.5 kg, whereas normal multiparas gain approximately 1 kg less. Most of the weight increase occurs in the second half of pregnancy [1, 2].

This average gestational weight gain, which is currently considered as physiologic, is markedly higher than norms that were established in the first part of this century, which led to needless restriction of salt and calories in many healthy gravidas. The currently accepted normal range for weight gain in pregnancy is comprised of large standard deviations around the mean value; thus it is not surprising that weight may increase barely or as much as twice the average, while gestation proceeds without complications.

An analysis of the components of weight gain in normal pregnancy, at 40 weeks of gestation, shows that the products of conception account for 39%, elevated maternal blood volume for 10%, and augmented extracellular, extravascular fluid for 13% of the total weight increase [2]. In gravidas who have not developed generalized edema, 60% of the total weight gain is due to retained water, less than 10% is caused by an increase in protein, and most of the remainder represents increments in maternal fat stores [2, 3].

2.2. Changes in fluid volumes in pregnancy

In normal pregnancy, 500–900 mmol sodium are retained and distributed between the products of conception and the maternal extracellular fluid volume [4].

Serial measurements of total body water show increases of 7–8 liters from week 10 to week 38 of pregnancy [3, 5]. Computations of the extracellular fluid component reveal a gain of more than 6 liters during gestation [6].

The extracellular fluid space is comprised of plasma and interstitial fluid. Several studies in normal primigravidas show that an increase in plasma volume begins in the first trimester, accelerates through midpregnancy, reaches its peak at week 32 of gestation, and remains at that level until delivery [7]. Mean plasma volume increases in normal pregnancy from 2.7 liters at week 13 to 3.7 liters at week 38 of gestation and falls to 2.5 liters 6–8 weeks after delivery.

The gestational increment in maternal interstitial fluid is greatest during the final trimester. It is presumably caused by a reduction in the plasma oncotic pressure, and by an increase in the ability of skin and subcutaneous tissues to absorb water, which may be due to pregnancy- and/or estrogen-induced changes in the hydration of the mucopolysaccharide ground substance [8–10]. It can be assumed that such increased interstitial fluid would not be mobilized by use of diuretics.

3. FACTORS THAT INFLUENCE SALT AND WATER RETENTION IN NORMAL AND PREECLAMPTIC PREGNANCY

Renal sodium handling is the main determinant of volume homeostasis. In the discussion of sodium metabolism in pregnancy it is therefore important to review hemodynamic and hormonal changes, as well as physical factors, that are associated with gestation and that may influence renal sodium excretion.

3.1. Glomerular filtration rate

In pregnancy the glomerular filtration rate increases as much as 50% above non-pregnant values [11] (see chapters 1 and 5). This results in an increment in the filtered load of sodium of 5000–10,000 mmol/day [12]. If enhanced filtration were not countered by a commensurate increase in tubular reabsorption of sodium, and if glomerulotubular balance were not maintained, massive sodium depletion would rapidly occur. Surprisingly, in gravidas, tubular sodium reabsorption not only equals but rather exceeds the increase in filtered load: an additional 3 mmol of sodium are reabsorbed daily in order to provide for the expanding maternal and fetal fluid compartments [11]. The increment in sodium reabsorption represents the largest functional adjustment of the kidney in pregnancy.

3.2. Hormonal changes

3.2.1. Progesterone

During the course of gestation, progesterone production increases and plasma levels of progesterone rise substantially [13]. Progesterone enhances sodium excretion in normal man [14]. Its natriuretic effect has been explained by the ability of progesterone to inhibit competitively the salt-retaining action of aldosterone and of other mineralocorticoids in the distal nephron. Administration of progesterone to patients with adrenal insufficiency blocks the sodium-retaining effects of aldosterone when progesterone is given subsequently while continuing aldosterone [15]. Progesterone also has vasodilator properties, however, including renal hemodynamic effects, that in themselves may favor natriuresis [16]. More recently it has been demonstrated that the saliuretic effect of progesterone is in part independent of the ability of this steroid to inhibit mineralocorticoid action and may be mediated by reducing sodium absorption in proximal segments of the nephron [17].

3.2.2. Aldosterone

Secretion rate, plasma levels, and urinary excretion of aldosterone increase substantially in normal pregnancy [13, 18, 19] (Figure 6-1). As aldosterone is not tightly bound to plasma proteins, one may assume that its rising plasma concentrations result in comparable increases in the level of the biologically active, free mineralocorticoid.

The increase in production and plasma concentration of aldosterone has been explained as a compensatory response to the increment in filtered sodium and to the elevation of progesterone, a steroid with natriuretic and vasodilatory effect [12].

The view that aldosterone levels rise in order to balance increases in glomerular filtration rate and/or progesterone secretion in pregnancy is based on the following considerations: When glomerular filtration is enhanced, assuming that the

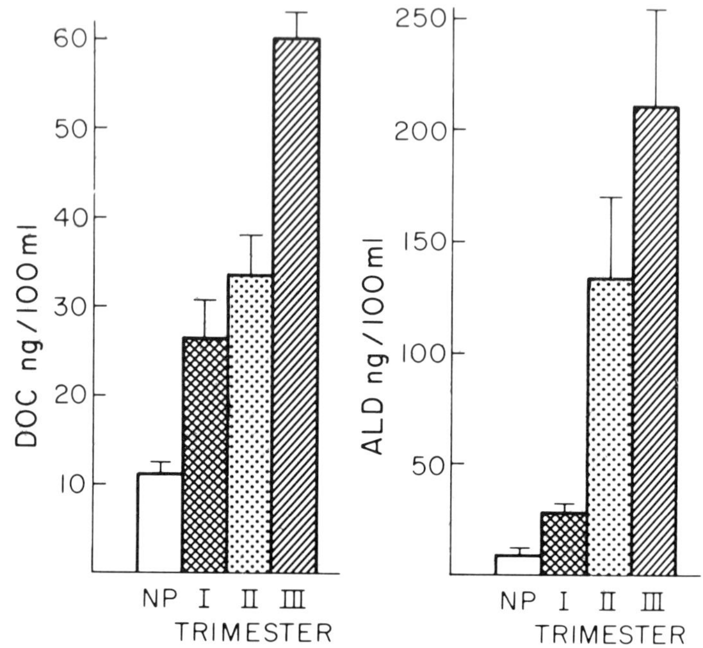

Figure 6-1. Mean plasma concentrations (±standard error) of desoxycorticosterone *(DOC)* and aldosterone *(ALD),* measured sequentially during pregnancy and three months postpartum. *NP,* nonpregnant. From Nolten et al. [19], by copyright permission of the C.V. Mosby Company.

glomerulotubular balance in the proximal renal tubule remains constant, more sodium will reach aldosterone-sensitive parts of the distal tubule and a compensatory increase in mineralocorticoid activity would prevent excessive natriuresis. Competitive inhibition of aldosterone in the distal nephron by progesterone would require a further increase in production of this mineralocorticoid in order to maintain sodium balance.

The assumption that the increase in aldosterone secretion is caused by the pregnancy-induced increment in progesterone is based on somewhat contradictory experimental data since not all researchers were able to demonstrate a positive correlation between plasma levels of aldosterone and progesterone in pregnant women [20, 21]. When progesterone was administered to women with a dead fetus but intact placenta, aldosterone production did, indeed, increase. Even when the given doses of progesterone equaled the amount of progesterone produced in pregnancy, however, the measured increment in aldosterone excretion was far less than that seen in normal gestation [22].

The high levels of renin and angiotensin II (AII) found in pregnancy are consistent with the assumption that the increased production of aldosterone is mediated by the renin–angiotensin system [23]. Numerous studies indicate that aldosterone secretion in pregnancy is regulated by normal mechanisms, and that elevated plasma aldosterone levels in gravidas are not excessive: secretion and excretion of aldosterone in pregnant women respond inversely to variations in sodium intake and rise even above their high baseline levels when the extracellular fluid volume is decreased by diuretics or when the effective blood volume is acutely reduced by a change of the gravida from the lateral recumbent to the supine upright position [18, 24, 25].

Moreover, pregnant women are quite sensitive to the sodium-retaining activity of administered mineralocorticoids, in spite of the elevation of plasma aldosterone that normally occurs in pregnancy [26]. Changes in salt and water balance observed during treatment with desoxycorticosterone acetate (DOCA) in a representative study resemble those in normal nonpregnant subjects [26] (figure 6-2). Initially there is intense sodium retention and associated weight gain, which subside after several days as volume expansion evokes the "escape" phenomenon. Contrarily, if pregnancy were associated with chronic volume hyperexpansion, because the high

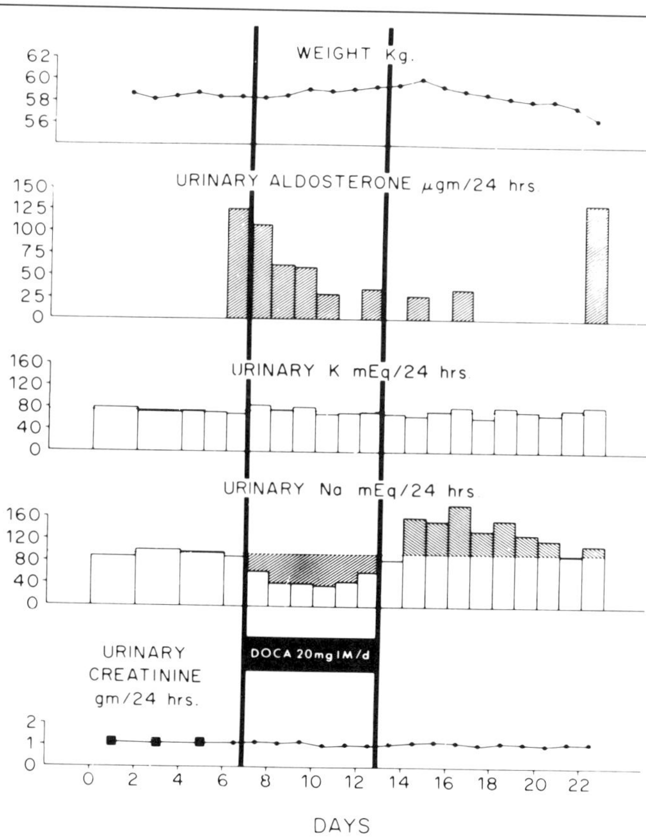

Figure 6-2. Metabolic and aldosterone responses to administered desoxycorticosterone acetate (DOCA), in a normal third-trimester pregnant woman. From Ehrlich and Lindheimer [26], by copyright permission of the American Society for Clinical Investigation.

aldosterone levels are in fact *excessive,* "escape" would already be operative at the onset of the study and the subject would be refractory to the sodium-retaining action of administered DOCA. Moreover, the fact that in this study increased excretion of aldosterone was suppressed by DOCA-induced volume expansion indicates that elevated aldosterone secretion in pregnancy is not autonomous, but remains sensitive to changes in volume.

As aldosterone production in pregnant women responds normally to physiologic stimuli and is apparently regulated by normal mechanisms, the conclusion is justified that aldosterone increases in normal gestation only to the extent necessary to maintain sodium balance and/or volume homeostasis. Therefore, if high maternal aldosterone levels were not maintained, salt loss and hypovolemia would be expected to occur. This hypothesis was tested by an experiment in which aldosterone excretion was decreased, without concomitant volume expansion, by administration of a heparinoid (R01-8307), which selectively impairs aldosterone production directly by undefined mechanisms [27]. As demonstrated by a representative study (Figure 6-3), the high baseline excretion of aldosterone decreased and natriuresis ensued when the heparinoid was given for a prolonged time. It is of importance that sodium loss occurred during treatment, when aldosterone excretion, although greatly diminished as compared with baseline levels, was still well above normal nonpregnant levels. After discontinuation of the heparinoid, natriuresis did not subside until aldosterone excretion had returned to its very high baseline levels. The observation that marked natriuresis occurs in the face of higher than normal aldosterone excretion supports the conclusion that increased aldosterone production is necessary to maintain sodium balance in pregnancy. It also suggests that in gravidas the action of aldosterone is opposed by rather potent saliuretic factors.

In several studies it was noted that, even when substantial cumulative sodium retention was maintained in pregnant women for an extended period by prolonged administration of a mineralocorticoid and/or high salt intake, aldosterone excretion and plasma renin activity, although markedly suppressed, were still significantly higher than in nonpregnant controls [26, 28]. Therefore, factors other than sodium loss and volume depletion must play a role in the elevation of plasma renin activity and aldosterone secretion that occurs in normal pregnancy. Plasma and urinary prostaglandin E may increase considerably in normal gestation [28]. Prostaglandin E not only acts as vasodepressor, it also enhances renin release [28]. Thus, elevated levels of prostaglandins in pregnancy may augment the activity of the renin–angiotensin–aldosterone system and thereby support sodium retention and simultaneously induce vascular refractoriness to the pressor effects of angiotensin, thereby maintaining the maternal blood pressure within the normal range. Moreover, studies in nonpregnant subjects suggest that vasodepressor prostaglandins enhance the response of the renin–angiotensin–aldosterone system to sodium restriction or to treatment with diuretics [29, 30]. Therefore, increased production of vasodepressor prostaglandins in pregnancy could also affect volume homeostasis by modulating the responsiveness of the renin–angiotensin–aldosterone system to volume depletion.

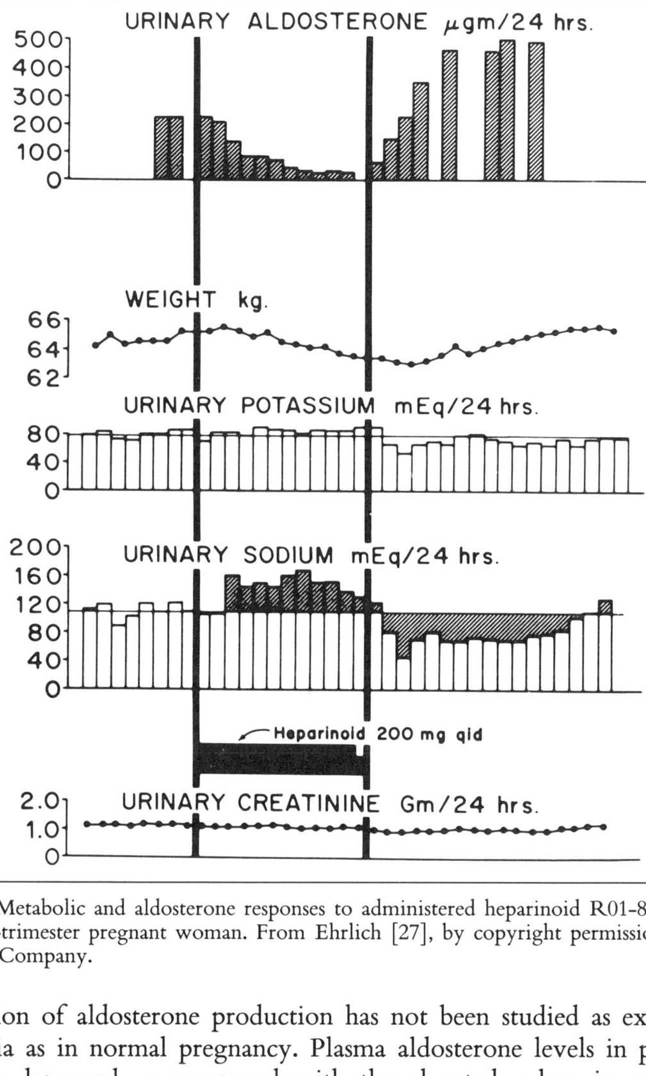

Figure 6-3. Metabolic and aldosterone responses to administered heparinoid R01-8307 in a normal third-trimester pregnant woman. From Ehrlich [27], by copyright permission of the C.V. Mosby Company.

Regulation of aldosterone production has not been studied as extensively in preeclampsia as in normal pregnancy. Plasma aldosterone levels in preeclamptic women are depressed, as compared with the elevated values in normotensive gravidas, but might still be inappropriately high in regard to the existing degree of sodium retention and could so contribute to the pathophysiologic consequences of preeclampsia [31].

3.2.3. Desoxycorticosterone

Secretion of the mineralocorticoid desoxycorticosterone (DOC) is markedly enhanced in normal gestation, as reflected by elevated levels of plasma DOC and augmented urinary excretion of its metabolic derivative, tetrahydro-DOC (THDOC) [19, 32, 33]. In the only reported study, where DOC production in pregnancy was measured by use of a urinary metabolite isotope-dilution method, the DOC production rate at term exceeded 8000 μg/day and fell to 174 μg/day three days post partum [32]. Sequential measurements of plasma DOC during the course of normal gestation show a steady rise in the first and second trimesters and an even more striking further increment in the third trimester, when mean plasma DOC concentrations reach levels that are more than five times higher than in the nonpregnant state [19] (figure 6-1).

In contrast to aldosterone, DOC is avidly bound to corticosteroid-binding globulin (CBG). Since concentrations of CBG also rise during pregnancy, it was not immediately apparent whether the increase in total plasma DOC in the maternal blood is associated with a rise in the unbound, biologically active DOC fraction. This question was addressed by measurements of the plasma-free DOC index, which reflects changes in the plasma levels of free DOC and which was found to be substantially higher in term gravidas than in nonpregnant controls [34]. This permits the conclusion that in gestation a marked increase in metabolically active, free DOC in the maternal circulation does indeed occur.

The small amount of DOC secreted in nonpregnant subjects is mainly a byproduct of cortisol biosynthesis. However, studies in third-trimester gravid women show a lack of synchrony between maternal diurnal patterns of plasma cortisol and DOC and also unresponsiveness of plasma DOC, not only to adrenal stimulation by ACTH and suppression by dexamethasone, but also to variations in the intake of salt [35, 36]. Therefore, it was assumed that increased DOC in late pregnancy does not arise from the maternal adrenal glands. Rather, a steep gradient between fetal and maternal DOC and DOC-SO_4 concentrations pointed to possible DOC production by the fetus [35]. Winkel et al. [37] showed that peripheral conversion of progesterone to DOC by 21-hydroxylation constitutes a major maternal source of DOC during gestation. MacDonald et al. [38] demonstrated that estrogens stimulate the activity of steroid 21-hydroxylase in such a manner that the transfer constant of conversion of plasma progesterone to DOC remains constant as pregnancy advances and as plasma concentrations of progesterone rise. Thus, the production rate of DOC in normal gestation would be proportional to the maternal plasma levels of progesterone. Extraadrenal conversion of progesterone to DOC may take place in the kidney, which is the major site of DOC action.

Cortisol, DOC, and progesterone are bound to CBG with high avidity. Consequently, changes in the plasma concentration of one steroid would be expected to directly influence protein binding and thereby the metabolically active free fraction of the others. This presumed interrelationship in the binding of steroid hormones to the increased levels of CBG that occur in pregnancy was investigated by measurements of plasma cortisol and DOC levels, plasma-free DOC index, and urinary THDOC excretion in third-trimester gravidas before and after adrenocortical stimulation [33, 34]: Although total plasma DOC failed to respond to ACTH, the plasma-free DOC index rose markedly due to displacement of DOC from CBG by the ACTH-induced increment in cortisol. Augmented THDOC excretion and cumulative sodium retention that occurred simultaneously with prolonged

ACTH stimulation, when aldosterone was depressed, were assumed to be consequent to the increment in biologically active free DOC that was displaced from its binding protein. Such plasma steroid-binding interactions have broad implications because they identify an additional mechanism, aside from those regulating secretion, whereby the biologic activity of steroids in plasma can be modulated.

Total plasma DOC levels determined in preeclamptic third-trimester women are not significantly different from those measured in normal gravidas [32]. However, concentrations of free DOC have not been measured in preeclampsia and it is conceivable that such determinations would reveal elevations not apparent from measurements of total plasma DOC concentrations.

A possible mechanism by which DOC activity might increase beyond the high levels of normal gestation was pointed out by Casey and MacDonald [39], who showed that, in pregnancy, conversion of DOC into its inactive metabolite, DOC-SO_4, can occur in the kidney, and that estrogens in large amounts may be necessary to effect optimal activity of the enzyme C-21 hydroxysteroid sulfotransferase that catalyzes this reaction. Impaired sulfurylation of DOC, formed in the kidney of primigravidas, could elevate DOC activity in the kidney and thereby be instrumental in the pathogenesis of pregnancy-induced hypertension and of salt retention of preeclampsia.

3.2.4. Estrogens

Estrogens, which increase during the course of gestation, are known to cause salt retention, possibly by stimulation of the renin–angiotensin–aldosterone system, that may be mediated by estrogen-induced increments in renin subtrate [40, 41]. The important role that estrogens play in enhancing the extraadrenal conversion of progesterone to DOC, and in promoting the metabolism of DOC into its inactive derivative DOC-SO_4, has been described above.

4. PHYSICAL FACTORS THAT INFLUENCE SODIUM METABOLISM IN PREGNANCY

4.1. Posture

Changes in posture markedly influence renal sodium handling in gravidas. The antinatriuretic effect of upright positioning is exaggerated in pregnant women [42]. In late gestation, even changes from lateral recumbency to supine–upright posture result in sodium retention associated with a concurrent increase in aldosterone excretion and plasma renin activity [25]. This renal adjustment to postural changes is not necessarily dependent upon an increase in aldosterone secretion or glomerular filtration rate, since it occurs even when these responses are prevented by prior induction of volume hyperexpansion [43]. The important influence of posture upon sodium excretion in pregnancy is underscored by the observation that normal third-trimester gravidas on a constant diet, who had previously maintained lateral recumbency for an extended time period, retained sodium for up to 72 h when they subsequently assumed the upright position [25]. These findings suggest that changes in physical activity patterns alone may lead to reversible fluid retention and weight gain, and, conversely, that lateral recumbent positioning of gravidas is a highly effective means of eliminating excessively retained fluid.

4.2. Circadian patterns of sodium excretion

Posture also might influence the circadian patterns of sodium excretion: in recumbent gravidas, sodium excretion rises in the morning hours toward a peak in the early afternoon and declines thereafter to a nighttime nadir [25]. In contrast, in ambulatory gravidas, sodium excretion frequently peaks at night [44]. This change in the pattern of circadian excretion might be explained by the salt-retaining effects of upright posture or of ambulation during the daytime that are more potent in pregnant women.

5. EFFECTS OF DIETARY SODIUM INTAKE IN NORMAL PREGNANCY

The current consensus seems to support the proposition that gravidas are subtle salt losers and are likely to develop signs of volume depletion when dietary sodium is restricted. It is noteworthy, however, that pregnancy may not be compromised in women belonging to certain Indian tribes of South America who live in an essentially salt-free culture. Pregnant women from these tribes show much higher levels of activity of the renin–angiotensin–aldosterone system than gravidas in neighboring tribes who have free access to dietary salt [45]. Although these observations might suggest that pregnant women are capable of satisfactorily accommodating extreme sodium restriction, questions regarding the outcome of pregnancy in this circumstance remain unanswered because fetal and neonatal parameters were not reported.

On the other hand, high sodium intake does not necessarily have adverse effects, as reflected by studies such as that by Robinson [46], who noted that weight gain and occurrence of edema or toxemia were not greater when pregnant women ingested a high salt diet. This study permits the conclusion that normal gravidas are able to deal with liberal sodium intake without developing clinical problems.

6. VOLUME HOMEOSTASIS AND SODIUM HANDLING IN PREECLAMPSIA: THE EFFECT OF INTRAVASCULAR VOLUME EXPANSION

Preeclamptic women usually present with generalized edema and a history of rapid weight gain. As compared with normal gravidas, these patients show contraction of the plasma volume, hemoconcentration, expansion of the interstitial fluid space, and increase in total body exchangeable sodium [11]. It is unknown by what mechanisms preeclamptic women retain sodium. Although the glomerular filtration rate may decrease by 25% or more, this abnormality alone would not serve as a satisfactory explanation for the noted sodium retention [11]. Aldosterone would be an unlikely cause, as plasma aldosterone typically decreases in preeclampsia [31]. To what degree enhanced peripheral conversion of progesterone to DOC, increased levels of metabolically active free DOC, or reduced production of prostaglandins with vasodilatory and natriuretic effects might contribute to sodium retention remains uncertain.

In contrast to normal pregnant women, toxemic gravidas presumably show impaired sodium excretion, and the occurrence of salt retention after parenteral sodium loading has been used as a criterion for the diagnosis of preeclampsia [47]. Preeclamptic gravidas were reported to have a decreased ability to concentrate urinary sodium, to show reduced sodium excretion rates, and to excrete a smaller than normal fraction of an infused sodium load [48, 49]. The validity of these findings has been questioned, however, because of problems in the design of the experimental protocols. Therefore, currently available information does not justify a recommendation for sodium restriction for pregnant hypertensive patients. In clinical practice, it is well known that preeclamptic gravidas resting in the lateral recumbent position often tolerate dietary sodium in excess of 100 mmol/day [12, 45, 49]. When given diuretics or when subjected to rigid salt restriction, these patients actually may develop sodium depletion [50].

7. THERAPEUTIC SODIUM RESTRICTION AND DIURETICS

In the past, diuretics and fluid restriction have been commonly prescribed for pregnant women, not only to treat symptomatic heart disease or as prophylaxis or therapy for preeclampsia, but also to alleviate excessive weight gain or to reduce asymptomatic edema. More recently, the majority of publications, as well as the report by the Ad Hoc Committee on Nutrition of the American College of Obstetricians and Gynecologists, have counseled against the practice of restricting sodium intake or prescribing diuretics during gestation as prophylaxis against toxemia [51–55]. The committee also indicated that regular restriction of sodium intake while administering diuretics on a long-term basis is potentially dangerous and has no place in the management of normal gravidas. It is therefore suitable to discuss some of these precautions in the light of current concepts of salt and water metabolism in pregnancy.

Maternal extracellular and intravascular fluid volumes increase markedly in pregnancy. Maternal volume receptors perceive these increments as normal. When this gestational expansion of extracellular fluid spaces is limited or prevented by salt restriction and/or diuretic therapy, a compensatory response of the renin–angiotensin–aldosterone system is evoked that is similar to that occurring in volume-depleted, nonpregnant individuals. It would be possible that diuretics or salt restriction might lead to a momentary exaggeration of the normal gestational tendency toward volume depletion, which would soon be corrected by compensatory responses. However, animal studies and observations in normal human pregnancy show that the stress of gestation and chronic salt restriction combined may exceed and even exhaust the adaptive capacity of the renin–angiotensin–aldosterone system and that under these conditions insidious salt wasting may occur [56]. Consequently, treatment with diuretics or salt restriction could lead to a reduction in the intravascular fluid volume, which might compromise placental perfusion. Indeed, it has been reported that such therapy will impair fetoplacental function, as reflected by a reduction in the metabolic and placental clearances of dehydroepiandrosterone sulfate [57]. Moreover, severe impairment of renal function, caused by salt depletion, has been described in preeclamptic gravidas [50, 58]. This complication could easily be misinterpreted as evidence of deterioration of preeclampsia, and the need for salt repletion and for discontinuation of diuretic therapy might then be ignored.

Earlier claims that prophylactic thiazide therapy reduces the incidence of preeclampsia have not been confirmed [11]. Rather, when diuretics were given to women without renal disease or hypertension, an increase in complications during labor and also in perinatal mortality was observed [52]. Furthermore, as preeclampsia can occur even without marked fluid retention, it is questionable whether removal of edema fluid would favorably influence the course of toxemia. Hemodynamic studies in women with severe preeclampsia and hypertension during labor and delivery suggest that a hyperdynamic, hypovolemic state exists in these patients [59, 60]. It must be assumed that additional volume depletion by use of diuretics in preeclampsia would decrease cardiac output and thereby compromise placental perfusion.

Since its benefit has not been proven, but its associated risks are well documented, the use of diuretics in pregnancy should be limited to the treatment of edema secondary to cardiac failure or impending acute renal failure [11]. Moreover, since restriction of dietary sodium has not been determined to prevent toxemia, but rather may result in complications of salt depletion, pregnant women should be permitted to salt their food to taste [61]. Adequate diuresis of asymptomatic edema, if seen necessary, can be achieved by bedrest in the lateral recumbent position, whereas suspected preeclampsia requires hospitalization, bedrest, and careful observation rather than administration of diuretics.

ACKNOWLEDGMENT

This work was supported by the Madison General Hospital Endocrine Research Fund.

REFERENCES

1. Thomson AM, Billewicz WZ: Clinical significance of weight trends during pregnancy. Br Med J 1:243–247, 1957.
2. Hytten FE: Weight gain in pregnancy. In: Hytten FE, Chamberlain G (eds) Clinical physiology in obstetrics. Oxford: Blackwell, 1980, p 193.
3. Pipe NGJ, Smith T, Halliday D, Edmonds CJ, Williams C, Coltart TM: Changes in fat, fat-free mass and body water in human normal pregnancy. Br J Obstet Gynaecol 86:929–940, 1979.
4. Hytten FE, Leitch I: The physiology of human pregnancy, 2nd edn. Oxford: Blackwell, 1971.
5. Hytten FE, Thomson AM, Taggart N: Total body water in normal pregnancy. J Obstet Gynaecol Br Commonw 73:553–561, 1966.
6. Chesley LC: A study of extracellular water changes in pregnancy. Surg Gynecol Obstet 76:-589–592, 1943.
7. Pirani BBK, Campbell DM, MacGillivray I: Plasma volume in normal first pregnancy. J Obstet Gynaecol Br Commonw 80:884–887, 1973.
8. Fekete S: The significance of mucopolysaccharides in the pathogenesis of toxemias of pregnancy. Acta Med Acad Sci Hung 5:293–308, 1954.
9. Rienits KG: The acid mucopolysaccharides of the sexual skin of apes and monkeys. Biochem J 74:27–38, 1960.
10. Langgard H, Hvidberg E: The composition of oedema fluid provoked by oestradiol and of acute inflammatory oedema fluid. J Reprod Fert [Suppl] 9:37–44, 1969.

11. Chesley LC: Hypertensive disorders in pregnancy. New York: Appleton-Century-Crofts, 1978.
12. Lindheimer MD, Katz AI: Kidney function and disease in pregnancy. Philadelphia: Lea and Febiger, 1977.
13. Weinberger MH, Kramer NJ, Peterson LP, Cleary RE, Young PCM: Sequential changes in the renin–angiotensin–aldosterone system and plasma progesterone concentration in normal and abnormal human pregnancy. In: Lindheimer MD, Katz AI, Zuspan FP (eds) Hypertension in pregnancy. New York: John Wiley and Sons, 1976, p 263.
14. Landau RL, Bergenstal DM, Lugibihl K, Kascht ME: The metabolic effects of progesterone in man. J Clin Endocrinol Metab 15:1194–1215, 1955.
15. Landau RL, Lugibihl K: Inhibition of the sodium retaining influence of aldosterone by progesterone. J Clin Endocrinol Metab 18:1237–1245, 1958.
16. Chesley LC, Tepper IH: Effects of progesterone and estrogen on the sensitivity to angiotensin II. J Clin Endocrinol Metab 27:576–581, 1967.
17. Oparil S, Ehrlich EN, Lindheimer MD: Effects of progesterone on renal sodium handling in man: relation to aldosterone excretion and plasma renin activity. Clin Sci Mol Med 49:139–147, 1975.
18. Watanabe M, Meeker CI, Gray MJ, Sims EAH, Solomon S: Secretion rate of aldosterone in normal pregnancy. J Clin Invest 42:1619–1631, 1963.
19. Nolten WE, Lindheimer MD, Oparil S, Ehrlich EN: Desoxycorticosterone in normal pregnancy. I. Sequential studies of the secretory patterns of desoxycorticosterone, aldosterone and cortisol. Am J Obstet Gynecol 132:414–420, 1978.
20. Ledoux F, Genest J, Nowaczynski W, Kuchel O, Lebel M: Plasma progesterone and aldosterone in pregnancy. Can Med Assoc J 112:943–947, 1975.
21. Smeaton TC, Andersen GJ, Fulton IS: Study of aldosterone levels in plasma during pregnancy. J Clin Endocrinol Metab 44:1–7, 1977.
22. Watanabe M, Meeker CI, Gray MJ, Sims EAH, Solomon S: Aldosterone secretion rates in abnormal pregnancy. J Clin Endocrinol Metab 25:1665–1670, 1965.
23. Weir RJ, Doig A, Fraser R, Morton JJ, Parboosingh J, Robertson JIS, Wilson A: Studies of the renin–angiotensin–aldosterone system, cortisol, DOC, and ADH in normal and hypertensive pregnancy. In: Lindheimer MD, Katz AI, Zuspan FP (eds) Hypertension in pregnancy. New York: John Wiley and Sons, 1976, p 251.
24. Ehrlich EN, Lugibihl K, Taylor C, Janulis M: Reciprocal variations in urinary cortisol and aldosterone in response to the sodium depleting influence of hydrochlorothiazide and ethacrynic acid in humans. J Clin Endocrinol 27:836–842, 1967.
25. Lindheimer MD, DelGreco F, Ehrlich EN: Postural effects on Na and steroid excretion and serum renin activity during pregnancy. J Appl Physiol 35:343–348, 1973.
26. Ehrlich EN, Lindheimer MD: Effect of administered mineralocorticoids or ACTH in pregnant women: attenuation of kaliuretic influence of mineralocorticoids during pregnancy. J Clin Invest 51:1301–1309, 1972.
27. Ehrlich EN: Heparinoid-induced inhibition of aldosterone secretion in pregnant women: the role of augmented aldosterone secretion in sodium conservation during normal pregnancy. Am J Obstet Gynecol 109:963–970, 1971.
28. Bay WH, Ferris TF: Factors controlling plasma renin and aldosterone during pregnancy. Hypertension 1:410–415, 1979.
29. Speckart P, Zia P, Zipser R, Horton R: The effect of sodium restriction and prostaglandin inhibition on the renin–angiotensin system in man. J Clin Endocrinol Metab 44:832–837, 1977.
30. Tan SY, Mulrow PJ: Inhibition of the renin–aldosterone response to furosemide by indomethacin. J Clin Endocrinol Metab 45:174–176, 1977.
31. Ehrlich EN: Mineralocorticoids in normal and hypertensive pregnancies. Semin Perinatol 2:-61–71, 1978.
32. Brown RD, Strott CA, Liddle GW: Plasma desoxycorticosterone in normal and abnormal human pregnancy. J Clin Endocrinol Metab 35:736–742, 1972.
33. Ehrlich EN, Biglieri EG, Lindheimer MD: ACTH induced sodium retention in pregnancy: role of desoxycorticosterone and corticosterone. J Clin Endocrinol Metab 38:701–705, 1974.
34. Nolten WE, Lindheimer MD, Oparil S, Rueckert PA, Ehrlich EN: Desoxycorticosterone in normal pregnancy. Am J Obstet Gynecol 133:644–648, 1979.
35. Nolten WE, Hughey Holt L, Rueckert PA: Desoxycorticosterone in normal pregnancy. III. Evidence of a fetal source of desoxycorticosterone. Am J Obstet Gynecol 139:477–482, 1981.
36. Nolten WE, Lindheimer MD, Oparil S, Rueckert PA, Ehrlich EN: Regulation of desoxycor-

ticosterone secretion in normal pregnancy. In: Beller FK, MacGillivray I (eds) Hypertensive disorders in pregnancy. Stuttgart: Georg Thieme, 1978, p 40.
37. Winkel CA, Milewich L, Parker CR Jr, Gant NF, Simpson ER, MacDonald PC: Conversion of plasma progesterone to deoxycorticosterone in men, nonpregnant and pregnant women, and adrenalectomized subjects: evidence for steroid 21-hydroxylase activity in nonadrenal tissues. J Clin Invest 66:803–812, 1980.
38. MacDonald PC, Cutrer S, MacDonald SC, Casey ML, Parker CR Jr: Regulation of extraadrenal steroid 21-hydroxylase activity: increased conversion of plasma progesterone to deoxycorticosterone during estrogen treatment of women pregnant with a dead fetus. J Clin Invest 69:469–478, 1982.
39. Casey ML, MacDonald PC: Metabolism of deoxycorticosterone and deoxycorticosterone sulfate in men and women. J Clin Invest 70:312–319, 1982.
40. Katz FH, Kappas A: The effects of estradiol and estriol on plasma levels of cortisol and thyroid hormone-binding globulins and on aldosterone and cortisol secretion rates in man. J Clin Invest 46:1768–1777, 1967.
41. Helmer DM, Judson WE: Influence of high renin substrate levels on renin–angiotensin system in pregnancy. Am J Obstet Gynecol 99:9–17, 1967.
42. Assali NS, Dignam WJ, Dasgupta K: Renal function in human pregnancy. II. Effects of venous pooling on renal hemodynamics and water, electrolyte and aldosterone excretion during normal gestation. J Lab Clin Med 54:394–408, 1959.
43. Lindheimer MD, Weston PV: Effect of hypotonic expansion on sodium, water, and urea excretion in late pregnancy: the influence of posture on these results. J Clin Invest 48:947–956, 1969.
44. Kalousek G, Hlavacek C, Nedoss B, Pollak VE: Circadian rhythms of creatinine and electrolyte excretion in healthy pregnant women. Am J Obstet Gynecol 103:856–867, 1969.
45. Oliver WJ, Neel JV, Grekin RJ, Cohen EL: Hormonal adaptation to the stresses imposed upon sodium balance by pregnancy and lactation in the Yanomama Indians, a culture without salt. Circulation 63:110–116, 1981.
46. Robinson M: Salt in pregnancy. Lancet 1:178–181, 1958.
47. Dieckmann WJ, Pottinger RE, Rynkiewicz LM: Etiology of pre-eclampsia–eclampsia. Am J Obstet Gynecol 63:783–791, 1952.
48. Chesley LC, Valenti C, Rein H: Excretion of sodium loads by nonpregnant and pregnant normal, hypertensive and preeclamptic women. Metabolism 7:575–588, 1958.
49. Sarles HE, Hill SS, Le Blanc AL, Smith GH, Canales CO, Remmers AR: Sodium excretion patterns during and following intravenous sodium chloride loads in normal and hypertensive pregnancies. Am J Obstet Gynecol 102:1–7, 1968.
50. Palomaki JF, Lindheimer MD: Sodium depletion simulating deterioration in a toxemic pregnancy. N Engl J Med 282:88–89, 1970.
51. Pitkin RM, Kaminetzky HA, Newton M, Pritchard JA: Maternal nutrition: a selective review of clinical topics. Obstet Gynecol 40:773–785, 1972.
52. Christianson R, Page EW: Diuretic drugs and pregnancy. Obstet Gynecol 48:647–652, 1976.
53. Gray MJ: Use and abuse of thiazides in pregnancy. Clin Obstet Gynecol 11:568–578, 1968.
54. Chesley LC: Disorders of the kidney, fluids, and electrolytes. In: Assali NS (ed) Pathophysiology of gestational disorders, New York: Academic Press, 1972, p 355.
55. Lindheimer MD, Katz AI: Sodium and diuretics in pregnancy. N Engl J Med 288:891–894, 1973.
56. Pike RL: Sodium requirement of the rat during pregnancy. In: Lindheimer MD, Katz AI, Zuspan FP (eds) Hypertension in pregnancy. New York: John Wiley and Sons, 1976, p 270.
57. Gant NF, Worley RJ: Hypertension in pregnancy: concepts and management. New York: Appleton-Century-Crofts, 1980.
58. Maclean AB, Doig JR, Aickin DR: Hypovolemia, preeclampsia and diuretics. Br J Obstet Gynaecol 85:597–601, 1978.
59. Benedetti TJ, Cotton DB, Read JC, Miller FC: Hemodynamic observations in severe preeclampsia with a flow-directed pulmonary artery catheter. Am J Obstet Gynecol 136:465–470, 1980.
60. Rafferty TD, Berkowitz RL: Hemodynamics in patients with severe toxemia during labor and delivery. Am J Obstet Gynecol 138:263–270, 1980.
61. Bremer TH: Human maternal–fetal nutrition. Obstet Gynecol 40:868–870, 1972.

7. HYPERTENSION COMPLICATING PREGNANCY

NORMAN F. GANT and JACK A. PRITCHARD

1. INTRODUCTION

Pregnancy may induce hypertension in previously normotensive women or aggravate hypertension in women who are already hypertensive. Generalized edema, proteinuria, or both, often accompany hypertension induced or aggravated by pregnancy. Convulsions may develop in association with the hypertensive state, especially in women whose hypertension remains undetected.

The hypertensive disorders in pregnancy are common complications of gestation and form one of the great triad of complications that continue to result in the majority of maternal deaths. Hypertensive disorders are an even more important cause of perinatal mortality and severe morbidity. How pregnancy per se incites or aggravates hypertensive vascular disease and associated complications remains unsolved despite decades of intensive research. These disorders remain among the most important unsolved problems in obstetrics.

What is apparent but frequently forgotten by the physician who cares for a gravida with hypertension is that he is caring for two patients with a combined life expectancy of 120 years—usually 50 additional years for the woman and 70 years for her fetus-infant. Thus, the reflex action to manage gravidas with hypertension in an identical pharmacologic manner as a nonpregnant patient can and often does endanger both the gravida and her fetus. These dangers can be reduced if the specific cause of the hypertension is properly identified, its pathophysiology is considered with respect to both patients, and appropriate therapy is applied. Thus it is imperative to recognize that hypertension induced by pregnancy is a different disease than coincidental hypertension (chronic hypertension) occurring during pregnancy.

In this chapter, a clinical classification of hypertension occurring during pregnancy is presented and clinical guides to diagnosis are made. The remaining sections of the chapter are devoted to a discussion of pregnancy-induced hypertension (PIH).

2. CLASSIFICATION OF HYPERTENSION COMPLICATING PREGNANCY

We have modified the classification of hypertension complicating pregnancy from that published in most text books. The reason for this modification is to try to separate hypertension generated by pregnancy from hypertension that merely coexists with pregnancy, yet emphasize that the presence of the latter enhances the frequency, and often the intensity, of the former:

A. Hypertension induced by pregnancy (pregnancy-induced hypertension, PIH)
   1. Without proteinuria or generalized, gross edema
   2. With proteinuria or generalized edema (preeclampsia)
      a. Mild
      b. Severe
   3. Eclampsia
B. Coincidental hypertension (chronic hypertension in pregnancy, CHP)
C. Hypertension worsened by pregnancy (pregnancy-aggravated hypertension)
   1. Superimposed preeclampsia
   2. Superimposed eclampsia

2.1. Pregnancy-induced hypertension (PIH)

Pregnancy-induced hypertension (PIH) is divided into three categories: (a) hypertension alone, (b) preeclampsia, and (c) eclampsia. The diagnosis of preeclampsia is based on the development of hypertension plus proteinuria, or edema that is generalized and overt, or both. Eclampsia is characterized typically by the abnormalities just cited plus convulsions that result as a consequence of the pregnancy-induced hypertension. Only rarely do these symptoms occur earlier than week 20 of gestation, and then most often only in cases of true hydatidiform mole or in cases with appreciable molar degeneration. Preeclampsia is almost exclusively a disease of the nulliparous woman. It more commonly affects the woman who is at the extremes of reproductive age, that is, a teenager or a woman over 35 years of age. The disease is occasionally seen, however, in the multipara with any of the following associated clinical conditions:

1. Multifetal pregnancy
2. Fetal hydrops

3. Vascular diseases, including essential chronic hypertension and diabetes mellitus
4. Coexisting renal diseases

The diagnosis of PIH is usually straightforward: The blood pressure is 140/90 or greater or there has been an increase of 30 mm Hg systolic or 15 mm Hg diastolic over baseline values on at least two occasions 6h or more apart.

Although the diagnosis of preeclampsia has traditionally required the identification of PIH plus proteinuria or generalized edema, many authorities concur that edema, even of the hands and face, is such a common finding in pregnant women that its presence should not validate the existence of preeclampsia any more than its absence should deny the diagnosis. Indeed, although Robertson [1] found that one-third of women developed generalized edema by week 38 of pregnancy, he was unable to show a significant statistical correlation between edema and hypertension. In another study, Friedman and Neff [2] reported that perinatal mortality was one-third lower in infants of women with edema alone compared with the general population. The edema of preeclampsia involves the face and hands and is present even after arising. A useful indicator of nondependent edema is the woman's complaint that her rings have become "too tight."

Proteinuria is an important sign of preeclampsia. Proteinuria is defined as the presence of 300 mg or more of protein in a 24-h urine collection or a protein concentration of 1 g/liter or more in at least two random urine specimens collected 6 h or more apart. It is important to note that the degree of proteinuria may fluctuate widely over any 24-h period, even in severe cases. Therefore, a single random sample may fail to detect significant proteinuria.

The combination of proteinuria and hypertension during pregnancy markedly increases the risk of perinatal mortality. McCartney and co-workers [3], in their extensive experience studying renal biopsy specimens of hypertensive pregnant women, invariably found that proteinuria was present when the glomerular lesion considered to be characteristic of preeclampsia was evident. It is important to recognize, however, that both proteinuria and alterations of glomerular histology develop late in the course of PIH. Evidence will be presented subsequently to show that preeclampsia becomes evident clinically only near the end of an often protracted, covert pathophysiologic process that may begin 3–4 months before hypertension appears. Therefore, even hypertension is a late manifestation in the pathophysiologic spectrum of preeclampsia—late enough, in fact, that once hypertension appears, the chance of perinatal survival is diminished.

When the blood pressure rises appreciably during the latter half of pregnancy it is perilous, to the fetus especially, not to take action, simply because proteinuria has not yet developed. Many clinicians have witnessed the onset of eclampsia before the onset of overt proteinuria. Thus, from both pathophysiologic and epidemiologic perspectives it is clear that hypertension is the *sine qua non* of preeclampsia and that, from the moment blood pressure begins to rise, both the fetus and the mother are at increased risk. Once the blood pressure exceeds 140/90 mm Hg, the diagnosis of PIH should be made and the patient treated accordingly. Proteinuria constitutes a sign of worsening hypertensive disease, and when the proteinuria is overt and persists, the risk to the fetus is increased even more.

2.2. Severity of pregnancy-induced hypertension

Pregnancy-induced hypertension is classified as mild or severe according to the frequency and intensity of the abnormalities listed in table 7-1. Importantly, the differentiation between severe and mild preeclampsia cannot be rigidly adhered to since an apparently mild case can rapidly become severe. Blood pressure alone is not always a dependable indication of severity, for an adolescent woman with a pressure of 145/85 mm Hg may develop convulsions, whereas some women with a blood pressure of 180/120 mm Hg do not. Fortunately, most women suffering from preeclampsia do not convulse. In some, the process is inherently mild and hence does not advance to the eclamptic stage. In others, suitable anticonvulsant treatment checks the process. In a third group, the termination of pregnancy either spontaneously or by intervention forestalls the development of convulsions, and the woman returns to normal after delivery.

Epigastric or right upper quadrant pain is presumed to be the result of hepatic edema and subcapsular hemorrhage that stretches the Glisson capsule. Rarely, the pain presages rupture of the liver, a rare but catastrophic complication of PIH. Hence, in this circumstance, prompt, definitive therapy is often indicated. Other signs of advanced PIH are overt thrombocytopenia, and hepatocellular dysfunction. They are likely to coexist. The etiology of impaired liver function in severely preeclamptic patients is unclear. Pritchard and associates [4] postulated that the thrombocytopenia results from platelet adherence to collagen exposed at sites of disrupted vascular endothelium. Brunner and Gavras [5] demonstrated that induction of hypertension by angiotensin-II infusion in experimental animals led to segmental constriction and dilation of arterioles with disruption of the vascular endothelium, especially in the dilated segments. They also found platelet adherence and fibrinogen deposited at the sites of denuded subendothelium. Using the scan-

Table 7-1. Indicators of severity of pregnancy-induced hypertension

Abnormality	Mild	Severe
Diastolic blood pressure	< 100 mm Hg	110 mm Hg or higher
Proteinuria	Trace to 1+	Persistent 2+ or more
Headache	Absent	Present
Visual disturbances	Absent	Present
Upper abdominal pain	Absent	Present
Oliguria	Absent	Present
Convulsions	Absent	Present
Serum creatinine	Normal	Elevated
Thrombocytopenia	Absent	Present
Hyperbilirubinemia	Absent	Present
SGOT elevation	Minimal	Marked
Fetal growth retardation	Absent	Obvious

ning electron microscope, Robertson and Khairallah [6] clearly identified platelet aggregates and fibrin strands adherent to the exposed subendothelial layer in rabbits treated with angiotensin II. Fetal growth retardation is less common with pregnancy-induced hypertension than with pregnancy-aggravated hypertension, but, when present, the physician should suspect that the disease process has been prolonged. The fetus in such a case can be in extreme jeopardy!

In neglected or, less often, fulminant cases of pregnancy-induced hypertension, eclampsia may develop. The seizures are grand mal in character. Seizures of eclampsia may first appear before labor, during labor, or postpartum. Any seizure occurring more than 48 h postpartum is more likely to be the consequence of some other lesion of the central nervous system.

2.3. Coincidental (chronic) hypertension

All chronic hypertensive disorders, regardless of their cause, appear to predispose the patient to the development of superimposed preeclampsia or eclampsia. These disorders can create a difficult problem of differential diagnosis and management in women who first present for obstetric care after week 20 of gestation. The diagnosis of coincidental hypertension is supported by the following findings: (a) a history of hypertension is (140/90 mm Hg or greater) antedating pregnancy or (b) discovery of hypertension (140/90 mm Hg or greater) before week 20 of pregnancy (with the exception of molar pregnancy noted above) or its persistence long after delivery. Additional historical factors that help support the diagnosis of coincidental hypertension are multiparity and the presence of hypertension in a previous pregnancy.

When the woman is not seen until the latter half of pregnancy, the diagnosis of chronic hypertension may be difficult to make because of the well-documented decrease in blood pressure that may occur during the second trimester and early in the third trimester of pregnancy in chronically hypertensive pregnant women. Thus a patient with chronic hypertensive disease who is seen for the first time at week 20 of pregnancy may have blood pressure that is within the normal range. During the third trimester, however, her blood pressure usually increases to or toward its former hypertensive level, which presents a diagnostic problem: Is this chronic (coexistent) hypertensive disease or is it pregnancy-induced hypertension? The physician is faced with a dilemma when a pregnant woman is not seen until the second half of pregnancy and at that time is normotensive, but subsequently demonstrates hypertension during the third trimester.

There are many diseases and syndromes associated with hypertension that may be encountered in pregnant women. Sims [7] proposed a classification of hypertension that is still useful, but essential hypertension is by far the most common of these diseases in pregnant women. McCartney [8], in his study of renal biopsies from women with "clinical preeclampsia," diagnosed chronic glomerulonephritis in 21% of the nulliparas and in 6.6% of the multiparas. Fisher and co-workers [9], however, did not confirm a high prevalence of chronic glomerulonephritis in their own patients.

It must be remembered that chronic hypertension is a dangerous disease whether the patient is pregnant or not. Specifically, chronic hypertension may lead to cardiovascular deterioration such as cardiac decompensation and cerebrovascular accidents. Finally, intrinsic renal damage may result from chronic hypertensive disease, or the hypertension itself may be the result of underlying chronic pyelonephritis or chronic glomerulonephritis. Additional dangers associated with chronic hypertension include the risk of developing pregnancy-aggravated hypertension and the risk of abruptio placentae. Several authors have reported that 5.7%–82% of pregnant women with chronic hypertension will develop superimposed PIH, depending on the criteria used to define superimposed PIH [8, 10–12]. Placental abruption has been reported to occur in 5%–10% of all chronically hypertensive pregnant women.

The fetus of the woman with chronic hypertension is, of course, subjected to additional risks, including growth retardation and intrauterine death. (For treatment of chronic hypertension in pregnancy, see chapter 8.)

2.4. Pregnancy-aggravated hypertension

Pregnancy-aggravated hypertension is the result of acute aggravation of the preexisting hypertension with the development of proteinuria and often gross edema. There may be a quick progression to eclampsia, which, unfortunately, may develop before week 30 of gestation. Diagnostic criteria include the following:

1. Documentation that the woman has chronic hypertension
2. Evidence of a superimposed, acute process as demonstrated by elevation of systolic blood pressure at least 30 mm Hg or of diastolic blood pressure at least 15 mm Hg above baseline on two occasions at least 6 h apart, and development of proteinuria, gross edema, or both

3. PREGNANCY-INDUCED HYPERTENSION

3.1. Pathophysiology

Vasospasm is basic to the disease process of pregnancy-induced hypertension. This concept, first advanced by Volhard [13], is based upon direct observation of small blood vessels in the nail beds, ocular fundi, and bulbar conjunctivae, and it has been surmised from histologic changes that are seen in various affected organs. In preeclampsia, Hinselmann [14], and later several others, noted alterations in the size of the arterioles in the nail bed, with evidence of segmental spasm that produced alternate regions of contraction and dilation. Even more striking changes have been identified in the bulbar conjunctivae; Landesman and co-workers [15] described marked arteriolar constriction, even to the extent that capillary circulation was intermittently abolished. Further evidence that vascular changes play an important role in pregnancy-induced hypertension is afforded by the frequency with which spasm of the retinal arterioles, commonly segmental, is found in this disorder.

The vascular constriction imposes a resistance to blood flow and accounts for the development of arterial hypertension. Vasospasm most likely exerts a noxious effect on the blood vessels themselves as well as the organs they supply. Circulation in the vasa vasorum is impaired, leading to damage of the vascular walls. Alternating segmental dilation that commonly accompanies the segmental arteriolar spasm probably contributes further to the development of vascular damage, since endothelial integrity may be compromised by stretch in the dilated segments. Moreover, angiotensin II appears to have a direct action on endothelial cells, causing them to contract. These events can create interendothelial leaks through which blood constituents, including platelets and fibrinogen, can pass and be deposited subendothelially [5]. The vascular changes, together with local hypoxia of the surrounding tissues, presumably lead to hemorrhage, necrosis, and other disturbances that have been observed at times with severe PIH. Deposition of fibrin is then likely to be prominent, as seen in fatal cases [16].

Normally, pregnant women develop refractoriness to the pressor effects of angiotensin II [17]. Increased vascular reactivity to pressor hormones in women with early preeclampsia has been identified by Raab and co-workers [18] and Talledo et al. [19] using either angiotensin II or norepinephrine, and by Dieckman and Michel [20] and Browne [21] using vasopressin. Subsequently, Gant and co-workers [22] demonstrated that increased vascular sensitivity to angiotensin II clearly preceded the development of PIH. In the primigravid women studied by them, refractoriness to the pressor effect of infused angiotensin II characterized normal pregnancy (figure 7-1). However, those women destined to develop PIH subsequently demonstrated a loss of the normal pregnancy refractoriness to angiotensin II some time before the onset of hypertension. Of all the normotensive women studied who at weeks 28–32 of gestation required more than 8 ng/kg/min of angiotensin II to develop a standardized pressor response, 91% remained normotensive throughout the remainder of the pregnancy. Conversely, among normotensive primigravid women who required for a pressor response less than 8 ng/kg/minute at weeks 28–32, 90% subsequently became overtly hypertensive. Similar results have been reported recently in 231 women studied by Öney and Kaulhausen in Germany [23].

Refractoriness to angiotensin II is not a generalized phenomenon, since aldosterone secretion is strikingly increased in pregnant women, and increased aldosterone secretion is modulated by the action of angiotensin II on the cells of the zona glomerulosa of the adrenal cortex. Based on the findings of a number of studies, Gant and co-workers [24], Cunningham and associates [25], and Everett and colleagues [26, 27] concluded that in pregnant women the blunted pressor response to angiotensin II was brought about by a specific decrease in responsiveness of the vasculature. Refractoriness to the pressor effects of angiotensin II begins early in pregnancy (figure 7-1) and in some women enormous amounts of angiotensin II are required to elicit a given pressor response. The refractoriness to angiotensin II appears to be mediated by the vascular tissue synthesis of a prostaglandin or prostaglandin-like substance, for example, prostacyclin or prostaglandin E_2. Indeed, the refractoriness to the pressor effect of angiotensin II in pregnant women can be

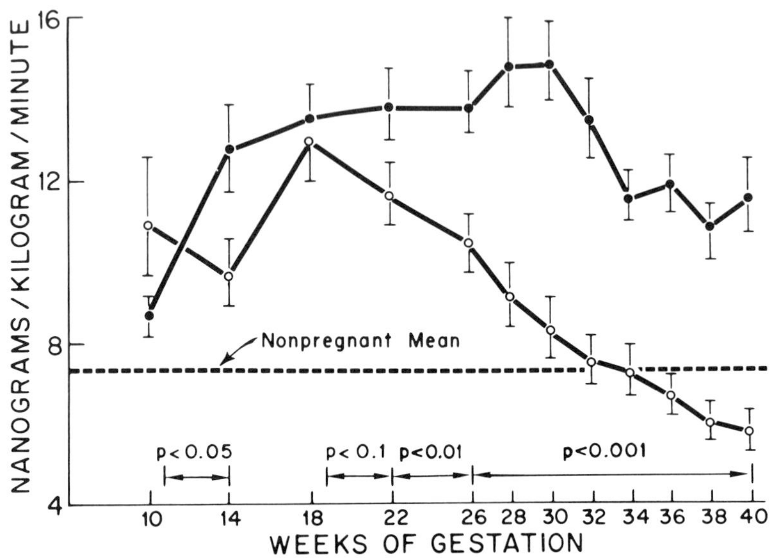

Figure 7-1. Comparison of the mean angiotensin II doses required to evoke a pressor response in 120 primigravidas who remained normotensive *(solid circles)* and 72 primigravidas who later developed pregnancy-induced hypertension *(open circles)*. From Gant et al. [22], by copyright permission of the American Society for Clinical Investigation.

abolished by the administration of the prostaglandin synthetase enzyme inhibitors, indomethacin and aspirin [26]. In some tissues, angiotensin-II action is mediated, at least in part, by promoting either the accelerated synthesis or the release of prostaglandins, or by both mechanisms. It is interesting to speculate that pregnancy brings about an increased capacity for prostaglandin formation in vascular tissue, normally with relatively greater synthesis of prostaglandins that induce vasodilation than of prostaglandins, e.g., prostaglandin $F_{2\alpha}$, that promote vasoconstriction.

3.2. Clinical aspects of hypertension with and without edema and/or proteinuria

The two especially important signs of PIH—hypertension and proteinuria—are abnormalities of which the pregnant woman is usually unaware. By the time she has developed symptoms, such as headache, visual disturbances, or epigastric pain, the disorder is almost always severe. Hence, the importance of prenatal care in the early detection and management of this complication becomes obvious.

The basic derangement in preeclampsia is vasospasm, especially of the arterioles. It is not surprising therefore that the most dependable warning sign of preeclampsia is a rise in blood pressure. The diastolic pressure is probably a more reliable prognostic sign than is the systolic, and any persisting diastolic pressure of 90 mm Hg or more is abnormal.

Another sign of development of PIH may be a sudden increase in weight. Indeed, excessive weight gain in some women is the first sign. Weight increase of about 1 pound per week is normal, but when weight gain exceeds much more than 2 pounds in any given week, or 6 pounds in a month, incipient preeclampsia must be suspected. Characteristic of preeclampsia is the suddenness of the excessive weight gain rather than an increase distributed throughout gestation. Sudden and excessive weight gain in gestation is attributable almost entirely to abnormal retention of fluid and is demonstrable, as a rule, before visible signs of nondependent edema, for example, swollen eyelids and puffiness of the fingers. In cases of fulminating preeclampsia or eclampsia, waterlogging may be extreme, and in such women a weight gain of 10 pounds or more within a week is not unusual [28].

Proteinuria varies greatly, not only from case to case, but also in the same woman from hour to hour. The variability points to a functional (vasospasm) rather than an organic cause. In early preeclampsia, proteinuria may be minimal or entirely lacking. In the more severe forms, proteinuria is usually demonstrable and may be as much as 10 g/liter. Proteinuria almost always develops later than the hypertension and usually later than excessive weight gain.

Headache is rare in milder cases, but is increasingly frequent in the more severe grades. In women who develop eclampsia, severe headache is a frequent forerunner of the first convulsion. It is often frontal, but may be occipital, and it is resistant to relief from ordinary analgesics.

Epigastric or right upper quadrant pain often is a symptom of severe preeclampsia and is indicative of imminent convulsions. It may be the result of stretching of the hepatic capsule possibly by edema and hemorrhage.

Visual disturbances ranging from a slight blurring of vision to blindness may accompany preeclampsia. Although such disturbances are thought by some to be of central origin, they are most likely attributable to retinal arteriolar spasm, ischemia, edema, and in rare cases actual retinal detachment. In general, the prognosis for such detachments is good, the retina reattaching, as a rule, within a few weeks after delivery. Hemorrhages and exudates are extremely rare in preeclampsia and when present are indicative most often of underlying chronic hypertensive vascular disease.

The prognosis for the mother and fetus depends to a considerable extent on the gestational age of the fetus, whether improvement follows hospitalization, when and how delivery is accomplished, and whether eclampsia supervenes.

The perinatal mortality rate is variably increased for pregnancies complicated by pregnancy-induced hypertension, as with the other hypertensive disorders. It is dependent primarily upon the time of onset and the severity of the disease. Much of the perinatal loss is the consequence of prematurity, either from early spontaneous labor or because of therapeutic interruption necessitated by the development of severe preeclampsia.

3.3. Prophylaxis and early treatment

Because women seldom notice the signs of incipient preeclampsia, the early detection of the disease demands careful observation at appropriate intervals, especially in women known to be predisposed to preeclampsia. The major predisposing factors are (1) nulliparity, (2) a familial history of preeclampsia–eclampsia, (3) multiple fetuses, (4) diabetes, (5) chronic vascular disease, (6) hydatidiform mole, and (7) fetal hydrops.

Rapid gain in weight any time during the latter half of pregnancy, or an upward trend in the diastolic blood pressure while still in the "normal" range, is ominous. Every woman should be examined at least weekly during the last month of pregnancy and every two weeks during the previous two months. At these visits, careful blood pressure measurements and weight checks of the woman are routine. All women should be advised to report immediately any of the well-known symptoms or signs of preeclampsia, such as headache, visual disturbances, and puffiness of hands or face. The reporting of any such symptoms, of course, calls for an immediate examination to confirm or exclude preeclampsia.

Obstetricians in the past often attempted to limit maternal weight gain to about 20 pounds, or even less, in the belief that preeclampsia can thereby be prevented. The total weight gain during pregnancy, however, probably has no relation to preeclampsia unless a large component of the gain is edema. Stringent restriction of weight gain is more likely to be detrimental rather than beneficial to both mother and fetus. The physician's scale, unfortunately, does not distinguish between the accumulation of edema fluid and the healthy deposition of fetal and maternal tissue.

Natriuretic drugs, such as chlorothiazide and its cogeners, have been severely overused. Although diuretics have been alleged to prevent the development of preeclampsia, the results of the studies by Kraus and co-workers [29], and others, cast doubt on their real value. The women studied by Kraus and associates took either a placebo or 50 mg of hydrochlorothiazide daily during at least the last 16 weeks of gestation. The incidences of preeclampsia were identical (6.67%) in the primigravid subjects who received hydrochlorothiazide and those who took the placebo. Moreover, the frequency of development of hypertension was not altered in multiparous women. The failure of natriuretic drugs in the prevention of preeclampsia raises serious doubt about the efficacy of rigid dietary restriction of sodium.

Thiazide diuretics and similar compounds are not used in the treatment or prophylaxis of PIH at Parkland Memorial Hospital. (Dallas) While there is no clear evidence that they are of any value, there is evidence that these agents can reduce renal perfusion as measured by creatinine clearance and, more important, probably reduce uteroplacental perfusion [30]. The thiazide diuretics can induce serious depletion of both sodium and potassium. Minkowitz and associates [31] and Menzies and Prystowsky [32] reported the findings of depletion of electrolytes and hemorrhagic pancreatitis in women who died following treatment of preeclampsia with chlorothiazide. Rodriguez and associates [33], moreover, found severe thrombocytopenia in some newborns whose mothers had received thiazide diuretics.

The basic objectives of management of any pregnancy complicated by PIH are (a) termination of the pregnancy with the least possible trauma to the mother and the fetus, (b) birth of an infant who subsequently thrives, and (c) complete restoration of the health of the mother.

In certain cases of preeclampsia, especially in women at or near term, all these objectives may be served equally well by one treatment, i.e., careful induction of labor and delivery. It cannot be emphasized too strongly, therefore, that the most important information that the obstetrician can possess for the successful management of pregnancy, and especially pregnancy that becomes complicated by hypertension, is precise knowledge of the age of the fetus.

Ambulatory treatment has no place in the management of pregnancy-induced or pregnancy-aggravated hypertension. Excluding young nulliparas, some women whose systolic blood pressure does not exceed 135 mm Hg and whose diastolic pressure does not exceed 85 mm Hg, and in whom proteinuria is absent, may be managed tentatively at home as long as the disease does not become more severe and fetal growth retardation is not a problem. Bedrest throughout the greater part of the day is essential. Moreover, these women should be examined twice weekly rather than weekly, and be instructed in detail about the reporting of symptoms. With minor elevations of blood pressure, the response to this regimen is often immediate, but the woman must be cooperative and the obstetrician wary.

The indication for hospitalization of women with preeclampsia is a systolic blood pressure of 140 mm or above or a diastolic pressure of 90 mm or above. For an intelligent continuing appraisal of the severity of the disease, upon admittance to the hospital systematic study should be instituted that includes the following:

1. An appropriate history and general physical examination followed by daily search for the development of such signs and symptoms as headache, visual disturbances, epigastric pain, and rapid weight gain
2. Weight measured on admittance and every two days thereafter
3. Urine screened for protein on admittance and subsequently at least every two days
4. Blood pressure readings with an appropriate size cuff every 4 h (except between midnight and morning, unless the midnight pressure has risen)
5. Measurements of plasma creatinine
6. Measurements of hematocrit, platelets, and serum SGOT
7. Frequent evaluation of fetal size by the same experienced examiner and by serial sonography if remote from term

Whenever observations so made serve to establish a diagnosis of severe preeclampsia (table 7-1), the management is prevention of seizures, control of blood pressure, and delivery.

Bedrest throughout much of the day is beneficial and ample, but not excessive, protein and calories should be included in the diet. Sodium and fluid intakes should be neither limited nor forced.

Phenobarbital administered in divided doses totaling 120–240 mg/day has been widely used for sedation. We do not do so. The possibility of adverse effects on the fetus from phenobarbital should be considered. The combination of phenobarbital and phenytoin given to the woman with epilepsy has been demonstrated to cause a reduction in vitamin-K-dependent coagulation factors in some fetuses. Moreover, phenobarbital has been reported to delay lung maturation, at least in the rabbit fetus [34].

The further management of PIH will depend upon (a) its severity as gauged by the presence or absence of the conditions cited in table 7-1, (b) the duration of gestation, and (c) the condition of the cervix. Fortunately, many cases prove to be sufficiently mild and near enough to term that they can be managed conservatively until labor commences spontaneously or until the cervix becomes favorable for induction of labor. Complete abatement of all signs and symptoms, however, is uncommon until after delivery. Almost certainly, the underlying disease persists until after delivery!

Occasionally, fulminant or neglected preeclampsia is encountered with blood pressure recordings in excess of 160/110 mm Hg, edema, and proteinuria. Headaches, visual disturbances, or epigastric pain are indicative that convulsions are imminent; oliguria resulting from preeclampsia is another ominous sign. Severe preeclampsia demands anticonvulsant and usually antihypertensive therapy followed by delivery. The prime objectives are to forestall convulsions, to prevent intracranial hemorrhage or serious damage to other vital organs, and to deliver an infant who, hopefully, survives and subsequently thrives.

In a more severe case of preeclampsia, as well as eclampsia, magnesium sulfate administered parenterally is a most valuable anticonvulsant agent, as attested to by the experience of many clinics over many years. Magnesium sulfate may be given intramuscularly by intermittent injection or intravenously by continuous infusion. At Parkland Memorial Hospital the dosage schedule for severe preeclampsia is the same as for eclampsia (table 7-2). Since the period of labor and delivery is a more likely time for convulsions to develop, all women suspected to have PIH are treated

Table 7-2. Magnesium sulfate dosage schedule for severe preeclampsia and eclampsia

1. Give 4 g of magnesium sulfate ($MgSO_4 7H_2O$, USP) intravenously at the rate of 1 g/min (20% solution).
2. Follow promptly with 10 g of 50% magnesium sulfate solution, one-half (5 g) injected deeply in the upper outer quadrant of both buttocks through a 3-inch long, 20-gauge needle. (Addition of 1.0 ml of 2% lidocaine minimizes discomfort.) If convulsions persist after 15 min or so, give up to 2 g more intravenously no faster than 1 g/min; if the woman is large, up to 4 g may be given slowly.
3. Every 4 h thereafter give 5 g of a 50% solution of magnesium sulfate injected deeply in the upper outer quadrant of alternate buttocks, but only after ascertaining the following:
   a. The patellar reflex is present.
   b. Respirations are not depressed.
   c. Urine output the previous 4 h was 100 ml or more.
4. Magnesium sulfate is discontinued 24 h after delivery.

at Parkland Memorial Hospital with intramuscular magnesium sulfate during labor and the early puerperium. Hydralazine (Apresoline), administered intravenously in appropriate doses intermittently, has proven to be an effective and safe antihypertensive agent. Its use is outlined in detail below.

To try to enhance fetal lung maturation, glucocorticoids have been administered by some to severely hypertensive pregnant women who need delivery and are thought to be remote from term. Several reports have appeared in which such treatment seemed not to worsen maternal hypertension, and a decrease in the incidence of respiratory distress syndrome and an improved fetal survival have been claimed. For example, Nochimson and Petrie [35] administered betamethasone to 20 severely hypertensive women and observed no untoward effect. Perinatal survival was 85.7%. Similar results have been reported by Semchyshyn and associates [36] and by Ruvinsky and colleagues [37].

We do not use corticosteroids in these circumstances for two reasons: (a) their administration poses potential risks to the mother and the fetus-infant, and (b) when the mother has severe pregnancy-induced hypertension requiring delivery, severe respiratory distress is uncommon in her neonate even when quite premature.

The cure for preeclampsia is the expulsion or removal of trophoblast, i.e., delivery. When the fetus is known or suspected to be premature, however, the tendency is widespread to temporize in the hope that a few more weeks in utero will reduce the risk to the infant of death or serious morbidity. Such a policy is justified in milder cases, but in severe preeclampsia, procrastination can prove to be ill-advised, since the preeclampsia itself may kill the fetus. Even for the fetus remote from term, the probability of fetal survival may be greater in a well-operated neonatal intensive care unit than when the fetus is left in utero.

Assessments of fetal well-being and placental function have been attempted especially when there is hesitation to deliver the fetus because of prematurity. Serial measurements of plasma or urinary estriol, or of placental lactogen, or the oxytocin challenge (contraction) test, or the fetal "biophysical profile" may result in abnormal results when the fetoplacental unit is compromised. To date, these tests have not been clearly demonstrated to provide valuable information otherwise unavailable for intelligent management of the pregnancy complicated by PIH.

Failure of the fetus to grow, as estimated clinically and by sonography, is an ominous sign of fetal jeopardy. Measurement of the *lecithin–sphingomyelin* (L/S) ratio in amnionic fluid may provide evidence of lung maturity, but it should be kept in mind during management of more severe cases that even when the L/S ratio is less than 2.0, respiratory distress may not develop and, when it does, most often it does not prove fatal.

With severe preeclampsia that does not improve after a few days of hospitalization as outlined above, termination of pregnancy is usually advisable for the welfare of both the mother and the fetus. Labor may be induced by administration of oxytocin. In severe cases, this procedure is often successful even when the cervix appears unfavorable for induction. Whenever it appears that induction of labor almost certainly will not succeed, or attempts at induction of labor are not fruitful, cesarean delivery for the more severe cases is the procedure of choice. In cases of severe preeclampsia and eclampsia with subarachnoid or epidural block, hypotension detrimental to the fetus, as well as the mother, may occur.

For a woman near term, with a soft, partially effaced cervix, even milder degrees of preeclampsia probably carry more risk to the mother and her fetus-infant than does induction of labor by carefully monitored oxytocin stimulation. This is not likely to be the case, however, if the preeclampsia is mild but the cervix is firm and closed, indicating that abdominal delivery might be necessary if pregnancy is to be terminated. The hazard of cesarean delivery may be greater than that of allowing the pregnancy to continue under close observation in the hospital until the cervix is more suitable for induction.

A high-risk pregnancy unit has been established at Parkland Memorial Hospital to provide care as just described. The results have been remarkable as originally reported by Gilstrap et al. [38]. Of 576 nulliparous women, usually teenage and often black, admitted to the unit because of hypertension remote from term, 545 remained for care until the pregnancy was terminated; the uncorrected perinatal mortality rate for this group was 0.9%. For the 31 who left the unit before delivery, although advised not to, the perinatal mortality was 13%! The mean birth weight of the infants whose mothers remained on the unit was 2974 g with 83% weighing 2500 g or more. Through 1983, more than 2000 women with mild to moderate early-onset pregnancy-induced hypertension have been so managed with equally good results! The cost of providing the relatively simple physical facility, modest nursing care, no drugs other than an iron supplement, and the very few laboratory tests that are essential is slight compared with the cost of neonatal intensive care. Moreover, the quality of the infant is very likely better.

After delivery there is usually rapid improvement, although, at times, the disease may worsen transiently. Eclampsia may develop any time during the first 24 h after delivery. After 24 h, eclampsia is rare in our now extensive experience. At Parkland Memorial Hospital, magnesium sulfate therapy instituted before or during parturition is continued for 24 h post partum with parenterally administered hydralazine given intermittently, if needed, to lower a diastolic blood pressure of 110 mm Hg or higher.

The woman may be discharged, even though still hypertensive, if there is evidence that severe hypertension is abating and she is otherwise well. Unless the hypertension persists at high levels during the puerperium, antihypertensive agents are not prescribed; instead, the woman is reevaluated in two weeks. Typically, but not always, hypertension induced by pregnancy will have dissipated during this period. If so, the episode of PIH does not mitigate against the use of oral contraceptives.

4. CLINICAL ASPECTS OF ECLAMPSIA

Eclampsia is an acute disorder characterized by clonic and tonic convulsions that are caused in some way by hypertension induced or aggravated by pregnancy. It is better to limit the diagnosis of eclampsia to convulsive cases, regarding fatal nonconvulsive cases of pregnancy-induced or pregnancy-aggravated hypertension as exceedingly severe preeclampsia.

4.1. Clinical course

Depending on whether the convulsion first appears before labor, during labor, or in the puerperium, eclampsia is designated as antepartum, intrapartum, or post partum. Eclampsia occurs most often in the last third of pregnancy and becomes increasingly frequent as term approaches. Nearly all cases of postpartum eclampsia appear within 24 h after delivery. In rare instances, eclampsia is said to have begun as late as one week after delivery, but cases in which the first convulsion is observed more than 48 h post partum should be regarded with skepticism.

Almost without exception, preeclampsia precedes the onset of convulsions. Isolated cases are occasionally cited in which an eclamptic convulsion is said to have occurred without warning in women who were apparently in good health. Usually such a woman had not been examined by her physician for some days or weeks previously, and she had neglected to report symptoms of preeclampsia. Headache, visual disturbance, and epigastric or right upper quadrant pain are symptoms that should incite grave concern. Apprehension, excitability, and hyperreflexia often precede the convulsion, although a convulsion may occur in their absence. An aura usually does not precede the convulsion.

Most often the first convulsion is the forerunner of other convulsions, which may vary in number from one or two in mild cases to 10–20, or even 100 or or more, in untreated severe cases. In rare instances, they follow one another so rapidly that the woman appears to be in a prolonged, almost continuous convulsion.

The duration of coma after a convulsion is variable. When the convulsions are infrequent, the woman usually recovers some degree of consciousness after each attack. As the woman arouses, a semiconscious combative state may ensue. In severe cases, the coma persists from one convulsion to another, and death may result before the patient awakens. In rare instances, a single convulsion may be followed by profound coma from which she never emerges, although, as a rule, death does not occur until after a frequent repetition of the convulsive attacks.

Respiration after an eclamptic convulsion is usually increased in rate and may be stertorous. The rate may reach 50 or more per minute in response presumably to hypercarbia from lactic acidemia, as well as varying intensities of hypoxia. Cyanosis may be observed in severe cases. Temperatures of 39.5°C or more are of very grave prognostic import. The cause of the fever is probably central.

Proteinuria is almost always present and frequently is pronounced. The output of urine is likely to be diminished and occasionally is entirely suppressed. On microscopic examination, various types of casts are found in abundance. Hemoglobinuria and hemoglobinemia may rarely be observed.

Some degree of edema is probably present in all women with eclampsia. Often, the edema is pronounced and, at times, massive, but it may be occult.

After delivery, an increase in urinary output is usually an early sign of improvement. The proteinuria and edema ordinarily disappear within a week. In most cases, but certainly not all, the blood pressure returns to normal within two weeks after delivery. The longer the hypertension persists after delivery, the more likely the hypertension is chronic.

In antepartum eclampsia, labor may begin shortly thereafter and progress rapidly to completion, sometimes before the attendants are aware that the woman is having effective uterine contractions. If the attack occurs during labor, the contractions may increase in frequency and intensity and the duration of labor may be shortened.

Occasionally, labor does not commence, convulsions cease, the coma disappears, and the woman becomes completely oriented. This improved state may continue for several days or longer, a condition known as intercurrent eclampsia. It has been claimed that such pregnancies may often return entirely to normal with complete subsidence of the hypertension and proteinuria, but such an event appears to have been rare. Although convulsions and coma may subside entirely and the blood pressure and proteinuria may decrease somewhat, such women usually continue to show substantial evidence of disease. It is likely that they have merely returned to the preeclamptic state and, after a few days of apparent improvement, are likely to convulse again. This second attack may be much more severe.

In fatal cases, pulmonary edema is common, especially during the terminal hours. Pulmonary edema also may be present in women who survive, but it is always a grave prognostic sign. Other signs of cardiac failure appear in the terminal stage of fatal eclampsia, especially cyanosis, a rising pulse rate, and a falling blood pressure.

In some women with eclampsia, death occurs suddenly, synchronously with or shortly after a convulsion, as the result of massive cerebral hemorrhage. In rare instances, hemiplegia may result from a sublethal cerebral hemorrhage. Eclampsia is followed very infrequently by psychosis in which the mother may become violent. The psychosis ordinarily lasts for 1–2 weeks. Chlorpromazine in carefully titrated doses has proved effective in the few cases of posteclampsic psychosis seen at Parkland Memorial Hospital. The prognosis in general is good, but occasionally there is preexisting mental illness.

Very infrequently, the woman finds herself blind as she begins to arouse from her coma. The disturbed vision, sometimes preceding the attack, is caused mainly by retinal edema, which usually disappears spontaneously. The blindness is sometimes central in origin [39], possibly caused by intense vasospasm of the distal posterior cerebral arteries. Rarely, detachment of the retina is observed. The blindness may persist for a few hours or for several weeks. Usually, however, the vision returns to normal within a week and the prognosis for sight is good.

4.2. Differential diagnosis

Generally, one is much more likely to make a diagnosis of eclampsia too frequently than to overlook the disease, because epilepsy, encephalitis, meningitis, cerebral tumor, acute prophyria, ruptured cerebral aneurysm, and even hysteria may simulate it. Consequently, such conditions should be borne in mind whenever convulsions or coma occur during pregnancy, labor, or the puerperium; and such conditions must be excluded before a positive diagnosis of eclampsia is made. Until eclampsia can be excluded, however, all pregnant women with convulsions should be considered to be eclamptic and kept under close observation on the obstetric service of the hospital.

4.3. Treatment of eclampsia

The basic treatment of eclampsia consists of control of convulsions and steps to effect delivery once the mother is free of convulsions and, hopefully, conscious. It is emphasized that, once delivery is accomplished, the pathologic changes of eclampsia per se ameliorate rapidly and subsequently are usually completely eradicated. This generalization holds true for the dysfunction of the central nervous system, for the liver, for the kidneys, and for any hematologic abnormalities, including thrombocytopenia and intense hemolysis!

4.4. Prognosis

The prognosis is always serious, for eclampsia is one of the most dangerous conditions with which the obstetrician must deal, although the maternal mortality rate in eclampsia has fallen notably in the past three decades. The maternal mortality rate reported since World War II for various methods of treatment has ranged from zero to as much as 17.5%. At the same time the perinatal mortality rate has ranged from 13% to 30% or more. Precise comparisons of perinatal mortality rates are difficult to make because of differences in the definition of stillbirth and neonatal deaths in different countries.

4.5. Eclampsia treatment at Parkland Memorial Hospital

Since 1955, standardized treatment applied uniformly to all cases of eclampsia at Parkland Memorial Hospital has consisted of (a) magnesium sulfate intravenously and intramuscularly to arrest convulsions and prevent their recurrence (b) intravenous hydralazine intermittently as necessary to lower diastolic blood pressure of 110 mm Hg or higher, and (c) steps initiated to effect delivery once the woman has regained consciousness [40]. The dosage schedule for magnesium sulfate is listed in table 7–2. This schedule, while empiric, has been tested extensively for both efficacy and toxicity. Delivery in the majority of cases has been accomplished vaginally; conduction anesthesia has been avoided. Neither diuretic nor osmotic agents in the form of hypertonic glucose, mannitol, or albumin have been used to treat eclampsia. Heparin has never been used! Through August 1983, 245 consecutive cases of eclampsia were so treated with one maternal mortality. Moreover, when congenital anomalies are excluded, all fetuses alive when treatment was initiated and who weighed 1800 g (4 lb) or more, survived.

The plan of management is presented in some detail.

4.5.1. Control of convulsions with magnesium sulfate

As soon as eclampsia has been established as the probable diagnosis, magnesium sulfate ($MgSO_4 \cdot 7H_2O$, USP) is administered as outlined in table 7-2. Magnesium sulfate so administered almost always promptly arrests the convulsions, but, very infrequently, another convulsion may soon appear. If the intravenous magnesium sulfate and intramuscular injections were completed within the 20 min before, however, then the subsequent convulsion usually is brief and does not recur. If the interval is much longer than 20 min, or if the convulsion recurs, 10 ml more of 20% magnesium sulfate solution (2 g) is given if the woman is unusually small; otherwise 20 ml of 20% magnesium sulfate (4 g) is injected intravenously over no less than 3 min. In the rare circumstance in which convulsions persist, sodium amobarbital (Sodium Amytal), up to 0.25 g, is slowly injected intravenously over a period of not less than 3 min.

Subsequent intramuscular injections of 10 ml of 50% solution of magnesium sulfate at 4-h intervals depend upon the patellar reflex being elicited just before each injection. If absent, which is very unlikely, the reflex is rechecked at half-hour intervals and the intramuscular dose of magnesium sulfate injected once the reflex is demonstrated. An active reflex ("hyperreflexia") is not an indication in our experience for increasing either the amount of magnesium sulfate injected or the frequency of the injection. The intramuscular injections are continued for 24 h after delivery. In the conscious patient, to minimize local discomfort, 1 ml of 2% lidocaine is added to the magnesium sulfate solution before injecting intramuscularly.

During the first hour or so of the postictal period, the eclamptic woman before fully regaining consciousness may occasionally demonstrate physical agitation that cannot be controlled by simple restraint. If this develops, to protect the mother from harming herself and her fetus, sodium amobarbital for sedation is injected intravenously in increments up to 0.25 g over not less than 3 min. Most often, however, the woman's confusion and agitation, as she regains consciousness, can be minimized by having an immediate member of the family at the bedside and by avoiding bright lights, loud noises, and numerous people in the room.

If respiratory depression were to develop, 10 ml of a 10% solution of calcium gluconate is given intravenously over 3 min. This has proved effective in two cases of eclampsia in which it was used at Parkland Memorial Hospital. The pharmacology and toxicology of magnesium sulfate are considered in more detail below.

4.5.2. Antihypertensive therapy

The intravenous injection of 4 g of magnesium sulfate produces a moderate lowering of blood pressure that most often is transient. Therefore, hydralazine is used to treat severe hypertension. Whenever the diastolic blood pressure reaches 110 mm Hg, hydralazine is administered as follows: A test dose of 5 mg is injected as a bolus intravenously and the blood pressure monitored every 5 min. If the diastolic pressure is not lowered to 90–100 mm Hg in 20 min, a 10-mg dose is similarly administered, and its effects monitored as described. This dose of hydralazine is repeated until the diastolic blood pressure is lowered to 90–100 mm Hg. The desired effect is most always achieved with 5–20 mg of hydralazine. Hydralazine is next given whenever the diastolic blood pressure again reaches 110 mm Hg.

Diazoxide has not been used at Parkland Memorial Hospital, nor is it recommended. The hypotensive response may be so great as to impair dangerously perfusion of vital organs, including the placenta. Unfortunately, if diazoxide is used in close proximity to other antihypertensive agents that act by direct peripheral vasodilation, profound and even fatal hypotension may ensue.

Metabolic derangements are commonly induced in the mother and the fetus by diazoxide, including edema from sodium and water retention, hyperglycemia, and hyperuricemia. Moreover, labor may be impaired by diazoxide, if not arrested.

4.5.3. Diuretics, hyperosmotic agents

Urinary output is monitored hourly. Mannitol, hypertonic dextrose, and albumin are not used at Parkland Memorial Hospital to try to mobilize edema fluid, to try to increase urinary output, or to expand the blood volume. Unless there is pulmonary congestion, diuretics are avoided, since oliguria reflects the intensity of the vasospastic disease, an intensification of the hypovolemia by blood loss at delivery, or both. If pulmonary edema were to develop, furosemide would be indicated and likely would be lifesaving.

In the absence of hemorrhage or hyponatremia, 5% glucose in lactated Ringer solution is administered intravenously at a rate of 60–120 ml/h.

4.5.4. Laboratory studies

Laboratory studies need not be extensive. Measurements of hemoglobin or hematocrit, leukocyte count, and platelet count, examination of a blood smear stained with Wright stain, and careful visual inspection of plasma for abnormal amounts of bilirubin, hemoglobin, or other heme pigments are performed. Plasma electrolytes are measured, although they are unlikely to be abnormal unless the woman previously has been treated vigorously with diuretics or has received oxytocin and appreciable volumes of aqueous glucose solution simultaneously. Hypocalcemia or hypercalcemia is rarely found. After a convulsion, the plasma bicarbonate concentration is variably reduced as the consequence of lactic acidemia and hyperventilation. The plasma creatinine concentration should be measured, but is not likely to be elevated markedly unless vigorous diuretic therapy has been administered elsewhere, or the disease has been unusually severe, or there is underlying renal disease.

4.5.5. Delivery

Steps are taken to initiate labor and effect delivery once the woman regains consciousness to the extent that she can be oriented as to time and place. Immediately after a convulsion, fetal bradycardia is common, most likely as the consequence of acidosis and hypoxia induced by the intense muscular activity, maternal apnea, and the already reduced uteroplacental perfusion. The generally favorable fetal outcomes at Parkland Memorial Hospital justify the policy of controlling the convulsions and providing oxygen, thereby allowing the mother and, in turn, the fetus to repair the metabolic derangement, rather than quickly performing a cesarean section. Once convulsions have been controlled and no other obstetric complications coexist or develop, there is no urgency for immediately effecting delivery, but neither is there reason for undue procrastination. Without obstetric contraindication to vaginal delivery, labor is induced with carefully administered intravenous oxytocin. Even when remote from term, the uterus often is responsive to oxytocin. Although very high plasma magnesium levels may impair myometrial contractility, the levels achieved with the dosage schedule described above do not. Labor has been induced successfully with oxytocin in 59 (83%) of 71 cases in which it was attempted at Parkland Memorial Hospital, including seven of ten cases in which fetal weight was less than 1000 g and all 20 in which the fetus weighed between 1000 and 2500 g [41]. The frequency, duration, and apparent intensity of uterine contractions and the fetal heart rate are monitored closely. Hyperstimulation is a constant danger and must be avoided.

Analgesia during labor is limited to 50–75 mg of meperidine and 25 mg of promethazine given intravenously or intramuscularly, with the meperidine repeated at intervals of 2 h or longer, and withholding administration during the 2 h before delivery. If the fetus is premature, meperidine and similar agents are to be avoided.

If oxytocin induction fails, or if there are obstetric contraindications to the use of oxytocin, cesarean section is performed.

Blood loss at and after delivery is less well tolerated by women with eclampsia. The maternal blood volume typically is appreciably less than with normal pregnancy, thereby increasing the dangers from blood loss. An abrupt fall in blood pressure at the completion of delivery or soon after most often indicates serious hypovolemia rather than immediate relief of the vasospastic disease! The oliguria from severe hypovolemia following hemorrhage is treated with blood and lactated Ringer solution and not with diuretics or hyperosmotic agents.

4.5.6. Anesthesia

Spinal, caudal, or lumbar epidural anesthesia is not used at Parkland Memorial Hospital for labor or delivery of the woman with eclampsia or preeclampsia because of the likelihood of hypotension from both regional sympathetic blockage and significant blood loss in the presence of an already shrunken blood volume. For most forceps deliveries, and for cesarean sections, general endotracheal anesthesia consists of the administration of a small dose of sodium thiopental, followed by nitrous oxide plus oxygen, and succinylcholine. Anesthesia is begun only after the woman has received 30 ml of milk of magnesia orally and the obstetric team is fully prepared to deliver the fetus vaginally or to incise the abdominal wall. While the amount of succinylcholine necessary for appropriate muscle relaxation usually is less for the woman who has received magnesium sulfate, this does not contraindicate the simultaneous use of these two agents. Pudendal block of local perineal and vaginal infiltration, supplemented with nitrous oxide, often provides satisfactory pain relief for episiotomy and spontaneous vaginal delivery.

4.5.7. Perinatal mortality

With this treatment regimen, the absolute perinatal mortality rate for 216 fetuses and newborns, including five sets of twins, of the 211 mothers with eclampsia before delivery was 15.7%, irrespective of fetal weight or duration of gestation, and including fetuses that were dead when the mother was brought to Parkland Memorial Hospital. Of the fetuses, 21 weighed less than 1000 g and six weighed less than 500 g. Every one of the fetuses survived of the 187 who were alive when the diagnosis of eclampsia was made, who were without congenital abnormalities incompatible with life, and who weighed 1800 g (4 pounds) or more at birth [40].

4.5.8. Pharmacology and toxicology of magnesium sulfate

Magnesium sulfate administered as described will practically always arrest eclamptic convulsions and prevent their recurrence. The initial intravenous injection of 4 g is used to establish promptly a therapeutic level that is then maintained by the nearly simultaneous intramuscular administration of 10 g of the compound, followed by 5 g intramuscularly every 4 h, as long as there is no evidence of potentially dangerous hypermagnesemia. With this dosage schedule, the plasma levels for magnesium that are achieved are therapeutically effective and range from 2 to 3 mmol/liter, compared with pretreatment plasma levels usually of less than 1 mmol/liter [42, 43]. Magnesium sulfate injected deeply into the upper outer quadrant of the buttocks, as described above, has not resulted in erratic absorption and, in turn, erratic plasma levels; indeed, the reverse has been true.

Recently, Graham and co-workers [44] reported on a prospective study in which a comparison between continuous intravenous magnesium sulfate and intramuscular magnesium sulfate was made. A total of 18 preeclamptic women received intramuscular magnesium sulfate as recommended by Pritchard [45]; 14 patients then received a 4-g intravenous loading dose of magnesium sulfate over 15 min. Following the intravenous loading dose, seven patients received a continuous intravenous maintenance dose of 1 g/h while the other seven patients received 2 g/h. All patients were of similar age, height, weight, and gestational state of pregnancy. There was no significant difference after 3 h of therapy between the mean magnesium levels observed after intramuscular magnesium sulfate and those observed following the intravenous regimen using a maintenance dose of 2 g/h. However, the intramuscular regimen resulted in serum magnesium levels that were significantly higher than those obtained with a continuous intravenous maintenance dose of 1 g/h. A similar result was reported by Sanders and Hayashi [46]. Both groups concluded that there appeared to be no therapeutic advantage to the intravenous route of administration except for the avoidance of pain at the intramuscular site of injection.

The patellar reflex disappears by the time the plasma magnesium level reaches 10 mq/liter, presumably as the consequence of a curariform action. This sign serves to warn of impending magnesium toxicity, since a further increase will lead to respiratory depression.

Parenterally injected magnesium is excreted rapidly through the maternal kidney; as the magnesium concentration in plasma increases, so does renal clearance. A fraction of the injected magnesium is deposited in bone.

In monkeys with angiotensin-induced hypertension late in pregnancy, Harbert and co-workers [47] demonstrated slightly increased uterine blood flow in response to the infusion of magnesium sulfate. At the same time, arterial blood pressure decreased minimally. More recently, Altura et al. [48] reported that, when isolated umbilical arteries and veins, obtained from normal infants at term, were incubated with 0–9.6 mmol of magnesium per liter, basal tension of the vessels increased in the absence of magnesium and decreased when the concentration of magnesium was increased. They also observed that the absence of magnesium significantly potentiated the contractile response of the vessels to bradykinin, angiotensin II, serotonin, and prostaglandin $F_{2\alpha}$. They concluded that their observation might help explain the favorable outcome observed in infants of preeclamptic women who receive magnesium sulfate therapy.

Somjen and co-workers [49] induced in themselves, by intravenous infusion, marked hypermagnesemia, achieving plasma levels to 15 meq/liter. Predictably, at such high plasma levels, respiratory depression developed that necessitated mechanical ventilation, yet there was little in the way of depression of the sensorium as long as hypoxia was prevented.

Borges and Gücer [50] provided convincing evidence that the magnesium ion has an effect on the central nervous system that is much more specific than generalized depression. They measured the effects of parenterally administered magnesium sulfate on epileptic neural activity induced in awake, undrugged subhuman primates. The infused magnesium sulfate suppressed neuronal burst firing and interictal electroencephalographic spike generation in neuronal populations rendered epileptic by topically applied pencillin G. The degree of cortical suppression increased as the plasma magnesium concentration increased and decreased as the magnesium level fell. Therefore, even though elevated concentrations of magnesium in plasma decrease acetylcholine release in response to motor nerve impulses, reduce motor end-plate sensitivity to acetylcholine, and decrease the motor end-plate potential, these actions do not account for, nor should they be implicated in, an explanation of the beneficial effects of magnesium sulfate in controlling the convulsions of eclampsia.

Magnesium ions in relatively high concentration will depress myometrial contractility in vivo and in vitro. With the regime described above and the plasma levels that have resulted, no evidence of depression of myometrial function has been observed beyond a transient decrease in activity during and immediately after the initial intravenous loading dose. Typically, as the cutaneous flushing from the intravenous dose disappeared, uterine activity returned to preinjection intensity. Magnesium ions administered parenterally to the mother cross the placenta promptly to achieve equilibrium between mother and fetus. Magnesium sulfate, given as a large single dose intravenously, but not with smaller doses, may transiently cause a loss of beat-to-beat variability in the fetal heart rate. [45].

The newborn infant may be depressed if severe hypermagnesemia exists at delivery. The kind of compromises that have been described by Lipsitz and English [51] to develop at times in the newborn after maternal continuous intravenous therapy with magnesium sulfate have not been observed by us [43] or by Green and associates [52]. The dosage schedule and route of administration described above, coupled with the safeguards observed before each injection, have effectively prevented worrisome adverse effects from hypermagnesemia in newborns at Parkland Memorial Hospital.

Indeed, Lipsitz [53] agreed with our observations after further study in which he found that infants were unlikely to be compromised when the mother had received magnesium sulfate according to the protocol for the treatment of eclampsia described above. The use of magnesium sulfate in PIH, its mechanisms of action, and its possible toxicity in mother and fetus-infant have been described in more detail elsewhere [45, 54].

4.5.9. Other treatment agents

A great variety of drugs have been used in the treatment of eclampsia and severe preeclampsia. We have had little personal experience with most of these drugs and/or other treatment regimen.

It should be pointed out that a tendency persists among some medical experts to group together for the purpose of treatment a variety of disease states that appear to have a common functional disturbance. So-called hypertensive encephalopathy is one that from time to time attracts interest and, in turn, incites recommendations for treatment broad in scope, without full appreciation of all the problems created by the disease or evoked by the proposed treatment. Too often, when eclampsia is included under the category of hypertensive encephalopathy, lack of concern for the impact of the recommended therapy on the fetus is apparent. Moreover, it is not unusual for the recommendations to have been based on little or no data.

The recurrent recognition of thrombocytopenia occasionally and, less often, of other changes in the coagulation mechanism, with or without evidence of abnormal erythrocyte destruction (microangiopathic hemolysis) has led to the recommendation of treatment with heparin, fresh whole blood, fresh frozen plasma, platelets, fibrinogen, and other specific clotting factors as necessary [55]. To date, insufficient numbers of cases have been reported to evaluate the merits, if any, of such therapy. In two reports, it was concluded that heparin did not prove effective in ameliorating the clinical course of established preeclampsia [56, 57].

We continue to look for such hematologic changes in the relatively large numbers of women with eclampsia and preeclampsia cared for at Parkland Memorial Hospital, but do not attempt treatment with heparin or with clotting factors other than those in blood-bank blood used at times to treat blood loss from hemorrhage at delivery. We have never used heparin in these circumstances because of fear of enhancing intracranial hemorrhage, on the one hand, and an appreciation that correction of the defects occurs promptly after delivery, on the other. The outcomes have been satisfactory, as already described. The safety of deliberate anticoagulation with heparin in the presence of severe hypertension is questionable and certainly cannot be recommended until much greater experience attesting to any benefits has been recorded.

4.5.10. Subsequent reproductive outcomes

Because of the catastrophic implications of eclampsia, women so affected and their families often are quite concerned over the prognosis for future pregnancies. Moreover, gloomy accounts have appeared repeatedly in the obstetric literature; hypertension, for example, has been reported to occur in as high as 78% of women who previously had eclampsia.

Chesley and co-workers [58], through meticulous, long-term follow-up studies of women with eclampsia at Margaret Hague Maternity Hospital between 1931 and 1952, have provided us with most useful information. For example, of 466 subsequent pregnancies in 189 of the eclamptic women, the fetal salvage was 76%, but much of the loss was early abortion. Of the pregnancies that continued to week 28 or longer, 93% resulted in infants that survived.

At Parkland Memorial Hospital, the subsequent reproductive performance of black women with eclampsia during their first pregnancy has been ascertained. Of 101 pregnancies, 11 aborted and 91 infants weighing 500 g or more were delivered. Four of the 91 succumbed, three of whom weighed less than 1000 g.

Of the subsequent pregnancies, 25% were complicated by hypertension in the 189 previously eclamptic women observed by Chesley et al. [59]. The hypertension, however, was severe in only 5%, while 2% were again eclamptic. Our experiences with previously eclamptic women are very similar.

Chesley and associates emphasized that many of the recurrences of elevated blood pressure represent nothing more than chronic hypertension. Some women do have normal blood pressures between pregnancies and at follow-up, but, in general, pregnancies after eclampsia are an excellent screening test for latent hypertensive disease. A large percentage of women who develop recurrences of hypertension during subsequent pregnancies ultimately become hypertensive, whereas the prevalence of ultimate hypertension is extremely low in those who are normotensive in later pregnancies.

Chesley and co-workers [60] traced to 1974 all but three of the 270 women surviving eclampsia at the Margaret Hague Maternity Hospital in 1931–1951. Women who had eclampsia in their first pregnancy carried 28 weeks or more have shown no increase over the expected number of remote deaths. In sharp contrast, women who had eclampsia as multiparas, the majority of whom undoubtedly had underlying chronic vascular disease, have shown three times the expected number of deaths.

4.5.11. Relation of preeclampsia–eclampsia to subsequent hypertension

Whether preeclampsia actually causes ensuing chronic hypertension has been a subject of debate. One point of view has been that preeclampsia and eclampsia represent an acute vascular disorder in the form of muscle spasm, which, if allowed to continue for several weeks, results in a permanent structural injury to the vascular wall through hypoxia. This injury becomes manifest by arteriolar fibrosis, consequent hypertension, and possible renal vascular damage. These findings led to the suggestion that permanent hypertension might be prevented by delivery of patients within two or three weeks after onset of preeclampsia. For some time, Chesley [12] was of this school, but reappraisal of his data led him to reverse his conclusions. The problem has been confused by the mistaken diagnosis of preeclampsia even in primigravid women who really had renal disease or essential hypertension. Many studies have included a substantial proportion of multiparas, few of whom actually had preeclampsia. Furthermore, nearly 40% of women with essential hypertension have significant drops in blood pressure during much of pregnancy. In many of them, normal pressures may be observed from early in gestation. Typically, the blood pressure rises again early in the third trimester, and some edema, with perhaps minimal proteinuria, may occur. Inasmuch as blood pressures before pregnancy are seldom known, the erroneous diagnosis of preeclampsia is likely to be made.

Many follow-up studies have been made of women thought to have had preeclampsia, and the frequency of chronic hypertension had ranged from 2% to more than 60%.

The results of the long-term follow-up studies reported by Chesley and associates [60], who have reexamined women repeatedly for up to 44 years after eclampsia in the first pregnancy, are indicative that the prevalence of hypertension is not increased over that in unselected women matched for age and race. Tillman [61] accumulated a series of 377 women whose blood pressures were recorded before, during, and at intervals after pregnancy. He could find no indication that normal, preeclamptic, or hypertensive pregnancies had any effect on the blood pressure at follow-up examination and concluded that preeclampsia neither causes residual hypertension nor aggravates preexisting hypertension. Interestingly, Chesley and co-workers [60] have identified diabetes to be 2.5–4.0 times the expected rate among women who previously had eclampsia.

ACKNOWLEDGMENT

This work was supported, in part, by US Public Health Service grant HD 08360.

REFERENCES

1. Robertson EG: The natural history of oedema during pregnancy. J Obstet Gynaecol Br Commonw 78:520–529, 1971.
2. Friedman EA, Neff RK: Pregnancy outcome as related to hypertension, edema, and proteinuria. In: Lindheimer MD, Katz AI, Zuspan FP (eds) Hypertension in pregnancy. New York: John Wiley, 1976, pp 13–22.
3. McCartney CP, Schumacher GFB, Spargo BH: Serum proteins in patients with toxemic glomerular lesion. Am J Obstet Gynecol 111:580–590, 1971.
4. Pritchard JA, Cunningham FG, Mason RA: Coagulation changes in eclampsia: their frequency and pathogenesis. Am J Obstet Gynecol 124:855–864, 1976.
5. Brunner HR, Gavras H: Vascular damage in hypertension. Hosp Pract 10:97–108, 1975.

6. Robertson AL, Khairallah PA: Effects of angiotensin II and some analogues on vascular permeability in the rabbit. Circ Res 31: 923–931, 1972.
7. Sims EAH: Pre-eclampsia and related complications of pregnancy. Am J Obstet Gynecol 107:-154–181, 1970.
8. McCartney CP: Pathological anatomy of acute hypertension of pregnancy. Circulation [Supply 2] 30: 37–42, 1964.
9. Fisher ER, Pardo V, Paul R, Hayashi TT: Ultrastructural studies in hypertension. IV. Toxemia of pregnancy. Am J Pathol 55:109–131, 1969.
10. Wellen I: Specific "toxemia," essential hypertension, and glomerulonephritis associated with pregnancy. Am J Obstet Gynecol 39:16–24, 1940.
11. Browne FJ, Dodds GH: Pregnancy in the patient with chronic hypertension. J Obstet Gynaecol Br Emp 49:1–17, 1942.
12. Chesley LC: Superimposed preeclampsia or eclampsia. In: Chesley LC (ed) Hypertensive disorders in pregnancy. New York: Appleton, 1978, pp 14, 302, and 482.
13. Volhard F: Die Doppelseitigen Haematogenen Nierenerkrankungen. Berlin: Springer, 1918.
14. Hinselmann H: Die Eklampsie. Boon: F Cohen, 1924.
15. Landesman R, Douglas RG, Holze E: The bulbar conjunctival vascular bed in the toxemias of pregnancy. Am J Obstet Gynecol 68:170–183, 1954.
16. McKay DG: Disseminated intravascular coagulation. New York: Harper and Rowe, 1965.
17. Abdul-Karim R, Assali NS: Pressor response to angiotonin in pregnant and nonpregnant women. Am J Obstet Gynecol 82:246–251, 1961.
18. Raab W, Schroeder G, Wagner R, Gigee W: Vascular reactivity and electrolytes in normal and toxemic pregnancy. J Clin Endocrinol 16:1196–1216, 1956.
19. Talledo OE, Chesley LC, Zuspan FP: Renin–angiotensin system in normal and toxemic pregnancies. III. Differential sensitivity to angiotensin II and norepinephrine in toxemia of pregnancy. Am J Obstet Gynecol 100: 218–221, 1968.
20. Dieckman WJ, Michel HL: Vascular–renal effects of posterior pituitary extracts in pregnant women. Am J Obstet Gynecol 33:131–137, 1937.
21. Browne FJ: Sensitization of the vascular system in pre-eclamptic toxemia and eclampsia. Br J Obstet Gynaecol 53:510, 1946.
22. Gant NF, Daley GL, Chand S, Whalley PJ, MacDonald PC: A study of angiotensin II pressor response throughout primigravid pregnancy. J Clin Invest 52:2682–2689, 1973.
23. Öney T, Kaulhausen H: The value of the angiotensin sensitivity test in the early diagnosis of hypertensive disorders of pregnancy. Am J Obstet Gynecol 142:17–20, 1982.
24. Gant NF, Chand S, Whalley PJ, MacDonald PC: The nature of pressor responsiveness to angiotensin II in human pregnancy. Obstet Gynecol 43:854–860, 1974.
25. Cunningham GC, Cox K, Gant NF: Further observations on the nature of pressor responsivity to angiotensin II in human pregnancy. Obstet Gynecol 146:581–583, 1975.
26. Everett RB, Worley RJ, MacDonald PC, Gant NF: Effect of prostaglandin synthetase inhibitors on pressor response to angiotensin II in human pregnancy. J Clin Endocrinol Metab 46:-1007–1010, 1978.
27. Everett RB, Worley RJ, MacDonald PC, Gant NF: Modification of vascular responsiveness to angiotensin II in pregnant women by intravenously infused 5α-dihydroprogesterone. Am J Obstet Gynecol 131:352–357, 1978.
28. Pritchard JA, MacDonald PC, Gant NF: Williams Textbook of obstetrics, 17th edn. New York: Appleton-Century-Crofts, 1984.
29. Kraus GW, Marchese JR, Yen SSC: Prophylactic use of hydrochlorothiazide in pregnancy. JAMA 198:1150–1154, 1966.
30. Gant NF, Madden JD, Siiteri PK, MacDonald PC: The metabolic clearance rate of dehydroisoandrosterone sulfate. III. The effect of thiazide diuretics in normal and future preeclamptic pregnancies. Am J Obstet Gynecol 123:159–163, 1975.
31. Minkowitz S, Soloway HB, Hall JE, Yermakov V: Fatal hemorrhagic pancreatitis following chlorothiazide administration in pregnancy. Obstet Gynecol 24:337–342, 1964.
32. Menzies D, Prystowsky H: Acute hemorrhagic pancreatitis following chlorothiazide administration in pregnancy. J Fla Med Assoc 54:564–565, 1967.
33. Rodriguez SU, Leikin SL, Hiller MC: Neonatal thrombocytopenia associated with antepartum administration of thiazide drugs. N Engl J Med 270:881–884, 1964.
34. Karotkin EH, Cashore WJ, Kido M, Redding RA, Douglas W, Stern L, Oh W: The inhibition

of pulmonary maturation in the fetal rabbit by maternal treatment with phenobarbital. Am J Obstet Gynecol 124:529–531, 1976.
35. Nochimson DJ, Petrie RH: Glucocorticoid therapy for the induction of pulmonary maturity in severely hypertensive gravid women. Am J Obstet Gynecol 133:449–451, 1979.
36. Semchyshyn S, Zuspan F, Cordero L: Cardiovascular response and complications of glucocorticoid therapy in hypertensive pregnancies. Am J Obstet Gynecol 145:530–533, 1983.
37. Ruvinsky ED, Douvas SG, Roberts WE, Martin JN, Rhodes PG, Harris JB, Morrison JC: Maternal administration of dexamethasone in severe pregnancy-induced hypertension. Am J Obstet Gynecol, 1984 (submitted for publication).
38. Gilstrap LC, Cunningham FG, Whalley PJ: Management of pregnancy-induced hypertension in the nulliparous patient remote from term. Semin Perinatol 2:73, 1978.
39. Nishimura RN, Koller R: Isolated cortical blindness in pregnancy. West J Med 137:335–337, 1982.
40. Pritchard JA, Cunningham FG, Pritchard SA: The Parkland Memorial Hospital protocol for treatment of eclampsia: evaluation of 245 cases. Am J Obstet Gynecol, 148:951, 1984.
41. Pritchard JA, Pritchard SA: Standardized treatment of 154 cases of eclampsia. Am J Obstet Gynecol 123:543–552, 1975.
42. Chesley LC, Tepper I: Plasma levels of magnesium attained in magnesium sulfate therapy for preeclampsia and eclampsia. Surg Clin North Am 353–367, 1957.
43. Stone SR, Pritchard JA: Effect of maternally administered magnesium sulfate on the neonate. Obstet Gynecol 35:574–577, 1970.
44. Graham JM, Sibai BM, McCubbin JH: A comparison of intravenous versus intramuscular $MgSO_4$ in preeclampsia. Am J Obstet Gynecol, 1984 (in press).
45. Pritchard JA: The use of magnesium sulfate in preeclampsia–eclampsia. J Reprod Med 23:-107–114, 1979.
46. Sanders R, Hayashi R: Intravenous versus intramuscular magnesium sulfate for preeclampsia [abstr 25]. Society for Gynecologic Investigation, 30th annual meeting, Washington DC, 17–20 March 1983.
47. Harbert GM Jr, Cornell GW, Thornton WN JR: Effect of toxemia therapy on uterine dynamics. Am J Obstet Gynecol 105:94–104, 1969.
48. Altura BM, Altura BT, Carella A: Magnesium deficiency-induced spasms of umbilical vessels: relation to preeclampsia, hypertension, growth retardation. Science 221:376–378, 1983.
49. Somjen G, Hilmy M, Stephen CR: Failure to anesthetize human subjects by intravenous administration of magnesium sulfate. J Pharmacol Exp Ther 154:652–659, 1966.
50. Borges LF, Gucer G: Effect of magnesium on epileptic foci. Epilepsia 19:81–91, 1978.
51. Lipsitz PJ, English IC: Hypermagnesemia in the newborn infant. Pediatrics 40:856–862, 1967.
52. Green KW, Key TC, Coen R, Resnik R: The effects of maternally administered magnesium sulfate on the neonate. Am J Obstet Gynecol 146:29–33, 1983.
53. Lipsitz PJ: The clinical and biochemical effects of excess magnesium in the newborn. Pediatrics 47:501–509, 1971.
54. Cruikshank DP, Pitkin RM, Reynolds WA, Williams GA, Hargis GK: Effects of magnesium sulfate treatment on perinatal calcium metabolism. I. Maternal and fetal responses. Am J Obstet Gynecol 134:243–249, 1979.
55. Beecham JB, Watson WJ, Clapp JF: Eclampsia, preeclampsia, and disseminated intravascular coagulation. Obstet Gynecol 43:576–585, 1974.
56. Bonnar J, Redman CWG, Denson KW: The role of coagulation and fibrinolysis in pre-eclampsia. In: Lindheimer MD, Katz AL, Zuspan FP (eds) Hypertension in pregnancy. New York: John Wiley, 1976, pp 85–93.
57. Howie PW, Prentice CRM, Forbes CD: Failure of heparin therapy to affect the clinical course of severe preeclampsia. Br J Obstet Gynaecol 82:711–717, 1975.
58. Chesley LC, Cosgrave RA, Annitto JE: A follow-up study of eclamptic women: fourth periodic report. Am J Obstet Gynecol 83:1360–1372, 1962.
59. Chesley LC, Annitto JE, Cosgrove RA: Prognostic significance of recurrent toxemia of pregnancy. Obstet Gynecol 23:874–881, 1964.
60. Chesley LC, Annitto JE, Cosgrove RA: Long-term follow-up study of eclamptic women: sixth periodic report. Am J Obstet Gynecol 124:446–459, 1976.
61. Tillman AJB: The effect of normal and toxemic pregnancy on blood pressure. Am J Obstet Gynecol 70:589–603, 1955.

8. TREATMENT OF CHRONIC HYPERTENSION IN PREGNANCY

VITTORIO E. ANDREUCCI, ANTONIO DAL CANTON, and DOMENICO RUSSO

1. INTRODUCTION

There is still controversy as to whether mild hypertension antedating pregnancy has to be treated in pregnant women. Some authors are against treatment since the possible benefit of normalizing blood pressure is not relevant to the brief span of gestation [1]. Others emphasize that treatment of chronic hypertension in pregnancy (CHP) reduces the occurrence of midtrimester abortions [2].

As mentioned in chapter 7, however, CHP, regardless of its cause, is a predisposing factor to the development of superimposed preeclampsia. Furthermore it may cause cardiac decompensation. Placental abruption, finally, is also more frequent in hypertensive pregnant women. We have therefore important indications for continuous treatment of essential hypertension during pregnancy. In principle, blood pressure equal to or greater than 140/90 must be treated.

2. EFFECTS OF ANTIHYPERTENSIVE THERAPY ON CEREBRAL BLOOD FLOW AND PLACENTAL BLOOD FLOW

Treatment of hypertension may affect both cerebral blood flow and placental blood flow. We know that cerebral blood flow is autoregulated, i.e., it remains constant for variation in mean arterial pressure (diastolic blood pressure plus one-third of differential blood pressure) between 70 and 150 mm Hg [3]. Above the upper limit and below the lower limit of this autoregulatory range, hypertensive encephalopathy and cerebral ischemia, respectively, may occur [1]. Patients with chronic hypertension have lower and upper limits of the autoregulatory range that are higher than normal [4]. Thus, chronic hypertensive patients are more tolerant of higher pressures but less tolerant of lower pressures than are normotensive subjects [1]. While treating hypertensive pregnant women, therefore, we should bear in mind that our aim is to reduce blood pressure to values at which cerebral blood flow is autoregulated.

The placental blood flow is not autoregulated; spiral arteries, in fact, cannot constrict or dilate actively. Studies in experimental animals suggest that placental blood flow depends only on arterial blood pressure [1]. Human placenta in healthy women functions normally over the range of variation of systemic blood pressure [1]. The occurrence of maternal hypotension may cause fetal bradycardia because of hypoxemia. Since placental blood flow is reduced in preeclampsia and a maternal syndrome similar to preeclampsia may be induced in experimental animals by reducing placental blood flow, excessive lowering of systemic blood pressure by antihypertensive drugs may theoretically induce preeclampsia.

3. CHOICE OF ANTIHYPERTENSIVE DRUGS

In 1978, a questionnaire survey was carried out in the United Kingdom and Ireland to determine how obstetricians were treating pregnant women with preexisting essential hypertension or preeclampsia [5]. As many as 1093 obstetricians answered the questionnaire. It was concluded that most obstetricians were administering sedatives in mild hypertension and were using antihypertensive drugs in severe hypertension; methyldopa and diuretics were the most widely used antihypertensive drugs [5].

In reviewing the worldwide literature we conclude that there is not yet adequate experience with the use of all medications available today for treating hypertension in pregnant hypertensive women.

Hereafter we will consider only those drugs that have been studied in hypertensive pregnant women. Unfortunately in most studies no distinction is made in testing the drugs between pregnancy-induced hypertension (PIH) and chronic hypertension in pregnancy (CHP).

3.1. Diuretics

Thiazides have been used in the past to prevent the development of preeclampsia. This prophylactic efficacy, however, has not been demonstrated [6]. Thus, when pregnant women were treated either with hydrochlorothiazide (50 mg daily) or with placebo during the last 16 weeks of gestation, there was no difference in the incidence of preeclampsia [7]. There is today a general agreement, therefore, that diuretics do not protect against preeclampsia [1].

It is still controversial, on the other hand, whether or not diuretics may cause damage to the mother or to the fetus or both. Thus, while some experts believe, as adequately proved by controlled trials, that the prophylactic use of diuretics does not modify perinatal mortality and that there is not an absolute contraindication of diuretics in pregnancy [1], others [8, 9] warn about the use of diuretics because of a reported increase both in complications during labor and in perinatal mortality [10].

Bearing in mind that (a) blood volume is commonly reduced not only in PIH but also in CHP, (b) hypovolemia seems to precede and probably cause preeclampsia, (c) diuretic therapy itself causes a reduction in blood volume, and (d) a decrease both in creatinine clearance and probably in uteroplacental perfusion has been demonstrated following diuretic treatment [11], in our opinion the use of diuretics in CHP may theoretically precipitate preeclampsia. Although not clearly stated, there seems to be a consensus in recent, specialized literature, because of this potentially dangerous effect, that the use of diuretics in pregnancy should be limited to emergencies, e.g., for treating left ventricular failure [1, 2, 8, 9, 12]. We agree with this advice completely.

In our opinion, even restriction of dietary sodium in women with CHP should be avoided for the same reasons. More than 25 years ago it was observed, in a large prospective study (including 2077 normal pregnant women), that the incidence of preeclampsia was reduced when pregnant women were placed on a high-salt diet in comparison with those on a low-salt diet [13].

3.2. Beta-adrenoreceptor blocking agents (beta-blockers)

These drugs have been widely used in pregnancy for treating idiopathic hypertrophic subaortic stenosis, hyperthyroidism, tachydysrhythmias, and hypertension [14].

3.2.1. Propranolol

There are, up to now, only a few prospective studies on the use of propranolol in the treatment of essential hypertension in pregnancy. When nine pregnant, severely hypertensive women were treated with propranolol (up to 240 mg daily) in combination with hydralazine and a diuretic, eight out of nine pregnancies ended without problems for the mothers and for their newborns [15].

Very interesting results have been obtained in women in whom previous pregnancies have been unsuccessful (abortions or stillbirths). One study involved 25 hypertensive women who had had 67 pregnancies, 32 (47.8%) of which had been unsuccessful; treatment of hypertension with propranolol (40–160 mg daily) throughout the subsequent pregnancies reduced the incidence of unsuccessful pregnancies to four out of 26 (15.4%)[16].

In another study, 13 hypertensive women, who had previously experienced 17 (44.8%) out of 38 unsuccessful pregnancies, were treated with propranolol (30–240 mg daily) and hydralazine throughout the subsequent 15 pregnancies; only one pregnancy was unsuccessful (6.7%), ending in a stillbirth [17].

It has been stated that treatment of pregnant women with propranolol is followed by respiratory distress in the neonate, increased perinatal mortality, and neonatal bradycardia or hypoglycemia. This statement, however, is based on anecdotal reports and on a retrospective study by chart review in which no information is given concerning other risk factors [18].

Actually, propranolol seems to be safe. No fetal malformations have been reported after maternal treatment with the drug, even when therapy was started before conception [15, 17]. No intrauterine fetal growth retardation and, only in single cases, transient neonatal bradycardia or hypoglycemia have been observed in the few prospective studies with propranolol in which neonatal data are available [14, 15, 17, 19].

3.2.2. Oxprenolol

Two major randomized controlled trials have been reported on the use of oxprenolol in treating hypertension (diastolic blood pressure equal to or greater than 95 mm Hg) in pregnant women. In both studies, oxprenolol was compared with methyldopa. In the first study [20], 26 patients were treated with oxprenolol (maximum daily dose, 200 mg) and 27 with methyldopa (maximum daily dose, 1 g); in 11 patients of the oxprenolol group and in seven patients of the methyldopa group, the addition of hydralazine was necessary to reduce blood pressure to less than 80 mm Hg. The results suggested a better outcome of pregnancy in the group treated with oxprenolol: better fetal growth, greater placental weight, and no neonatal death (two neonatal deaths in the methyldopa group). [20].

In the second study [21], 50 patients were treated with oxprenolol (maximum daily dose, 640 mg) and 50 with methyldopa (maximum daily dose, 3 g); in six patients of the oxprenolol group and in two patients of the methyldopa group, hydralazine had to be added to reduce blood pressure to less than 95 mm Hg. The results did not show any significant difference in the outcome of pregnancy between the two groups. In particular, birth weight, placental weight, and head circumference were not significantly different; there were no stillbirths in either group [21]. Unfortunately in both trials there was no indication of the number of patients with essential hypertension.

3.2.3. Metoprolol

A prospective study on the effect of metoprolol in hypertensive pregnant women has been performed with 198 patients (about one-third had preeclampsia) who had been unresponsive to thiazides [22]. The patients were divided in two groups: the 101 patients of one group received metoprolol (50–200 mg twice daily) either alone or (in 44 patients) associated with hydralazine; the 97 of the other group received hydralazine (up to 200 mg daily); the patients of both groups continued the thiazide throughout the study. There were 13 fetal or perinatal deaths in the hydralazine group and only three in the metoprolol group; no neonatal bradycardia or hypoglycemia was observed. Unfortunately there was no distinction in the study between PIH and CHP [22].

3.2.4. Atenolol

In a randomized, double-blind prospective study of 120 pregnant women with PIH, atenolol was compared with placebo [23]. The drug, given once daily, was effective in correcting hypertension at a daily dosage of 100 mg in 17 women and 200 mg in the rest. Growth retardation, neonatal hypoglycemia, respiratory distress syndrome, and hyperbilirubinemia had the same incidence in the atenolol and in the placebo groups. Only neonatal bradycardia was commoner in the atenolol newborns, without causing clinical problems [23].

Since uterine activity is under adrenergic control, beta-adrenergic blockade might enhance uterine activity and cause premature labor [24]. A large amount of experience with beta-blockers has been reassuring on this point [25]. Thus, no mention of such a side effect can be found in recent important reviews [1, 14].

It may be concluded that in general the maternal and perinatal outcome of therapy with beta-blockers is excellent. Unfortunately the available prospective controlled studies have been performed in heterogeneous populations including both essential (CHP) and pregnancy-induced (PIH) hypertension, so that we do not know whether the good results occur in either or both of these types of hypertension [14]. Moreover, the long-term effects on the growing child still have to be evaluated [1].

3.3. Labetalol

Labetalol is an alpha- and beta-adrenoreceptor antagonist now widely used for treating hypertension. It has been used in pregnancy both for emergency therapy intravenously and for oral long-term treatment. After intravenous injection, labetalol has been shown to decrease promptly the blood pressure without causing maternal tachycardia, headache, or other side effects [26–29]. Even though the drug does not affect placental blood flow or fetal heart rate [30], it appears to cause side effects in newborns [31].

Oral labetalol has been used for treating hypertension during pregnancy. The safety of the drug with respect to maternal and perinatal outcome has been demonstrated [32]. A long-term follow-up is still needed to determine the safety for newborns.

3.4. Hydralazine

Hydralazine has been widely used to treat hypertension in pregnancy, both by intravenous or intramuscular administration for acute therapy and per os. The drug causes vasodilatation by a direct effect on peripheral arterioles. Cerebral blood flow and intracranial pressure will increase [33, 34], thereby accounting for the frequent occurrence of headache. Reflex tachycardia in response to vasodilatation is also frequent and thus may exaggerate the physiologic hyperdynamic state of pregnancy. Other side effects of hydralazine include restlessness, anxiety, nausea, vomiting, and epigastric pain that may mimic impending eclampsia [1].

It seems that hydralazine reduces placental function in pregnant women with chronic hypertension [35]. Fetuses of hypertensive women treated with hydralazine have been reported to be growth retarded [36, 37]. Since the vasodilatation caused by the drug is responsible for an increase in sympathetic tone that may cause a reduction in placental blood flow, Redman [1] suggests using hydralazine in patients already on methyldopa; this may retard the sympathetically mediated response to the drug, thereby preventing fetal distress.

3.5. Calcium antagonists: nifedipine

The contraction of skeletal, smooth, and cardiac muscle cells depends on the increased intracellular concentration of calcium ions. Drugs that block the inward calcium ion current from extracellular space are referred to as *calcium antagonists.* Nifedipine is a drug with selective activity for vascular cells and therefore has been widely used in recent years for treating hypertension.

Up to now there is only one report on the use of nifedipine in pregnancy-associated hypertension [38]. The drug, given in the peripartum period, resulted in a decrease in blood pressure by 26/20 mm Hg within 20 min; no adverse effects were observed in the fetuses; maternal side effects were mainly headache and cutaneous flushing [1, 38].

We should bear in mind that magnesium ions may potentiate the effects of calcium antagonists [39]. This is important when using calcium channel blockers in patients treated with magnesium sulfate for eclampsia [1].

3.6. Methyldopa

Methyldopa remains the best, safest antihypertensive medication for chronic hypertension in pregnant women [1]. Prolonged treatment of severe hypertension with this drug in pregnancy has been successful [40]. Furthermore, controlled trials of the use of methyldopa either alone [41] or with a diuretic [42] for mild hypertension in pregnancy have resulted in improved perinatal outcome. Treatment of mild hypertension with methyldopa also reduces the frequency of severe hypertensive episodes during gestation [43]. Dosage of the drug is the usual dosage recommended for nonpregnant patients and may vary from 750 mg to 4 g/day [1].

Methyldopa crosses the placenta and is found in fetal plasma [44]. Neonatal blood pressure after maternal treatment is significantly reduced, but becomes normal within the first five days of life [45].

The results of long-term follow-up on the effects of maternal therapy with methyldopa on the growth and development of children have been reported recently [46]. As many as 195 children born to hypertensive women, half of whom had been treated with methyldopa (in a randomly control trial of methyldopa therapy) [41], were followed from birth for up to 7½ years. No significant differences were observed between the children in the treated and untreated groups in standing and supine blood pressures or in mean intelligence quotients, despite a reduction in head circumference in sons of women who entered the trial between weeks 16 and 20 of gestation [46].

4. CONCLUSION

In our opinion, women with chronic hypertension (all forms of systemic hypertension preceding gestation) have to continue their antihypertensive treatment when they become pregnant. Special attention in the choice of drugs is, however, necessary.

Methyldopa remains the drug of choice, being the safest for both mother and child. Hydralazine may be used, preferably in association with methyldopa.

Beta-blockers and labetalol seem to be safe, but require further controlled trials and long-term follow-up.

Ganglion-blocking agents are undesirable; they may cause meconium ileus in the fetus.

Low-salt diets and diuretics should be avoided, since they may further decrease the already reduced blood volume. Diuretic therapy may be useful in an emergency (e.g., cardiac failure).

Despite a questionnaire survey carried out in 1978 in the United Kingdom and Ireland that has shown that 21.1% of 1093 obstetricians would continue clonidine when a patient with moderately severe hypertension becomes pregnant, no trial has been reported in recent literature concerning efficacy and safety of this drug.

Calcium antagonists in pregnancy deserve further evaluation. Experience with captopril (the converting-enzyme inhibitor) in pregnant women is still lacking.

REFERENCES

1. Redman CWG: The management of hypertension in pregnancy. Semin Nephrol 4:270–282, 1984.
2. Rubin PC: Hypertension occurring during pregnancy. In: Robertson JIS (ed) Handbook of hypertension, vol 2: Clinical aspects of secondary hypertension. Amsterdam: Elsevier, 1983, pp 304–318.
3. Strandgaard S, Olesen J, Skinhoj E: Autoregulation of brain circulation in severe arterial hypertension. Br Med J 1:507–510, 1973.
4. Strandgaard S: Autoregulation of cerebral blood flow in hypertensive patients: the modifying influence of prolonged antihypertensive treatment in the tolerance to acute, drug-induced hypotension. Circulation 53:720–727, 1976.
5. Chamberlain GVP, Lewis PJ, De Swiet M, Bulpitt CJ: How obstetricians manage hypertension in pregnancy. Br Med J 1:626–629, 1978.
6. Chesley LC: Hypertensive disorders in pregnancy. New York: Appleton-Century-Crofts, 1978.
7. Kraus GW, Marchese JR, Yen SSC: Prophylactic use of hydrochlorothiazide in pregnancy. JAMA 198:1150–1154, 1966.
8. Nolten WE, Ehrlich EN: Sodium metabolism in normal pregnancy and in preeclampsia. (Chapter 6 in this volume.)
9. Gant NF, Pritchard JA: Hypertension complicating pregnancy. (Chapter 7 in this volume.)
10. Christianson R, Page EW: Diuretic drugs and pregnancy. Obstet Gynecol 48:647–652, 1976.
11. Gant NF, Madden JD, Siiteri PK, MacDonald PC: The metabolic clearance rate of dehydroisoandrosterone sulfate. III. The effect of thiazide diuretics in normal and future preeclamptic pregnancy. Am J Obstet Gynecol 123:159–163, 1975.
12. Davison JM: Renal function during normal pregnancy and the effect of renal disease and preeclampsia. (Chapter 5 in this volume.)
13. Robinson M: Salt in pregnancy. Lancet 1:178–181, 1958.
14. Rubin PC: Beta-blockers in pregnancy. N Engl J Med 305:1323–1326, 1981.
15. Tcherdakoff P, Colhard M, Berrard E, Kraft C, Dupay A, Bernante JM: Propranolol in hypertension during pregnancy. Br Med J 2:670, 1978.
16. Eliahou HE, Silverberg DS, Reisin E, Romem I, Mashrach S, Serr DM: Propranolol for the treatment of hypertension in pregnancy. Br J Obstet Gynaecol 85:431–436, 1978.
17. Bott-Kanner G, Schweitzer A, Reisner SH, Joel-Cohen SJ, Rosenfeld JB: Propranolol and hydralazine in the management of essential hypertension in pregnancy. Br J Obstet Gynaecol 87:110–114, 1980.
18. Lieberman BA, Stirrat GM, Cohen SL, Beard RW, Pinker GD, Belsey E: The possible adverse effect of propranolol on the fetus in pregnancies complicated by severe hypertension. Br J Obstet Gynaecol 85:678–683, 1978.

19. Tcherdakoff P: Bêta-bloquants et hypertension artérielle de la femme enceinte. Nouv Press Med 7:2807–2809, 1978.
20. Gallery EDM, Saunders DM, Hunyor SN, Györy AZ: Randomised comparison of methyldopa and oxprenolol for treatment of hypertension in pregnancy. Br Med J 1:1591–1594, 1979.
21. Fidler J, Smith V, Fayers P, De Swiet M: Randomised controlled comparative study of methyldopa and oxprenolol in treatment of hypertension in pregnancy. Br Med J 1:1927–1930, 1983.
22. Sandström BO: Antihypertensive treatment with the adrenergic beta-receptor blocker metoprolol during pregnancy. Gynecol Obstet Invest 9:195–204, 1978.
23. Rubin PC, Butters L, Clark DM, Reynolds B, Sumner DJ, Steedman D, Low RA, Reid JL: Placebo-controlled trial of atenolol in treatment of pregnancy-associated hypertension. Lancet 1:431–434, 1983.
24. Harden TP, Stander RW: Effects of adrenergic blocking agents and catecholamines in human pregnancy. Am J Obstet Gynecol 102:226–235, 1968.
25. Redman CWG: Treatment of hypertension in pregnancy. Kidney Int 18:267–278, 1980.
26. Lamming GD, Broughton Pipkin F, Seymonds EM: Comparison of the alpha and beta blocking drug labetalol, and methyldopa in the treatment of moderate and severe pregnancy-induced hypertension. Clin Exp Hypertens 2:865–895, 1980.
27. Lunell NO, Hjemdahl P, Fredholm BB, Nisell H, Persson B, Wager J: Circulatory and metabolic effects of a combined alpha- and beta-adrenocepor blocker (labetalol) in hypertension of pregnancy. Br J Clin Pharmacol 12:345–348, 1981.
28. Garden A, Davey DA, Dommisse J: Intravenous labetalol and intravenous dihydralazine in severe hypertension in pregnancy. Clin Exp Hypertens 1:371–383, 1982.
29. Rubin PC, Butters L, Kelman AW: Labetalol disposition and concentration–effect relationship during pregnancy. Br J Clin Pharmacol 15:465–470, 1983.
30. Lunell NO, Nylund L, Lewander R: Acute effect of an antihypertensive drug, labetalol, on uteroplacental blood flow. Br J Obstet Gynaecol 89:640–644, 1982.
31. Woods DL, Malan AF: Side effects of labetalol in newborn infants. Br J Obstet Gynaecol 90:876, 1983.
32. Redman CWG: Controlled trial of the treatment of hypertension in pregnancy: labetalol compared with methyldopa. In: Riley A, Symonds EM (eds) The investigation of labetalol in the management of hypertension in pregnancy. International Congress series 591. Amsterdam: Excerpta Medica, 1982, pp 101–110.
33. McCall ML: Cerebral circulation and metabolism in toxemia of pregnancy: observations on the effects of veratrum viride and Apresoline (1-hydrazinophthalazine). Am J Obstet Gynecol 66:1015–1030, 1953.
34. Overgaard J, Skinhoj E: A paradoxical cerebral hemodynamic effect of hydralazine. Stroke 6:402–404, 1975.
35. Gant NF, Madden JD, Siiteri PK, MacDonald PC: The metabolic clearance rate of dehydroisoandrosterone sulfate. IV. Acute effects of induced hypertension, hypotension and natriuresis in normal and hypertensive pregnancies. Am J Obstet Gynecol 124:143–148, 1976.
36. Vink GJ, Moodley J, Philpott RH: Effect of dihydralazine on the fetus in the treatment of maternal hypertension. Obstet Gynecol 55:519–522, 1980.
37. Vink GJ, Moodley J: The effect of low-dose dihydralazine on the fetus in the emergency treatment of hypertension in pregnancy. S Afr Med J 62:475–477, 1982.
38. Walters BNJ, Redman CWG: Treatment of severe pregnancy-associated hypertension with the calcium antagonist nifedipine. Br J Obstet Gynaecol 91:330–336, 1984.
39. Turlapaty PDM, Weiner R, Altura BM: Interactions of magnesium and verapamil on tone and contractility of vascular smooth muscle. Eur J Pharmacol 74:263–272, 1981.
40. Kincaid-Smith P, Bullen M, Mills J: Prolonged use of methyldopa in severe hypertension in pregnancy. Br Med J 1:274–276, 1966.
41. Redman CWG, Beiling LJ, Bonnar J, Ounsted MK: Fetal outcome in a trial of antihypertensive treatment in pregnancy. Lancet 2:753–756, 1976.
42. Leather HM, Humphreys DM, Baker P, Chadd MA: A controlled trial of hypotensive agents in hypertension in pregnancy. Lancet 2:488–490, 1968.
43. Redman CWG, Beilin LJ, Bonnar J: Treatment of hypertension in pregnancy with methyldopa: blood pressure control and side effects. Br J Obstet Gynaecol 84:419–426, 1977.

44. Jones HMR, Cummings AJ: A study of the transfer of alpha-methyldopa of the human foetus and newborn infant. Br J Clin Pharmacol 6:432–434, 1978.
45. Whitelaw A: Maternal methyldopa treatment and neonatal blood pressure. Br Med J 283:471, 1981.
46. Cockburn J, Moar VA, Ounsted M, Redman CWG: Final report of study on hypertension during pregnancy: the effects of specific treatment on the growth and development of the children. Lancet 1:647–649, 1982.

9. PROTEINURIA DURING PREGNANCY

PRISCILLA S. KINCAID-SMITH, ROBYN A. NORTH, GAVIN J. BECKER, and
KENNETH F. FAIRLEY

1. PATHOPHYSIOLOGY OF PROTEINURIA DURING PREGNANCY

In healthy nonpregnant adults, 30–130 mg of protein is excreted in the urine each day, the upper limit of normal being 150 mg/24 h [1]. This consists of albumin, small proteins such as ceruloplasmin, and various globulins. The filtration of a protein molecule is dictated by a variety of factors. These include the glomerular capillary wall structure and charge, the molecule's size, charge and configuration, and hemodynamic factors. Most protein in the ultrafiltrate is reabsorbed in the renal tubules. The renal tubules also secrete some proteins, in particular Tamm Horsfall protein. The combined effect of glomerular filtration, tubular reabsorption, and tubular secretion determines the net urinary protein excretion.

As there have been few studies of the pathophysiology of proteinuria in pregnancy, we initially review the pathophysiology of proteinuria in the nonpregnant state.

1.1. Mechanisms of proteinuria: structure and functional considerations in the normal kidney

1.1.1. The glomerular filtration barrier

The glomerular capillary wall consists of three layers: the endothelium, with multiple fenestrae (50–100 nm in diameter); the glomerular basement membrane (GBM), with its central lamina densa, subendothelial lamina rara interna, and subepithelial lamina rara externa; and epithelial cells, with their interdigitating foot processes attached to the lamina rara externa [2, 3] (figure 9–1). The gaps between the foot processes are bridged by slit diaphragms. The diaphragms consist of a central filament, with connecting parallel rods creating a series of rectangular pores 4×14 nm in cross section.

All three layers of the glomerular capillary wall carry a negative charge. The presence of anionic moieties in the wall has been demonstrated by electron-microscopic studies showing that cationic reagents bind to these structures [3–8]. This negative charge has been attributed to the presence of sialoglycoproteins and proteoglycan rich in sulfate groups in the cell coats, the slit diaphragm, and the glomerular basement membrane [5, 9, 10], and results in an electrostatic barrier to macromolecules [11, 12].

The site at which this sieving occurs has been a matter of contention, confused by studies using tracer molecules that vary in charge as well as molecular weight and by conducting experiments under different hemodynamic circumstances [13–16]. It is likely that all layers of the capillary wall contribute to the barrier, the depth that a molecule penetrates being influenced by both its size and charge. The inner GBM is probably the major site at which anionic species are retarded, whereas cationic molecules are predominantly retarded at the epithelial slit diaphragms [8, 11, 17, 18].

1.1.2. Molecular size selectivity

Small uncharged molecules with radii equal or below that of inulin (1.4 nm) pass relatively freely into the ultrafiltrate [11]. As the molecular size increases, passage

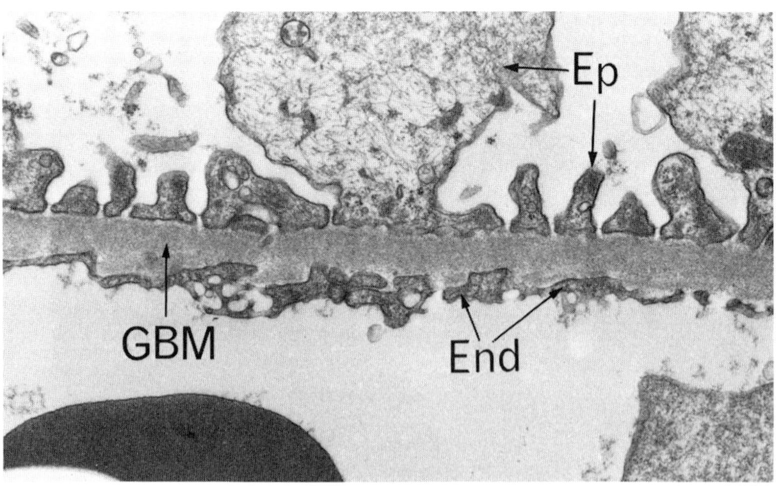

Figure 9-1. Glomerular capillary wall: *Ep,* epithelial cell with foot process; *GBM,* glomerular basement membrane; and *End,* endothelial cell layer.

through the glomerular capillary wall is retarded [11, 19]. The upper limit seems to be around 4.2 nm, since minimal amounts of dextran, a neutral polysaccharide of variable molecular weight, is filtered once this size is exceeded.

1.1.3. Charge selectivity

Chang et al. [20] noted that glomerular permeability to albumin, which is negatively charged, is reduced compared with neutral dextran of the same molecular size (3.6 nm), while anionic dextran sulfate (3.6 nm) has a fractional clearance similar to that of albumin. Bohrer and co-workers [21] showed that the cationic dextran polymer, diethylaminoethyl dextran, has a greater fractional clearance than does neutral dextran. These and other studies support the theory that the electrostatic interaction between the charged macromolecules and the anionic sites in the glomerular capillary wall play an important role in determining filtration. In simple terms, the negatively charged glomerular capillary wall is less permeable to negatively charged molecules, such as albumin, than to positively charged molecules, resulting in a "charge-selective barrier" [1, 11].

1.1.4. Molecular configuration

Venkatachalam and Rennke [3] proposed that the molecular configuration is also important in filtration of macromolecules by the glomerular capillary wall. They found that the glomerular capillary wall was significantly more permeable to molecules with a flexible configuration, such as neutral dextran, than to protein molecules of a similar size and charge.

1.1.5. Hemodynamic factors

Blood flow to the glomerulus influences the filtration characteristics of the glomerular capillary wall. There is an inverse relationship between the glomerular plasma flow and fractional clearance of macromolecules. Both the size and the charge of the macromolecules alter the degree to which hemodynamic factors can affect filtration [22, 23].

1.1.6. Tubular protein reabsorption

Although the glomerular capillary wall is an effective barrier, small amounts of protein pass into the urinary space [1, 24, 25]. Most of the filtered proteins, including albumin, insulin, growth hormone, vasopressin, adrenocorticotrophic hormone, glucagon, and parathyroid hormone, are reabsorbed and degraded within the tubular cells [1, 26–29].

1.1.7. Tubular protein secretion

A mucoprotein, with no plasma equivalent, was reported in the urine by Tamm and Horsfall in 1952 [30]. It is secreted by the loop of Henle, distal convoluted tubules, and collecting ducts [31] and is the major protein component in urinary casts [32, 33]. In the nephrotic syndrome there may be a slight increase in Tamm Horsfall protein associated with heavy proteinuria [34].

1.2. Renal damage and proteinuria

Proteinuria is a hallmark of renal injury. It occurs either when the glomerulus fails to be an effective barrier, when the filtered proteins are not reabsorbed in the proximal tubule, or when a combination of both factors exist. In most cases, significant proteinuria largely results from increased glomerular permeability.

1.2.1. Glomerular proteinuria

In an attempt to predict the type of underlying glomerular disease, many investigators have assessed glomerular permeability by using the ratio of the clearance of a small molecule, such as albumin or transferrin, to clearance of a large molecule, such as globulin. Glomerular proteinuria can thus be described as either "highly selective" or "nonselective" [35]. When the clearance ratio of IgG to albumin (or transferrin) is less than 0.1, it is considered to be highly selective proteinuria, whereas it is defined as a nonselective pattern when the ratio is greater than 0.5. Highly selective proteinuria is typical of minimal-change glomerulonephritis in children, but in adults the test is much less useful and renal biopsy is required to establish the diagnosis [35, 36].

What are the underlying changes in the glomerular capillary wall that result in a decrease in the filtration barrier? Two major schools of thought exist, though they are not mutually exclusive. The first considers that the morphologic changes in damaged glomeruli lead to the formation of "larger pores" and hence proteinuria. Several other investigators [4, 5, 21, 37–39] have shown an association between a decrease in anionic sites in the glomerular capillary wall and the development of proteinuria. In renal disease models in rats, this occurs in aminonucleoside nephrosis [4, 5] after infusion of polycations that neutralize the negative charges [37–39], and in nephrotoxic serum nephritis [21, 40]. Patients with significant proteinuria due to glomerular disease have also been shown to have reduced anionic moieties in glomerular capillary walls [41].

Reduction in polyanions has been demonstrated in glomeruli with the morphologic appearance of foot process fusion [6, 39], endothelial and epithelial cell detachment from the GBM [6], and membranous glomerulonephritis [40].

In brief, loss of anion moieties in the glomerular capillary wall might have two major sequelae. First, there is a decrease in charge-selective barrier, resulting in anionic proteins, such as albumin, leaking into the urine. Second, this loss of fixed negative charges may actually lead to morphologic alterations in the glomerular capillary wall structure and development of "enlarged pores," through which larger proteins such as IgG may pass [12, 18]. The precipitating event resulting in the decrease in polyanions is a matter of conjecture at present.

Additionally, in experimental models, coincidentally induced coagulation changes and hemodynamic factors may also be important [23, 24].

In pregnancy, glomerular proteinuria occurs in preeclampsia and in patients with a variety of preexisting renal diseases, including glomerulonephritis, reflux nephropathy, and diabetic nephropathy.

1.2.2. Tubular proteinuria

Impaired tubular reabsorption of filtered protein molecules results in low molecular weight proteinuria. This pattern of abnormal protein excretion occurs in a diverse group of tubulointerstitial diseases. Tubular proteinuria is uncommon during pregnancy and rarely causes concern.

1.3. Proteinuria in normal pregnancy

In normal pregnancy, there is a striking change in both renal blood flow and glomerular filtration rate (GFR), which both increase by 25%–50%, reaching a maximum during the second trimester. This increase in GFR is accompanied by a slight increase in urinary protein secretion such that proteinuria is not considered abnormal until it exceeds 300 mg in 24 h [43].

Strenuous exercise, exposure to cold, emotional stress, and postural changes can all potentially induce significant transient proteinuria [44]. Any of the above may cause increased urinary protein excretion in normal pregnant women.

1.4. Detection and quantitation of proteinuria

There are a variety of tests used to detect proteinuria [45]. Traditionally, checking for turbidity after boiling and addition of acetic acid, or the addition of sulfosalicylic acid have been used as sensitive semiquantitative ward tests for proteinuria. The need for special equipment and the possibility of false-positive results (e.g., with turbid urine, radiologic contrast media, and some drugs) have largely lead to their replacement by various dipstick tests for protein that are convenient and can be combined with other valuable indicators (e.g., for pH, glucose, and blood). The dipstick are based on a color change in tetrabromophenol blue when protein is added, and are more sensitive to albumin than other proteins such as globulin, Bence Jones, and Tamm Horsfall protein. They are sensitive and semiquantitative over a range from about 0.05–20.0 g/liter, a similar range as with the turbidity tests.

Obviously, since these are all dependent on urine concentration, their ability to detect significant proteinuria depends partly on the state of diuresis in the patient. In general, however, they are sufficiently sensitive to detect significant proteinuria in most cases, and are particularly reliable if first morning specimens are tested.

The accurate quantitation of urinary protein excretion can be made on a carefully collected 24-h specimen, a valuable investigation in patients suspected of renal disease, usually combined with a creatinine clearance, that will indicate renal function and allow estimation of the adequacy of the urine collection by reference to the amount of creatinine excreted per 24 h (usually 7–17 mmol/day in the steady state). More recently, use of the ratio between urinary albumin and creatinine concentrations has been recommended as a method for estimating glomerular permeability without the need for timed urine specimens (which are difficult to collect) or blood tests (which also can be troublesome in obese patients) [46].

1.5. Investigation of proteinuria during pregnancy

When proteinuria is detected in a pregnant woman, a 24-h urine protein level should be measured. It is important to remember that in preeclampsia the level of proteinuria may vary markedly from day to day. The aggressiveness with which proteinuria is investigated in pregnancy depends on the gestation at presentation and the presence or absence of hypertension. A woman presenting prior to 20 weeks with proteinuria, with or without hypertension, is more likely to have underlying renal disease than is a primigravida presenting late in the third trimester with proteinuria and hypertension.

Pregnant women with proteinuria should have a careful clinical assessment for evidence of renal disease or essential hypertension. In particular, blood pressure, weight gain, and the presence of edema should be noted. Investigations including blood urea and uric acid, creatinine clearance, careful urine microscopy, and urine culture should be performed. In measuring blood pressure and renal function, one needs to take into account the fact that normally blood pressure falls during pregnancy, particularly in the second trimester, and the glomerular filtration increases during pregnancy. If the GFR fails to increase, this may indicate significant renal disease. In some cases, renal ultrasound, single-exposure intravenous urography, or other renal imaging may be required to define the lesion.

It is becoming increasingly clear that, not only the distinction among various forms of glomerulonephritis usually requires renal biopsy, but also that in many cases the distinction among preeclampsia, preeclampsia in a patient with glomerular disease, and worsening of glomerular disease can be difficult to determine without tissue diagnosis.

In most situations in the second and third trimesters, a biopsy result will not influence management, and hence the biopsy is usually postponed until six months after delivery, when the pregnancy-related changes will have largely resolved. When a woman presents with significant proteinuria in early pregnancy, however, and has evidence of an underlying glomerulonephritis on urine microscopy, our usual practice is to do a renal biopsy to guide us in our management. In our experience with over 300 renal biopsies during pregnancy, the only complication was macroscopic hematuria in one patient, which resolved spontaneously.

2. PROTEINURIA RELATED TO PREECLAMPSIA

In 1827, Richard Bright [47] boiled a teaspoon of urine from patients with edema and discovered "albuminous urine." The obstetrician, John Lever [48] wrote in 1843, "I particularly noted the great similarity that presented in her appearance and that of patients labouring under anasarca with the 'morbus Brightii' and it was with this in view that we proceeded to examine the condition of her urine. We extracted the urine from the bladder by catheter and found it to be highly charged with albumin. . . . I was led to suppose that the albuminous condition of the urine depended upon some transient cause, probably connected with the state of gestation itself." In 1843, Simpson [49] simultaneously taught on puerperal convulsions and the presence of albuminous urine. They are jointly acknowledged for identifying this as a separate entity occurring in pregnancy, and not just a manifestation of nephritis.

Since then, preeclampsia (gestational hypertension and proteinuria) has become a well recognized complication of pregnancy, but the signs of preeclampsia occur in several separate disease processes. They occur in "true idiopathic" preeclampsia, which is generally considered a first-pregnancy phenomenon, resolving with delivery and not associated with long-term maternal morbidity. Proteinuria and hypertension also occur in pregnant women with underlying essential hypertension and in women with renal disease. In this second group, increased proteinuria may occur as a consequence of the normal physiologic changes of pregnancy, as a result of superimposed preeclampsia, or as a consequence of coincidental increased renal disease activity.

In women with preeclampsia the underlying pathologic process cannot always be identified on clinical grounds. Fisher et al. [50] found that, of 176 women considered "toxemic" during gestation, only 76% of the primigravidas and 24% of the multigravidas had the isolated lesions of preeclampsia on renal biopsy. In a recent prospective study [51], 59 women with severe preeclampsia prior to week 37 were carefully investigated postpartum. Underlying renal disease was found in 60% of both the primigravida and multiparous patients.

Difficulty in separating the different patient groups on clinical grounds has meant that they are often studied collectively, which this has lead to considerable confusion in the literature.

2.1. Pathophysiology of proteinuria in preeclampsia

The proteinuria related to preeclampsia is glomerular in origin and has been found to be of intermediate or poor selectivity [52–56]. The urinary protein pattern has not been shown to be useful as a predictor of underlying renal disease or chronic hypertension in an individual woman with preeclampsia [50, 52, 55, 57].

Fisher et al. [50] presented data showing the severity of proteinuria correlated with the severity of the renal lesion in patients with preeclampsia. The morphologic changes occurring in the glomerulus and contributing to the defective filtration barrier in preeclampsia will be discussed later.

To our knowledge, no studies on the "charge" characteristics of the glomerular capillary wall in preeclampsia have been reported. It is well established [58] that vascular reactivity is increased in preeclamptic women compared with normal pregnant women. This may result in fluctuations in renal blood flow, which in turn may alter the effective filtration barrier in the glomerulus.

2.2. Clinical characteritics of proteinuria in preeclampsia

Significant proteinuria in pregnancy has been defined by the Committee on Terminology of the American College of Obstetricians and Gynecologists as either a urinary protein concentration of greater than 0.3 g in 24 h or greater than 1 g/liter in a random sample. Occasionally, normal pregnant women may develop this degree of proteinuria and, at least from a researcher's point of view, this level may be too low and a 24-h urinary protein of 0.5 g may be more appropriate.

Usually mild to moderate proteinuria occurs in preeclamptic patients, but heavy proteinuria (up to 20 g/24 h) may occur [59–61]. In 1970, Studd et al. [62] suggested that preeclampsia was the commonest cause of nephrotic syndrome in pregnancy. This has been confirmed by Fisher and colleagues [50, 59], who reviewed postpartum renal biopsies from women with proteinuria in the nephrotic range.

Characteristically, the degree of proteinuria in preeclampsia fluctuates markedly from day to day [63, 64]. It has been proposed that this results from alterations in the renal blood flow [65]. Proteinuria may also fluctuate with the level of physical activity, diminishing during rest and increasing with normal daily activities.

Proteinuria usually develops after week 20, although in an occasional patient, glomerular lesions, virtually diagnostic of preeclampsia, may be seen in renal biopsies carried out before week 20. Early onset of preeclampsia is more likely to indicate underlying renal disease or some other predisposing factor, such as a twin pregnancy. Proteinuria is a late manifestation in the course of preeclampsia. Chesley [65] studied 206 primiparous women with eclampsia and found that 58.2% presented with hypertension and 33.6% with hypertension and proteinuria, and that proteinuria preceded hypertension in 8.2%.

2.2.1. Relationship to hypertension and edema

No correlation has been found between the degree of proteinuria and the severity of the hypertension [59, 66, 67]. Similarly, Friedman and Fox [68] found no definite relationship between the level of proteinuria and the presence of edema.

2.2.2. Proteinuria in eclampsia

Eclampsia is usually associated with moderate to heavy proteinuria, but Chesley [65] found that 2.5% of 199 women showed no proteinuria in the day or two before they convulsed. In a few women, initially admitted to hospital with preeclampsia, the proteinuria had decreased to a trace by the time they had seizures.

2.3. Clinical investigation in preeclampsia

2.3.1. Serum protein levels

Maternal serum protein concentrations are altered in preeclampsia. Albumin, transferrin and IgG are lower than in normal pregnancy and macroglobulin and lipoproteins are elevated [69]. The serum albumin of the fetus is maintained even in the presence of severe maternal hypoalbuminemia, but hypogammaglobulinemia can occur.

2.3.2. Urine microscopy

As with other features of preeclampsia, there is marked variability in the urinary microscopic findings among individuals with preeclampsia. The red blood cell count is often elevated, and a glomerular pattern of bleeding (figure 9–2), as

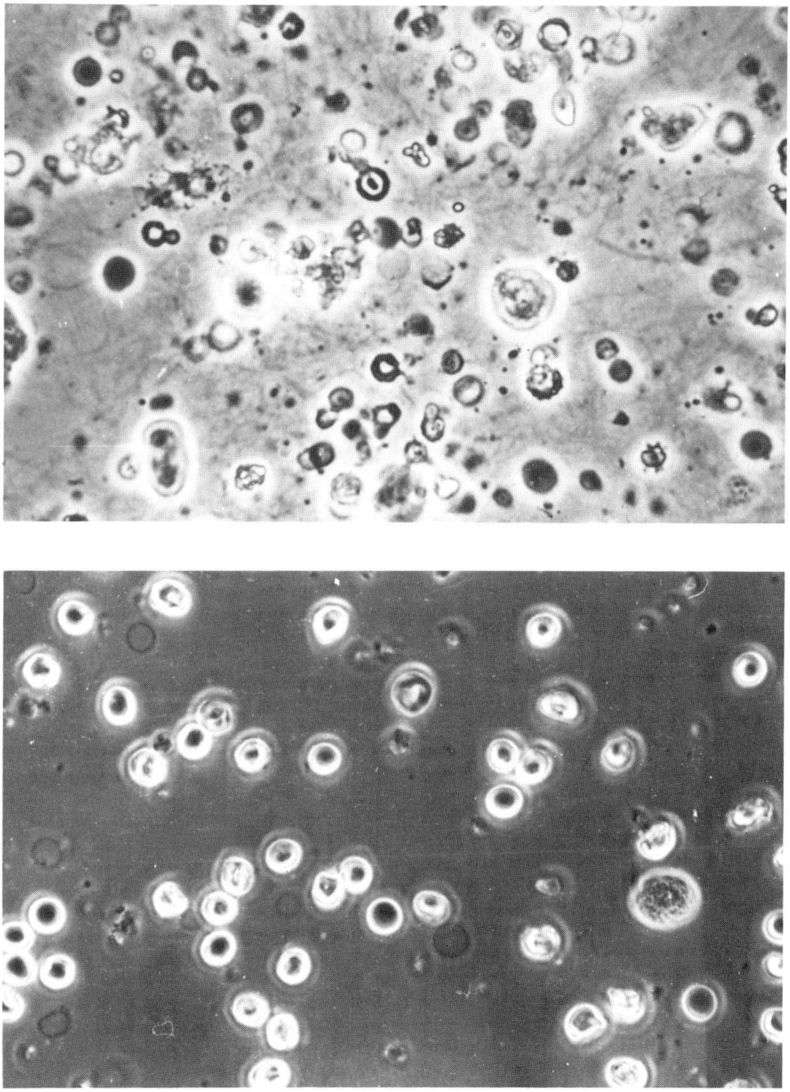

Figure 9-2. Morphologic features of glomerular and nonglomerular hematuria. **(a)** Glomerular bleeding—dysmorphic urinary red cells with gross variation in size and shape (phase-contrast microscopy). **(b)** Nonglomerular bleeding—uniform size and shape (2–3 populations only) of urinary red cells (Phase-contrast microscopy).

described by Fairley and Birch [70], is seen. In a recent review of 60 preeclamptic patients in our institution, five of whom had glomerulonephritis on renal biopsy, 45% had microscopic glomerular hematuria, with a median count of 16,000 cells/ml. Hyaline casts are common, many may be granular, and occasionally red blood cell casts are seen in women who on follow-up after pregnancy have no evidence of an underlying glomerulonephritis. Other findings include fat particles (a nonspecific marker of glomerular damage) and an occasional oval fat body. Usually there is gradual resolution of these urinary microscopic findings over three months after delivery, but occasionally diminishing microscopic hematuria and fat particles may persist for months.

2.3.3. Renal biopsy: the glomerular lesions in preeclampsia

There are some differences in findings by different groups in relation to morphologic changes in glomeruli that accompany preeclampsia. This is surprising because the changes are striking and can be recognized at a glance by an experienced pathologist. The changes that we have described previously [71–75] have been largely confirmed by some authors [76, 77] but not by others [80]. Certain aspects of the glomerular lesion, such as endothelial cell swelling and vacuolization with foam cell formation, have been much more prominent in some series [78, 79]. The timing of the biopsy could well affect this, and a postpartum biopsy, in our experience, is more likely to show this change. Many of the biopsy series in which it is best recorded were done at this time, during resolution of the lesion, rather than at the time at which the patients presented during pregnancy.

Basement membrane changes in the acute stage can mimic those of mesangiocapillary glomerulonephritis with reduplication of the basement membrane. Even more characteristic is a "chain-like" lesion. These changes resolve after pregnancy but may take months to do so. The swelling of endothelial cells originally described as a lesion in preeclampsia [79] was subsequently shown to be a mesangial cell change [76]. In our experience this change is more prominent during resolution of the glomerular lesion.

A very characteristic change is the presence of subendothelial and mesangial deposits of fibrin or fibrin-like material [71–73]. Sheehan [78] failed to find these, perhaps because his studies were carried out on autopsy material when postpartum fibrinolytis could have occurred.

Granules in epithelial cells within the Bowman space have been recognized more recently as a feature of preeclampsia [74, 75] (figure 9-3). The percentage of glomeruli showing these cells correlates well with the degree of preeclampsia (figure 9-4) and hence probably with the degree of proteinuria in preeclampsia. These cells are rarely seen, however, in patients with proteinuria in pregnancy unless preeclampsia develops (figure 9-5). They are also not seen in biopsies done at a time remote from the episode of preeclampsia and are rare in other forms of proteinuria. They may closely resemble the peripolar cells described by Ryan et al. [81], which are a prominent feature in a toxemia model in pregnant sheep [82]. These cells appear to secrete droplets into the Bowman space and may well have

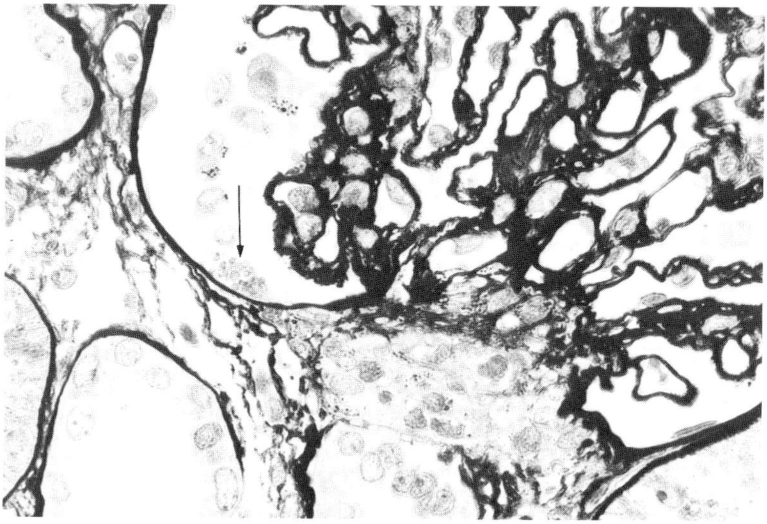

Figure 9-3 Granulated epithelial cells. A glomerulus in a biopsy taken four days after delivery from a patient with membranous glomerulonephritis. A granulated epithelial cell *(arrow)* is present in a peripolar situation (Silver Masson).

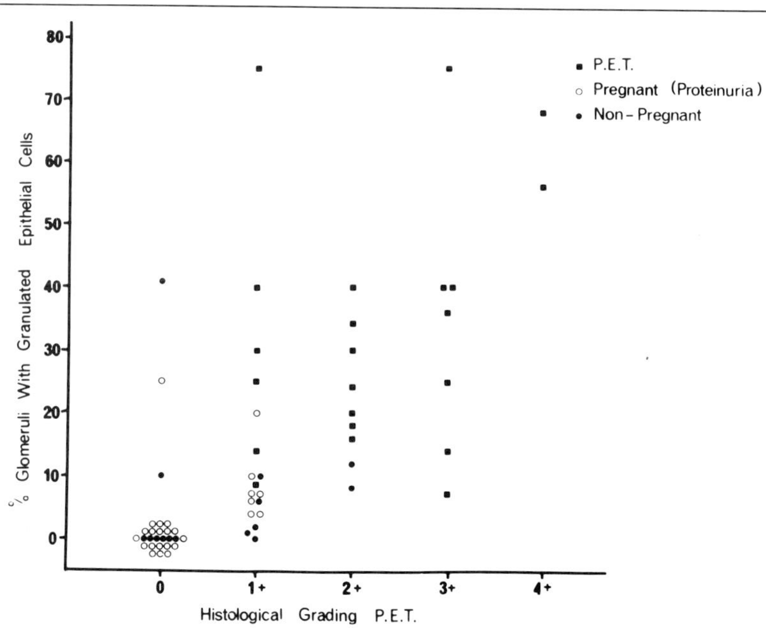

Figure 9-4. Granulated epithelial cells in preeclampsia—correlation with severity. The histologic severity of preeclampsia correlates with the percentage of glomeruli with granulated epithelial cells. Also shown are the results in second biopsies from 15 of the 22 patients with preeclampsia taken at a time remote from the pregnancy, and those of patients with proteinuria in pregnancy. Granulated epithelial cells were rarely observed except in the context of preeclampsia. *PET,* preeclamptic toxemia.

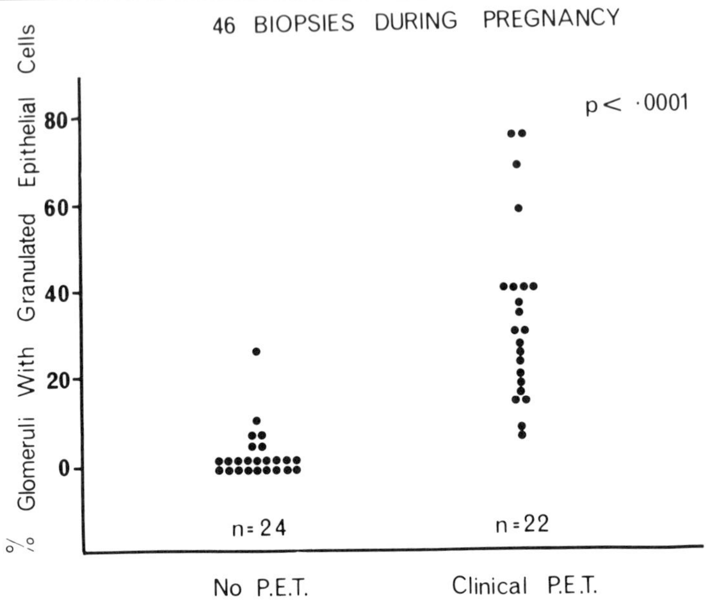

Figure 9-5. Granulated epithelial cells in clinical preeclampsia. Blind histologic evaluation of biopsies taken during pregnancy from patients with and without clinical evidence of preeclampsia. *PET,* preeclamptic toxemia. Only one biopsy from a patient without clinical evidence of PET showed any granulated epithelial cells and these were present in only 20% of glomeruli in this biopsy.

a secretory role rather than an absorptive one as would be expected if they were so-called hyaline resorption droplets.

2.4. Proteinuria and fetal outcome in preeclampsia

Several studies have shown that the presence of proteinuria has an adverse effect on fetal outcome [59, 60, 67, 83–85]. Lin et al. [85] found that proteinuria of 3.5 g/24 h or greater was associated with intrauterine growth retardation, but the role of prolonged hypertension in these patients was not clear. Studd and Blainey [60] reported that, in women with the nephrotic syndrome, maternal hypoalbuminemia correlated with low birth weight.

Proteinuria, with or without edema, is associated with a significant increase in perinatal death rate [67, 83]. The presence of hypertension with proteinuria results in a further increase in perinatal mortality. Friedman and Neff [84] analyzed the perinatal mortality in 38,000 pregnancies and found that the presence of 1+ proteinuria occurring with a diastolic blood pressure of 85 mm Hg or greater was associated with higher fetal mortality (rate ratio of fetal mortality, 7.2). This was nearly double that occurring in patients with 2+ proteinuria alone (rate ratio, 4.1) or only a diastolic blood pressure of 95 mm Hg or greater (rate ratio, 4). Lin et al. [85] reported increased perinatal mortality in women with hypertension and heavy proteinuria, particularly if on renal biopsy the underlying lesion was preeclampsia not glomerulonephritis. On the other hand, women with nephrosclerosis, who were hypertensive but rarely had heavy proteinuria, usually had a successful fetal outcome.

2.5. Resolution postpartum

To our knowledge there are no adequate prospective studies reporting the resolution of proteinuria related to preeclampsia after delivery. In general, however, there is considerable variation between individuals but, in patients with "true idiopathic" preeclampsia, our usual experience is that proteinuria resolves over a few days to two weeks, often associated with a diuresis. If the patient has underlying renal disease, the level of proteinuria may decrease in the postpartum period, but may not completely resolve. As mentioned previously, the renal biopsy abnormalities associated with preeclampsia may take several months to resolve completely.

3. PROTEINURIA AS A MANIFESTATION OF UNDERLYING RENAL DISEASE

3.1. Idiopathic glomerular disease

Glomerular disease is by far the commonest form of renal lesion in the community. Urinary erythrocytes of the type that occur in glomerular disease are found in over 6% of healthy subjects [86]. Few screening studies of populations have been done and followed by renal biopsy, but what evidence is available suggests that 2% of normal subjects have glomerulonephritis [87]. In two centers where biopsies are frequently performed, underlying renal disease has been noted in 41% [88] of patients with preeclampsia and glomerulonephritis was detected in 38% of patients with proteinuria detected during pregnancy [89]. There was no particular "selection" in either series and these figures suggest that almost half the women presenting with preeclampsia or with proteinuria (including preeclampsia) during pregnancy have underlying renal disease, most commonly glomerulonephritis.

The types of glomerular disease in a consecutive series of 123 patients who presented with proteinuria in pregnancy [89] are shown in table 9-1. The two commonest lesions were membranous glomerulonephritis (19%) and focal and segmental proliferative glomerulonephritis (17%). Only three of 47 patients had diffuse mesangial proliferative glomerulonephritis which, in an age-matched group of women biopsied in this unit, is by far the commonest lesion (table 9-2).

This difference in frequency of focal and segmental lesions in biopsies carried out during pregnancy is better illustrated within one group of patients with glomerulonephritis, namely, those with mesangial IgA nephropathy [90]. Table 9-3 shows that the percentage of biopsies showing focal and segmental lesions is far higher in biopsies carried out in women during or immediately after pregnancy than in other women. Most of these segmental lesions were those of hyalinosis and sclerosis, a relatively infrequent (10%) lesion in nonpregnant women with mesangial IgA nephropathy. This finding suggests that focal and segmental glomerular lesions appear during pregnancy in patients with mesangial IgA nephropathy. We

Table 9-1. Glomerulonephritis in patients presenting with proteinuria in pregnancy [89]

	Number	Percentage
Minimal lesions (previous history available)	4	9
Membranous	9	19
Diffuse proliferative		
Endocapillary	2	4
Mesangial	3	6
Mesangiocapillary	6	13
Focal and segmental		
Proliferative	8	17
Hyalinosis	6	13
Sclerosis	2	4
Other		
Familial	2	4
Lupus	5	11
Total	47	100

Table 9-2. Morphologic classification of women, aged 15–40 years, with glomerulonephritis biopsied 1982–1983

	Number	Percentage
Minimal abnormalities	24	8
Membranous	22	7
Diffuse Proliferative		
Endocapillary	4	1
Mesangial non-IgA	104	32
Mesangial IgA	78	25
Mesangiocapillary	12	4
Focal and Segmental		
Proliferative	2	1
Hyalinosis and sclerosis	17	5
Other		
Familial	3	1
Lupus	50	16
Total	316	100

have also observed this in biopsies performed during pregnancy in other forms of glomerulonephritis (figure 9-6).

The origin of these lesions is uncertain, but they closely resemble "hyaline thrombi" seen in lupus nephritis where they are the result of intravascular coagulation. There is other evidence of activated intravascular coagulation in pregnancy [91–93] and this may well be the result of this. At times these glomerular thrombi seen during pregnancy are frankly fibrinoid.

The course of pregnancy in patients with idiopathic glomerulonephritis is re-

Table 9-3. Focal and segmental hyalinosis and sclerosis in biopsies in women with mesangial IgA nephropathy [90]

	Biopsies during pregnancy and early postpartum Period	Other biopsies
Focal and segmental hyalinosis	8	6
No focal and segmental hyalinosis	4	61
Total	12	67

Chi square = 21.52; $p < 0.005$.

corded in surprisingly small numbers of patients. The three largest series are the 54 patients reported by Katz et al. [94], our own series of 105 patients [75], and the recent study by Surian et al. [95], which included 66 patients with primary glomerulonephritis. The forms of glomerulonephritis in these series are presented in table 9-4, where clearly somewhat different histologic classifications exist, making comparison difficult.

The outcome in pregnancy in these studies is summarized in table 9-5. These studies indicate a higher proportion of patients in our series in whom deterioration in renal function occurred during pregnancy. It is not surprising that the results are different in these studies, since they reflect differences in patient selection. Our patients are largely referred when renal problems arise during pregnancy whereas,

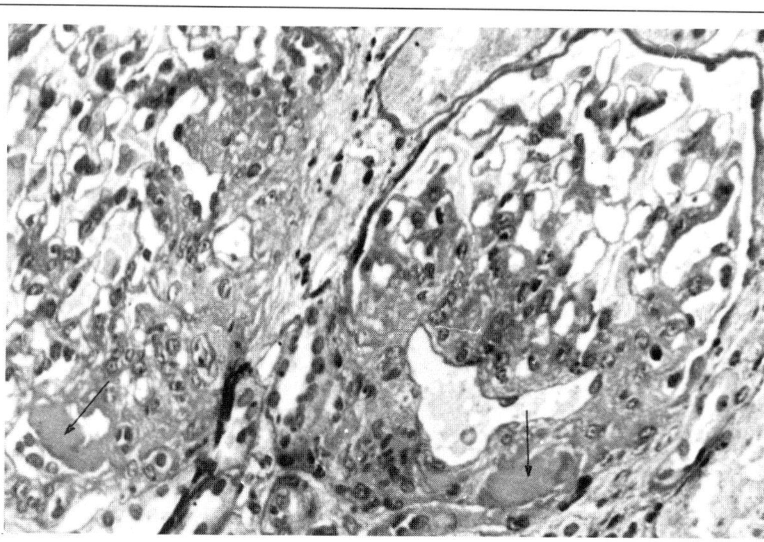

Figure 9-6. Focal and segmental hyalinosis. The lesions of focal and segmental hyalinosis *(arrow)* seen at four months of pregnancy in a woman with underlying membranous glomerulopathy. Such lesions were not seen in a biopsy taken two years before pregnancy and had largely resolved by ten weeks postpartum (PAS).

Table 9-4. Morphologic categories of glomerulonephritis in pregnant women

	Katz et al. [94]		Melbourne [75]	Surian et al. [95]	
Diagnosis	Patients	Pregnancies	Patients	Patients	Pregnancies
Minimal change (lipoid nephrosis, Katz et al.)	3	6	—	2	2
Focal and segmental proliferative (non-IgA) (focal glomerulonephritis, Katz et al.)	12	26	13	—	—
Focal glomerulosclerosis	1	1	—	19	25
Diffuse mesangial proliferative (non-IgA) (diffuse glomerulonephritis, Katz et al.)	26	33	47	—	—
Mesangial IgA	1	1	25	21	29
Membranous	7	10	11	7	8
Mesangiocapillary (membranoproliferative, Katz et al., Surian et al.)					
Type I	3	3	5	14	18
Type II	1	1	4	1	1
Acute glomerulonephritis	—	—	—	2	2
Total	54	81	105	66	85

in the other studies, approximately 30% of patients had known preexisting renal disease. Katz et al. [94] included women who had renal biopsies as a routine follow-up to preeclampsia and in none of the 70 pregnancies in which renal function was measured before conception was the mother's plasma creatinine concentration greater than 124 μmol/liter (1.4 mg/dl). It is likely that our group is biased toward patients with more severe underlying renal disease.

If we extracted the details of the course of pregnancy in the thousands of women with glomerulonephritis who attend our department, we suspect the results would be even better than those recorded by Katz et al. [94]. An example of this is shown in table 9-6 in which we record the details of pregnancies in all women with dense-deposit disease seen in our unit over 20 years. Very few problems arose during pregnancy.

3.2. Systemic lupus erythematosus (SLE)

This increasingly common disease particularly affects young women; hence probably more has been written about pregnancy in lupus than in any other renal condition. Our experience, last summarized over ten years ago [96], is that there is little risk of pregnancy in quiescent lupus, either to the baby or the mother. The corollary is that, if lupus nephritis is adequately managed before patients become pregnant, they do well. On the other hand, pregnancy in the presence of active renal disease is dangerous for both mother and child.

Proteinuria is one of the more common features of SLE, which should be considered if systemic illness, such as joint pains and rashes, or microhematuria and impaired renal function are also found. Diagnosis depends on demonstration of circulating antinuclear antibodies, but a renal biopsy is frequently necessary to determine the severity and nature of the renal lesion, since the glomerular lesions seen in SLE are extremely varied. With treatment, even florid lesions can be healed before or even during pregnancy. High-dose steroids (on the order of 1 mg/kg/day) are the mainstay of treatment, though in exceptional cases we have combined this with plasma exchange, antiplatelet agents, heparin, and cytotoxic agents during pregnancy (figure 9-7).

In the last few years, several large series of patients with SLE and lupus nephropathy in pregnancy have provided valuable information on the effect of SLE on the fetus and the mother [97–103].

3.2.1. Effect of lupus nephropathy on the fetus

The fetal outcomes in four large recent series [97–100] are shown in table 9-7. After exclusion of therapeutic abortion, the fetal survival varies from 74% to 85%. In patients with inactive disease, only a slight reduction in the likelihood of a successful outcome can be shown [97], with fetal survival rates of 88%–100%. However, clinical activity prior to conception results in a decrease in fetal survival to 73%–75% with spontaneous abortion, prematurity, and stillbirth all contributing to poor fetal outcome.

Similarly, diagnosis in pregnancy or the early postpartum period was associated with a reduction in live births in all series, with a successful outcome in 57%–75% of pregnancies.

Some studies have investigated the link between proteinuria, impaired renal function, and fetal loss. Hayslett and Lynn [97] found 50% fetal loss in patients with plasma creatinine levels of 133 μmol/liter (1.5 mg/dl) or more, while Fine et al. [98] reported 46% fetal loss if creatinine clearance was less than 100 ml/min. Fine et al. [98] also found that proteinuria in excess of 300 mg/day was associated with a reduced fetal survival of 62%. Importantly, Hayslett and Lynn [97] separately analyzed patients with heavy proteinuria (> 3.0 g/day) with and without severe renal impairment. There were nine live births among ten nephrotic gravidas with a serum creatinine of 133 μmol/liter (1.5 mg/dl) or less, and only two live births among five uninterrupted pregnancies in patients with nephrotic syndrome and impaired renal function. The authors commented that this was in keeping with previous studies showing a good prognosis for nephrotic syndrome in pregnancy, providing hypertension and renal insufficiency are absent.

Surprisingly, in these large reviews, heart block in the neonate, a known compli-

Table 9-5. Effect of pregnancy on renal function in women with glomerulonephritis

Diagnosis (see Table 9-4)	Katz et al. (1980) [94]			Melbourne (1983) [75]			Surian et al. (1984) [95]		
		Decreased renal function[a]			Decreased renal function[b]			Decreased renal function[c]	
	Total patients	Pregnancy and postpartum	Permanent	Total patients	Pregnancy	Permanent	Total pregnancies	Pregnancy and postpartum	Permanent
Minimal change	3	0	0	—	—	—	2	0	0
Focal and segmental proliferative (non-IgA)	12	2	2	13	4	2 1 transplanted 1 year	—	—	—
Focal glomerulo-sclerosis	1	0	1 ESRF 8 yrs	—	—	—	25	0	0
Diffuse mesangial proliferative (non-IgA)	26	12	5 2 transplanted, 7 mths, 3 yrs	25	5	0	—	—	—

Table 9-5. (continued)

	Katz et al. (1980) [94]			Melbourne (1983) [75]			Surian et al. (1984) [95]		
		Decreased renal function[a]			Decreased renal function[b]			Decreased renal function[c]	
Diagnosis (see Table 9-4)	Total patients	Pregnancy and postpartum	Permanent	Total patients	Pregnancy	Permanent	Total pregnancies	Pregnancy and postpartum	Permanent
Mesangial IgA	1	0	0	24	9	2 both ESRF 8 mths, 4 yrs	29	0	0
Membranous	7	0	0	7	2	2 1 ESRF 5 yrs	8	1	0
Mesangio-capillary	4	1	0	9	3	3 2 died < 3 mths 1 ESRF 8 yrs	19	2	2 1 ESRF < 18 mths
Acute glomerulo-nephritis	—	—	—	—	—	—	2	0	0

[a]BUN $\geq$ 25 mg/dl ($\geq$ 8.92 mmol/liter) or serum creatinine > 1.5 mg/dl (> 133 μmol/liter) or increased 50% or more above prepregnancy in any of these two measurements.
[b]Serum creatinine > 110 μmol/liter (> 1.24 mg/dl) or serum urea > 8.4 mmol/liter (> 50 mg/dl) or a rise during pregnancy of serum creatinine > 20 μmol/liter (> 0.23 mg/dl) or serum urea > 0.5 mmol/liter (> 3 mg/dl).
[c]Increase in serum creatinine of more than 50% over initial value.

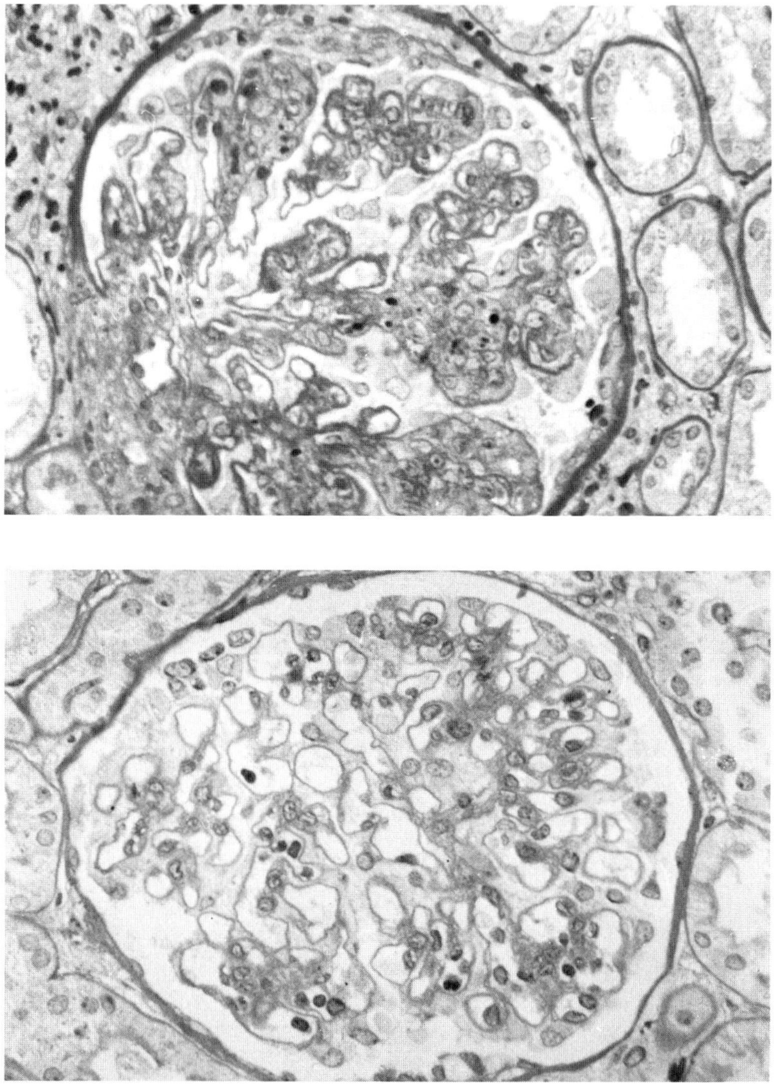

Figure 9-7. Diffuse proliferative lupus glomerulonephritis in pregnancy. **(a)** Severe mixed diffuse proliferative and membranous glomerulonephritis at 26 weeks of pregnancy in a woman with SLE on no treatment for two years. Proteinuria and edema noted at eight weeks. **(b)** Resolution of proliferative changes in repeat biopsy six days after delivery of a live baby at 33 weeks. Treatment had been with high-dose prednisolone, plasma exchange, and antiplatelet agents (PAS).

Table 9-6. Complications of pregnancy in dense-deposit disease [75][a]

Number of pregnancies	Hypertension	Deterioration[b] in function	Increase in[c] plasma urate
14	11/11	0/14	1/14

[a]Seven of our total experience of 16 women with dense-deposit disease experienced 14 pregnancies.
[b]Rise in plasma creatinine to > 110 μmol/liter (> 1.24 mg/dl) or by > 20 μmol/liter (> 0.23 mg/dl).
[c]Rise in plasma urate to > 8.4 mg/dl (> 0.5 mmol/liter).

Table 9-7. Fetal outcome in pregnancy in patients with SLE

			% Fetal survival (therapeutic abortions excluded)				
			Preexisting SLE				
	Pregnancies (patients)	Therapeutic abortions	Overall	Active	Inactive	SLE diagnosed in pregnancy/ postpartum	All patients
Hayslett and Lynn (1980) [97]	65 (47)	11%	76	73	88	63	74
Lieb (1981) [98]	58 (44)	22%	—	—	—	—	78
Jungers et al. (1982) [99]	35 (23)	14%	87	75	100	57	80
Varner et al. (1983) [100]	38 (31)	11%	88	—	—	75	85

cation of SLE [104], was very uncommon. The relationship between abortion and the presence of lupus anticoagulant, which has recently been highlighted [105], was also not revealed. Clearly, further prospective studies into the true incidence of heart block and the relationship between lupus anticoagulant and fetal loss are required.

3.2.2. Effect of pregnancy on SLE

It has long been known that pregnancy is likely to be associated with an exacerbation of SLE and lupus nephropathy. Recent series confirm this. Moreover they correct an earlier impression that the postpartum period was the only time of risk since, in many cases, SLE first became clinically apparent or was increased in activity during pregnancy.

Hayslett and Lynn [97] found that an exacerbation occurred in 32% of pregnancies in SLE begun during clinical remission. Most exacerbations occurred during pregnancy. In patients with clinically active disease during the six months before conception, 48% deteriorated, 40% remained unchanged, and 12% improved. SLE was first diagnosed during pregnancy in a further 19% of their patients. Overall, 48% of pregnancies were associated with clinical deterioration. They commented, however, that in some cases this apparent worsening may have been partly due to increased proteinuria, with the increased GFR of pregnancy.

The Necker Hospital (Paris) group [99] also found a high frequency of disease exacerbation with pregnancy. Worsening occurred in 27% of patients in remission, 47% of patients with disease activity, and 26% of their cases first presented during pregnancy or the postpartum period—remarkably similar figures to those reported by Hayslett and Lynn [97]. Overall, 66% of their patients diagnosed before or related to pregnancy experienced an exacerbation of disease again, most commonly during pregnancy.

The UCLA series [98] highlighted postpartum (24–72 h) exacerbations including skin rash, fever, and arthritis that occurred in 31% of patients not receiving steroids and much less frequently (9.5%) in patients treated during late pregnancy. They therefore endorsed a previous recommendation [106] that high-dose steroids during the delivery and three weeks postpartum are important.

Imbasciati and his group [103] drew attention to acute anuric renal failure occurring after delivery. They reported three healthy women who developed proteinuria and hypertension in late pregnancy, then worsened after delivery with anuria, fever, leukopenia, and thrombocytopenia leading to the diagnosis of SLE. Six of the 19 patients in their series had severe postpartum exacerbations, usually before the diagnosis and effective treatment had been established.

Follow-up of the 47 patients of Hayslett and Lynn [97] over a mean of 8.9 years from the onset of the disease (at a mean age of onset of 20.4 years) revealed only five (10.6%) of the patients either dead or in renal failure. This overall survival compares favorably with other studies of lupus nephropathy, suggesting that pregnancy in most women did not deleteriously affect the overall prognosis.

3.2.3. Summary

Our experience and the picture in the literature is therefore as follows:

1. If good remission of SLE has been achieved for at least six months prior to pregnancy, a successful outcome should result. However, exacerbation during pregnancy is common and requires adequate treatment. In our hands, high-dose steroids, anticoagulation and, in occasional cases, plasma exchange and immunosuppression have been used. The benefits of the treatment outweigh potential disadvantages to the fetus or mother.
2. Pregnancy should be deferred in patients with active disease until good clinical remission has been achieved, since high fetal losses occur in this group. Persistent impairment of renal function (plasma creatinine exceeding 133 μmol/liter (1.5 mg/dl) is indicative of a likely poor fetal and maternal outcome.
3. There is a subgroup of women in whom SLE is first diagnosed in pregnancy. If they are inadequately treated, fetal and maternal survival can be poor. Postpartum exacerbation in inadequately treated cases can be catastrophic.

3.3. Reflux nephropathy

Proteinuria is a common manifestation of this disease in adults, being found in approximately 45% of adult women at presentation [107]. The disorder, alternatively termed chronic atrophic pyelonephritis, is one of the commonest renal diseases in the community, yet few studies have addressed its relationship to pregnancy. Since the underlying abnormality, vesicoureteric reflux, is congenital, the disease always antedates pregnancy; yet nearly 20% of affected women first present with pregnancy-related symptoms, usually urinary infection, proteinuria, or hypertension [107]. It is, in fact, the commonest underlying lesion in patients with bacteriuria in pregnancy [108].

A high proportion of women with reflux nephropathy experience pregnancy-related complications. In our early series of 37 women with the disease [109] who had experienced 85 pregnancies, 59 (69%) of these were complicated, usually by urinary tract infection (UTI), hypertension, proteinuria, or edema.

If hypertension and UTI are controlled adequately, pregnancy has no permanent deleterious effect on the vast majority of patients with this disease.

We have found that, in the presence of impaired renal function, however, pregnancy can lead to acceleration of renal functional deterioration. In a ten-year prospective study of reflux nephropathy in adults [107], we observed six pregnancies extending beyond 12 weeks in women whose plasma creatinine concentration exceeded 200 μmol/liter (2.25 mg/dl). All six experienced rapid renal functional deterioration, despite adequate control of blood pressure, resulting in end-stage renal failure in four within two years of delivery. A similar group of 14 women with plasma creatinine concentrations between 200 and 400 μmol/liter (2.25 and 4.50 mg/dl) experienced slow renal functional decline, with the exception of four patients who developed accelerated hypertension related to noncompliance or loss from follow-up. In the absence of pregnancy or accelerated hypertension, none of ten patients reached end-stage renal failure in less than seven years.

The reason for the deleterious effect is unclear, although there are several possibilities. We have previously suggested that the vascular lesions, such as those which occur in postpartum renal failure and may be seen in preeclampsia [71–75], might contribute to this rapid deterioration. This would help to explain continued deterioration after delivery before such lesions had time to resolve. More recently, it has been suggested that pregnancy might accelerate the focal and segmental glomerular hyalinosis and sclerosis lesions seen in reflux nephropathy [110]. Certainly, acceleration of this lesion may occur in IgA glomerulonephritis [92] and in the primary form of focal glomerular sclerosis [111]. If so, it is possible that the so-called hyperfiltration seen in pregnancy with enhanced renal perfusion and glomerular filtration might contribute.

3.4. Diabetic glomerulosclerosis

Though there are many studies of pregnant diabetics, less is known of the effect of pregnancy on diabetic glomerulopathy. Up to 45% of insulin-dependent diabetics excrete more than normal amounts of albumin in the urine, though this is usually not detectable with routine screening tests [112]. This has been termed microalbuminuria [112, 113] and has been shown to be associated with a 20-fold increased risk of developing diabetic nephropathy [114].

Deckert et al. [115] have proposed that the initial event leading to increased albumin excretion is a reduction in the charge-selective barrier, due to a decrease in glomerular basement membrane sialic acid [116] and heparin sulfate [117]. This is consistent with the finding that reversible microalbuminuria occurs in patients with poor diabetic control [118, 119].

These factors may contribute in part to increased proteinuria in pregnant insulin-dependent diabetics, but renal hemodynamic changes of pregnancy must also be important. The latter are particularly relevant in women with significant diabetic glomerular sclerosis, where the increased glomerular filtration rate may aggravate the "hyperfiltration" already present.

The most comprehensive study on the course of pregnancy in women with clinical diabetic nephropathy is that reported by Kitzmiller et al. [120]. Of the 35 women studied, four had spontaneous abortions and five had elective abortions. In most of the remaining 26 women, proteinuria significantly increased during pregnancy, exceeding 6 g/24 h in 58%; 23 women were followed up after delivery, and proteinuria halved in 64%, remained unchanged in 32%, and increased in 4%. Jovanovic and Peterson [121] found a similar increase in proteinuria during pregnancy in eight women with diabetic nephropathy, though in all the proteinuria returned to prepregnancy levels after delivery.

Kitzmiller's group [120] did not report prepregnancy creatinine clearance levels, but found no deterioration from the first to the third trimester in 16 out of 17 women. A total of 23 women who had continued their pregnancies past weeks 24 were followed up after delivery. Although most had stable renal function, three progressed to severe renal failure within 1–2 years. All three had elected to continue their pregnancy despite hypertension, low creatinine clearance (< 70 ml/min), and azotemia at the onset of gestation. A further two of the six women who aborted early with low creatinine clearance, hypertension, and azotemia progressed to end-stage renal failure within two years. Jovanovic and Peterson [121] reported no decrease in renal function in any of eight women, all of whom had creatinine clearances of 45–70 ml/min prior to pregnancy. It is likely that their plasma creatinine levels would have been close to the normal range.

In neither study did perinatal outcome correlate with severity of proteinuria alone. Kitzmiller et al. [120] found a poorer perinatal outcome, however, when severe proteinuria was associated with hypertension and markedly impaired renal function.

3.5. Polycystic kidney disease

Although this disease is uncommon, it is responsible for 5%–10% of patients entering maintenance dialysis–transplant programs [122, 123] and accordingly has been well studied. Although severe proteinuria is uncommon, trace amounts at least are usually present. The diagnosis can be made easily, even in pregnancy, by abdominal palpation, family history, and finally renal ultrasound revealing multiple bilateral cysts.

Studies of patients with polycystic kidney disease (PCK) suggest that the majority experience few problems, and patients with normal renal function commonly experience several pregnancies before the PCK disease is detected, hence perpetuating this genetic condition. A recent survey by Milutinovic and colleagues [124] retrospectively compared 76 women with PCK with 61 women with a family history of PCK, but normal kidneys. They found no significant impairment of fertility in the PCK group. Not surprisingly, however, patients with PCK were more likely to be hypertensive and to experience complications in pregnancy (37% compared with 13% of controls). Of PCK patients, 32% were hypertensive before or during pregnancy (6% of controls) and, of these, 20% first became hypertensive in the third trimester. Preeclampsia occurred in two (3%) of the PCK patients and none of the controls. No apparent effect of pregnancy on the natural history of PCK was observed, since increased numbers of pregnancies were not associated with a higher incidence of renal failure. It is important to realize that their study group was detected by screening relatives of patients with PCK and no mention is made of renal function at the time of the pregnancies, hence most patients probably had good renal function at the time of the pregnancies.

Since the disease is usually characterized by slow renal functional deterioration, any evidence of rapid deterioration related to pregnancy is of interest. We have reported acceleration of renal functional impairment from a blood urea of 130 mg/dl to 380 mg/dl (217 mmol/liter to 635 mmol/liter) and end-stage renal failure related to pregnancy in a patient with PCK [125]. A survey of the literature reveals only two other patients with PCK and severe renal functional impairment. In the first [126], a patient with a plasma creatinine of 330 μmol/liter (3.73 mg/dl) at week 20 of gestation, delivered a live baby, though creatinine clearance fell from 30 to 20 ml/min and remained at that level four months postpartum. The second patient in the series from Katz and his colleagues [94] had a maximum plasma creatinine of 220 μmol/liter (2.50 mg/dl) at some stage in pregnancy, a postpartum plasma creatinine of 190 μmol/liter (2.15 mg/dl) postpartum, and did not reach end-stage renal failure until six years later.

On such scanty information it is difficult to give any conclusion, but overall it appears that, even in the presence of significant functional impairment, women with PCK usually tolerate pregnancy well.

3.6. Analgesic nephropathy

Analgesic nephropathy usually does not become clinically evident until middle life, hence is uncommonly associated with pregnancy, although we have seen patients presenting with pregnancy-related bacteriuria. Because the analgesics may have other toxic effects on the conceptus, both through direct toxicity and alteration of prostaglandin metabolism, a variety of effects such as infertility, postmaturity, preeclampsia, and congenital abnormality have been described in patients taking excessive quantities.

3.7. Scleroderma

The dramatic adverse effect of pregnancy on renal scleroderma is sufficient to warrant discussion of this rare disease. Johnson and his colleagues [127] reported deterioration in the systemic manifestations of scleroderma in 39% of cases. If renal scleroderma is present, the outlook is even more grave with malignant hypertension and rapid deterioration in renal function usually occurring [128]. The fulminating malignant hypertension that occurs is associated with intrarenal lesions that closely resemble idiopathic postpartum thrombotic microangiopathy. The prognosis is so grave that termination should be considered at the first sign of renal abnormality in pregnant patients with scleroderma.

4. PREGNANCY IN PATIENTS WITH KNOWN RENAL DISEASE

In most cases, renal disease should not be regarded as a contraindication to pregnancy. The general consensus is that, in the absence of hypertension or significant renal functional impairment, pregnancy poses few risks to the mother and only a slight risk to the fetus. However, an occasional woman will follow an unpredictable course during pregnancy and the postpartum period, leading to permanent renal impairment.

The presence of renal functional impairment should be regarded as a major risk factor. In our experience, patients with reflux nephropathy and plasma creatinine concentrations exceeding 200 μmol/liter (2.25 mg/dl) commonly suffer severe renal functional decline during pregnancy and pursue an accelerated postpartum course toward end-stage renal failure. Grossman and colleagues [129] found that 25% of patients with plasma creatinine concentrations exceeding 1.4 mg/dl (124 μmol/liter) suffered an irreversible decline in renal function during pregnancy. On available information it would seem wise, therefore, to give a very guarded prognosis to women with renal functional impairment who wish to become pregnant. Active SLE and scleroderma are two multisystem diseases where pregnancy is contraindicated.

4.1. Management of pregnancy

The vast majority of patients with renal disease who become pregnant have good renal function and are normotensive. They often develop reversible complications during pregnancy, however, and need close observation. Women with impaired renal function and/or poorly controlled hypertension should be advised of the increased risks of fetal loss and possible acceleration of their renal disease. If these women decide to continue with their pregnancy, they need joint supervision by obstetrician and nephrologist. The single most useful measure is the maintenance of good blood pressure control, even if this requires long periods of hospitalization for rest and adjustment of medications. Renal function should be monitored carefully, using plasma urea and creatinine, creatinine clearance, and the plasma uric acid concentration. The latter is an especially needed measurement in pregnancy, since it often rises early in the course of preeclampsia, probably due to enhanced tubular reabsorption. Urine microscopy is repeated frequently in patients with abnormal sediment and, in all patients, urinary protein excretion should be monitored. In patients with renal impairment, anemia can be troublesome and we readily transfuse such patients, keeping the hemoglobin above 10 g/dl.

At some stage during pregnancy the patient may develop worsening blood pressure, proteinuria, and/or rising blood urea, creatinine, and uric acid. Clearly, if the pregnancy has progressed to fetal viability, this constitutes an indication for delivery. The dilemma occurs in patients in whom this syndrome occurs earlier in pregnancy, since it is usually progressive and results in fetal loss.

In patients in whom termination is not to be carried out, we have used systemic heparin therapy [130] and plasma exchange in successful attempts to prolong pregnancy in this situation [131, 132].

5. FOLLOW-UP OF PATIENTS WITH PROTEINURIA IN PREGNANCY

Since the proteinuria and hypertension associated with preeclampsia usually resolve postpartum, it is essential that in all cases adequate postpartum recovery is documented. Should either persist beyond several months, detailed investigation for underlying renal disease is warranted, particularly if further pregnancies are contemplated. Other indications for postpartum investigation include recurrent preeclampsia, early-onset preeclampsia, and persisting abnormalities of the urinary sediment.

In most cases, we defer detailed investigation for approximately six months, presuming there is no postpartum renal functional impairment. This is compatible with the care of the neonate by the mother and also allows substantial resolution of both the pyelographic dilatation seen in pregnancy and the renal biopsy changes attributable to preeclampsia that can cause confusion in diagnosis. We find renal biopsy a good indicator of the likelihood of hypertension in subsequent pregnancies. Prominent vascular lesions are particularly useful in this regard [72, 74].

REFERENCES

1. Kassirer JP, Gennari FJ: Laboratory investigations of renal function. In: Earley LE, Gottschalk CW (eds) Strauss and Welt's diseases of the kidney, 3rd edn. Boston: Little, Brown and Company, 1979, pp 41–92.
2. Heptinstall RH: Pathology of the kidney. Boston: Little, Brown and Company, 1983, pp 17–25.
3. Venkatachalam MA, Rennke HG: The structural and molecular basis of glomerular filtration. Circ Res 43:337–347, 1978.
4. Caulfield JP, Farquhar MG: Loss of anionic sites from the glomerular basement membrane in aminonucleoside nephrosis. Lab Invest 39:505–512, 1978.
5. Michael AF, Blau E, Vernier RL: Glomerular polyanion: alteration in aminonucleoside nephrosis. Lab Invest 23:649–657, 1970.
6. Seiler MW, Rennke HG, Venkatachalam MA, Cotran RS: Pathogenesis of polycation-induced alterations ("fusion") of glomerular epithelium. Lab Invest 36:48–60, 1977.
7. Latta H, Johnston WH, Stanley TM: Sialoglycoproteins and filtration barriers in the glomerular capillary wall. J Ultrastruct Res 51:354–376, 1975.
8. Kanwar YS, Farquhar MG: Anionic sites in the glomerular basement membrane: in vivo and in vitro localization to the laminae rarae by cationic probes. J Cell Biol 81:137–153, 1979.
9. Spiro RG: Studies on the renal glomerular basement membrane: preparation and chemical composition. J Biol Chem 242:1915–1922, 1967.

10. Mohos SC, Skoza L: Glomerular sialoprotein. Science 164:1519–1521, 1969.
11. Brenner BM, Hostetter TH, Humes HD: Molecular basis of proteinuria of glomerular origin. N Engl J Med 298:826–833, 1978.
12. Kanwar YS: Biology of disease: biophysiology of glomerular filtration and proteinuria. Lab Invest 51:7–21, 1984.
13. Graham RC, Karnovsky MJ: Glomerular permeability: ultrastructural cytochemical studies using peroxidases as protein tracers. J Exp Med 124:1123–1133, 1966.
14. Farquhar MG, Wissig SL, Palade GE: Glomerular permeability. I. Ferritin transfer across the normal glomerular capillary wall. J Exp Med 113:47–65, 1961.
15. Venkatachalam MA, Cotran RS, Karnovsky MJ: An ultrastructural study of glomerular permeability in aminonucleoside nephrosis using catalase as a tracer protein. J Exp Med 132:-1168–1180, 1970.
16. Farquhar MG: The primary glomerular filtration barrier: basement membrane or epithelial slits? Kidney Int 8:197–211, 1975.
17. Rennke HG, Cotran RS, Venkatachalam MA: Role of molecular charge in glomerular permeability: tracer studies with cationized ferritins. J Cell Biol 67:638–646, 1975.
18. Cotran RS, Rennke HG: Anionic sites and the mechanisms of proteinuria. N Engl J Med 309:1050–1052, 1983.
19. Pappenheimer JR: Passage of molecules through capillary walls. Physiol Rev 33:387–417, 1953.
20. Chang RLS, Deen WM, Robertson CR, Brenner BM: Permselectivity of the glomerular capillary wall. III. Restricted transport of polyanions. Kidney Int 8:212–218, 1975.
21. Bohrer MP, Baylis C, Humes HD, Glassock RJ, Robertson CR: Permselectivity of the glomerular capillary wall: facilitated filtration of circulating polycations. J Clin Invest 61:72–78, 1978.
22. Chang RLS, Ueki IF, Troy JL, et al.: Permselectivity of the glomerular capillary wall to macromolecules. II. Experimental studies in rats using neutral dextran. Biophys J 15:887–906, 1975.
23. Ryan GB, Karnovsky MJ: Distribution of endogenous albumin in the rat glomerulus: role of hemodynamic factors in glomerular barrier function. Kidney Int 9:36–45, 1976.
24. Dirks JH, Clapp JR, Berliner RW: The protein concentration in the proximal tubule of the dog. J Clin Invest 43:916–921, 1964.
25. Oken DE, Flamenbaum W: Micropuncture studies of proximal tubule albumin concentrations in normal and nephrotic rats. J Clin Invest 50:1498–1505, 1971.
26. Bourdeau JE, Carone FA: Protein handling by the renal tubule. Nephron 13:22–34, 1974.
27. Bourdeau JE, Carone FA, Ganote CE: Serum albumin uptake in isolated perfuse renal tubules: quantitative and electron microscope radioautographic studies in three anatomical segments of the rabbit nephron. J Cell Biol 54:382–398, 1972.
28. Van Liew JB, Buentig W, Stolte H, Boylan JW: Protein excretion: micropuncture study of rat capsular and proximal tubule fluid. Am J Pathol 219:299–305, 1970.
29. Maunsbach AB: Absorption of I^{125}-labelled homologous albumin by rat kidney proximal tubule cells. J Ultrastruct Res 15:197–241, 1966.
30. Tamm I, Horsfall FL: A mucoprotein derived from human urine which reacts with influenza, mumps and Newcastle disease viruses. J Exp Med 95:71–96, 1952.
31. Pollak VE, Arbel C: The distribution of Tamm Horsfall mucoprotein (uromucoid) in the human nephron. Nephron 6:667–672, 1969.
32. Rutecki GJ, Goldsmith C, Schreiner GE: Characterization of proteins in urinary casts. N Engl J Med 284:1049–1052, 1971.
33. McQueen EG: The nature of urinary casts. J Clin Pathol 15:367–373, 1962.
34. McKenzie JK, Patel R, McQueen EG: The excretion rate of Tamm-Horsfall urinary mucoprotein in normals and in patients with renal disease. Aust Ann Med 13:32–39, 1964.
35. Blainey JD, Brewer DB, Hardwicke J, Soothill JF: The nephrotic syndrome. Q J Med [New Ser] 29:235–251, 1960.
36. Joachim GR, Cameron JS, Schwartz M, Becker EL: Selectivity of protein excretion in patients with the nephrotic syndrome. J Clin Invest 43:2332–2346, 1964.
37. Kelley VE, Cavallo T: Glomerular permeability: transfer of native ferritin in glomeruli with decreased anionic sites. Lab Invest 39:547–553, 1978.
38. Barnes JL, Radnik RA, Gilchrist EP, Venkatachalam MA: Size and charge selective permeability defects induced in glomerular basement membrane by a polycation. Kidney Int 25:11–19, 1984.

39. Hunsicker LG, Shearer TP, Shaffer SJ: Acute reversible proteinuria induced by infusion of the polycation hexadimethrine. Kidney Int 20:7–17, 1981.
40. Border WA, Ward HJ, Kamil ES, Cohen AH: Induction of membranous nephropathy in rabbits by administration of an exogenous cationic antigen. J Clin Invest 69:451–461, 1982.
41. Blau EB, Haas JE: Glomerular sialic acid and proteinuria in human renal disease. Lab Invest 28:447–481, 1973.
42. Editorial: Charge and the kidney. Lancet 2:732, 1984.
43. Davison JM: The kidney in pregnancy: a review. J R Soc Med 76:485–501, 1983.
44. Abuelo JG: Proteinuria: diagnostic principles and procedures. Ann Intern Med 98:186–190, 1983.
45. Kark RM, Lawrence JR, Pollak VE, et al.: A primer of urinalysis, 2nd edn. New York: Harper and Row, 1963.
46. Barratt M: Proteinuria. Br Med J 287:1489–1490, 1983.
47. Bright R: Report of medical cases, vol 1. London: Longmans Green, 1827.
48. Lever JCW: Guy's Hospital reports 495, 1843.
49. Simpson JY: London Edinburgh J Med Sci 1015, 1843.
50. Fisher KA, Luger A, Spargo BH, Lindheimer MD: Hypertension in pregnancy: clinical–pathological correlations and remote prognosis. Medicine (Baltimore) 60:267–287, 1981.
51. Ihle BU, Long P, Oats J: Renal disease and preeclampsia (PET) [abstr]. In: Proceedings of the 4th world congress, International Society for the Study of Hypertension in Pregnancy, 1984, p 76.
52. Studd J: The origin and effects of proteinuria in pregnancy. J Obstet Gynaecol Br Commonw 80:872–883, 1973.
53. MacLean PR, Paterson WG, Smart GE, et al.: Proteinuria in toxaemia and abruptio placentae. J Obstet Gynaecol Br Commonw 79:321–326, 1972.
54. Simanowitz MD, MacGregor WG, Hobbs JR: Proteinuria in preeclampsia. J Obstet Gynaecol Br Commonw 80:103–108, 1973.
55. Robson JS: Proteinuria and the renal lesion in preeclampsia and abruptio placantae. In: Lindheimer MD, Katz AI, Zuspan FP (eds) Hypertension in pregnancy. New York: John Wiley and Sons, 1976, pp 61–73.
56. Wood SM, Burnett D, Studd J: Selectivity of proteinuria during pregnancy assessed by different methods. In: Lindheimer MD, Katz AI, Zuspan FP (eds) Hypertension in pregnancy. New York: John Wiley and Sons, 1976, pp 75–83.
57. Lorincz AB, McCartney CP, Pottinger RE, Li KH: Protein excretion patterns in pregnancy. Am J Obstet Gynecol 82:252–259, 1961.
58. Gant NF, Worley RJ, Everett RB, MacDonald PC: Control of vascular responsiveness during human pregnancy. Kidney Int 18:253–258, 1980.
59. Fisher A, Ahuja S, Luger A, Spargo BH, Lindheimer MD: Nephrotic proteinuria with preeclampsia. Am J Obstet Gynecol 129:643–646, 1977.
60. Studd JW, Blainey JD: Pregnancy and the nephrotic syndrome. Br Med J 1:276–280, 1969.
61. First MR, Ooi BS, Jao W, Pollak VE: Pre-eclampsia with the nephrotic syndrome. Kidney Int 13:166–177, 1978.
62. Studd JWW, Blainey JD, Bailey DE: Serum protein changes in the pre-eclampsia–eclampsia syndrome. J Obstet Gynaecol Br Commonw 77:796–801, 1970.
63. Chesley LC: The variability of proteinuria in the hypertensive complications of pregnancy. J Clin Invest 18:617–620, 1939.
64. Lindheimer MD, Katz AI: Kidney function and disease in pregnancy. Philadelphia: Lea and Febiger, 1977, p 102.
65. Chesley LC: Hypertensive disorders in pregnancy. New York: Appleton-Century-Crofts, 1978.
66. McEwan HP: Investigation of proteinuria in pregnancy by immunoelectropheresis. J Obstet Gynaecol Br Commonw 75:289–294, 1968.
67. De Alvarez RR: Proteinuria relationships. Prog Clin Biol Res 7:169–191, 1976.
68. Friedman EA, Fox BH: Evaluation of criteria. Prog Clin Biol Res 7:215–247, 1976.
69. Studd JWW, Shaw RW, Bailey DE: Maternal and fetal serum protein concentration in normal pregnancy and pregnancy complicated by proteinuric pre-eclampsia. Am J Obstet Gynecol 114:582–588, 1972.
70. Fairley KF, Birch DF: Hematuria: a simple method for identifying glomerular bleeding. Kidney Int 21:105–108, 1982.
71. Kincaid-Smith P: The similarity of lesions and underlying mechanism in pre-eclamptic toxaemia

and post-partum renal failure. In: Kincaid-Smith P, Mathew TH, Becker EL (eds) Glomerulonephritis. New York: John Wiley and Sons, 1973.
72. Kincaid-Smith P: The kidney: a clinicopathological study. Oxford: Blackwell, 1975.
73. Kincaid-Smith P: Participation of intravascular coagulation in the pathogenesis of glomerular and vascular lesions. Kidney Int 7:242–253, 1975.
74. Kincaid-Smith P: Modifications in glomeruli and arterioles in pregnancy and the post-partum period. In: Sammour MB, Symonds EM, Zuspan FP, El-Tomi N (eds) Pregnancy hypertension. Cairo: Ain Shams University Press, 1982, pp 333–338.
75. Kincaid-Smith P: The kidney in pregnancy. In: Becker GJ, Atkins RC, Kincaid-Smith P (eds) Proceedings of the 2nd Asian Pacific Congress of Nephrology, Melbourne, 1983. Maryborough, Australia: Dominion Press–Hedges and Bell, 1984, pp 228–236.
76. Spargo BH, Seymour AE, Ordonez NG: Renal biopsy pathology with diagnostic and therapeutic implications. New York: John Wiley and Sons, 1980, pp 316–328.
77. Churgh J, Sobin LH: Renal disease: classification and atlas of glomerular diseases. Tokyo: Igaku-Shoin, 1982.
78. Sheehan HL: Renal morphology in pre-eclampsia. Kidney Int 18:241–252, 1980.
79. Spargo B, McCartney CP, Winemiller R: Glomerular capillary endotheliosis in toxemia of pregnancy. Arch Pathol 68:593, 1959.
80. Spargo B, Lichtig C, Luger AM, Katz AI, Lindheimer MD: The renal lesion in pre-eclampsia. In: Lindheimer MD, Katz AI, Zuspan FP (eds) Hypertension in pregnancy. New York: John Wiley and Sons, 1976, pp 129–138.
81. Ryan GB, Coghlan JP, Scoggins BA: The granulated peripolar epithelial cell: a potential secretory component of the renal juxtaglomerular complex. Nature 277:655–656, 1979.
82. Hill PA, Coghlan JP, Scoggins BA, Ryan GB: Ultrastructural changes in the sheep renal juxtaglomerular apparatus in response to sodium depletion or loading. Pathology 15:463–473, 1983.
83. Vollman RF: Study design, population and data characteristics. Prog Clin Biol Res 7:89–121, 1976.
84. Friedman EA, Neff RK: Pregnancy outcome as related to hypertension, edema and proteinuria. In: Lindheimer MD, Katz AI, Zuspan FP (eds) Hypertension in pregnancy. New York: John Wiley and Son, 1976, pp 13–22.
85. Lin CC, Lindheimer MD, River P, Moawad AH: Fetal outcome in hypertensive disorders of pregnancy. Am J Obstet Gynecol 142:255–260, 1982.
86. Fairley KF, Birch DF: Unpublished observations.
87. Lim CH, Woo KT, Pwee HS, Edmondson RPS, Chiang GSC: The results of screening for proteinuria and microscopic haematuria in 16 year old National Service registrants. In: Becker GJ, Atkins RC, Kincaid-Smith P (eds) Proceedings of the 2nd Asian Pacific Congress of Nephrology, Melbourne, 1983. Maryborough, Australia: Dominion Press–Hedges and Bell, 1984, pp 175–182.
88. Lindheimer MD, Fisher KA, Spargo BH, Katz AI: Hypertension in pregnancy: a biopsy study with long-term follow-up. Contrib Nephrol 25:71–77, 1981.
89. Kincaid-Smith P, Fairley KF: The differential diagnosis between pre-eclamptic toxaemia and glomerulonephritis in patients with proteinuria during pregnancy. In: Lindheimer MD, Katz AI, Zuspan FP (eds) Hypertension in pregnancy. New York: John Wiley and Sons, 1976, pp 157–168.
90. Whitworth ja, Kincaid-Smith P, Fairley KF: The outcome of pregnancy in mesangial IgA nephropathy. In: Proceedings of the 2nd Congress of International Society for Study of Hypertension in Pregnancy. Cairo: Ain Shams University Press, 1982, pp 403–408.
91. McKay DG: Chronic intravascular coagulation in normal pregnancy and pre-eclampsia. Contrib Nephrol 25:108–119, 1981.
92. Thorburn J, Drummond MM, Whigham KA, et al.: Blood viscosity and haemostatic factors in late pregnancy, pre-eclampsia and fetal growth retardation. Br J Obstet Gynaecol 89:117–122, 1982.
93. Prentice CRM: Coagulopathy of pre-eclampsia. In: Lewis PJ (ed) Prostacyclin in pregnancy. New York: Raven, 1983, pp 175–181.
94. Katz AI, Davison JM, Hayslett JP, Singson E, Lindheimer MD: Pregnancy in women with kidney disease. Kidney Int 18:192–206, 1980.
95. Surian M, Imbasciati E, Cosci P, et al.: Glomerular disease and pregnancy: a study of 123

pregnancies in patients with primary and secondary glomerular diseases. Nephron 36:101–105, 1984.
96. Fairley KF, Whitworth JA, Kincaid-Smith P: Glomerulonephritis and pregnancy. In: Kincaid-Smith P, Mathew TH, Becker EL (eds) Glomerulonephritis: morphology, natural history and treatment. New York: John Wiley and Sons, 1973, pp 997–1011.
97. Hayslett JP, Lynn RI: Effect of pregnancy in patients with lupus nephropathy. Kidney Int 18:207–220, 1980.
98. Fine LG, Barnett EV, Danovitch M, Nissenson AR, et al.: Systemic lupus erythematosus in pregnancy. Ann Intern Med 94:667–677, 1981.
99. Jungers P, Dougados M, Pelissier C, et al.: Lupus nephropathy and pregnancy. Arch Intern Med 142:771–776, 1982.
100. Varner MW, Meehan RT, Syrop CH, et al.: Pregnancy in patients with systemic lupus erythematosus. Am J Obstet Gynecol 145:1025–1040, 1983.
101. Zulman JI, Talal N, Hoffman GS, Epstein WV: Problems associated with the management of pregnancies in patients with systemic lupus erythematosus. J Rheumatol 7:37–49, 1980.
102. Houser MT, Fish AJ, Tagatz GE, et al.: Pregnancy and systemic lupus erythematosus. Am J Obstet Gynecol 138:409–413, 1980.
103. Imbasciati E, Surian M, Bottino S, et al.: Lupus nephropathy and pregnancy: a study of 26 pregnancies in patients with systemic lupus erythematosus and nephritis. Nephron 36:46–51, 1984.
104. Chameides L, Truex KC, Vetter V, et al.: Association of maternal systemic lupus erythematosus with congenital complete heart block. N Engl J Med 297:1204–1207, 1977.
105. Hughes GRV: Thrombosis, abortion, cerebral disease and lupus anticoagulant. Br Med J 27:1088, 1983.
106. McGee CD, Makowski EL: Systemic lupus erythematosus in pregnancy. Obstet Gynecol 107:1008–1012, 1970.
107. Kincaid-Smith PS, Bastos M, Becker GJ: Reflux nephropathy in the adult. Contrib Nephrol 39:94–101, 1984.
108. Kincaid-Smith P, Bullen M: Bacteriuria in pregnancy. Lancet 1:7382–7399, 1965.
109. Kincaid-Smith P, Becker GJ: Reflux nephropathy in the adult. In: Hodson J, Kincaid-Smith P (eds) Reflux nephropathy. New York: Masson, 1979, pp 21–28.
110. Brown RS: Case 18-1984. N Engl J Med 310:1176–1181, 1984.
111. Taylor J, Novak R, Christiansen R, Sorensen ET: Focal sclerosing glomerulopathy with adverse effects during pregnancy. Arch Intern Med 158:1695–1696, 1978.
112. Viberti GC, Wiseman M, Redmond S: Microalbuminuria: its history and potential for prevention of clinical nephropathy in diabetes mellitus. Diabetic Nephropathol 3:79–82, 1984.
113. Viberti GC, Mackintosh D, Bilous RW, Pickup JC, Keen H: Proteinuria in diabetes mellitus: role of spontaneous and experimental variation of glycemia. Kidney Int 21:714–720, 1982.
114. Viberti GC, Jarratt RJ, Mahmud U, Hill RD, Argyropoulos A, Keen H: Microalbuminuria as a predictor of clinical nephropathy in insulin-dependent diabetes mellitus. Lancet 1:1430–1432, 1982.
115. Deckert T, Feldt-Rasmussen B, Mathiesen ER, Baker L: Pathogenesis of incipient nephropathy: a hypothesis. Diabetic Nephropathol 3:83–88, 1984.
116. Wahl P, Deppermann D, Hasslacher C: Biochemistry of glomerular basement membrane of the normal and diabetic human. Kidney Int 21:744–749, 1982.
117. Parthasarathy N, Spiro RG: Effect of diabetes on the glycosaminoglycan component of the human glomerular basement membrane. Diabetes 31:738, 1982.
118. Morgensen CE: Urinary albumin excretion in early and long-term juvenile diabetes. Scand J Clin Lab Invest 28:183–187, 1971.
119. Parving H-H, Noer I, Deckert T, et al.: The effect of metabolic regulation on microvascular permeability to small and large molecules in short-term juvenile diabetics. Diabetologia 12:-161–166, 1976.
120. Kitzmiller JL, Brown ER, Phillippe M, et al.: Diabetic nephropathy and perinatal outcome. Am J Obstet Gynecol 141:741–750, 1981.
121. Jovanovic L, Peterson CM: Is pregnancy contraindicated in women with diabetes mellitus. Diabetic Nephropathol 3:36–38, 1984.
122. Disney APS (ed): Seventh report of the Australian and New Zealand Transplant Registry, 1984.
123. Wing AJ, Boyer M, Brunner FP, et al.: Combined report on regular dialysis and transplantation

in Europe, XIII, 1982. In: Davison AM, Guillou PJ (eds) Proc EDTA–ERA. London: Pitman, 1983.
124. Milutinovic J, Fialkow PJ, Agoda LY, et al.: Fertility and pregnancy complications in women with autosomal dominant polycystic kidney disease. Obstet Gynecol 61:566–570, 1983.
125. Kincaid-Smith P, Fairley KF, Bullen M: Kidney disease and pregnancy. Lancet 2:1155–1159, 1967.
126. Katz M, Guagliorello J, Young BK: Severe polycystic kidney disease in pregnancy. Obstet Gynecol 53:119–123, 1979.
127. Johnson TR, Banner EA, Winkelman RK: Scleroderma and pregnancy. Obstet Gynecol 23:-467–469, 1964.
128. Karlen JR, Cook WA: Renal scleroderma and pregnancy. Obstet Gynecol 44:349–354, 1974.
129. Grossman SD, Madias NE, Sou SM: Pregnancy in women with moderate renal insufficiency [abstr]. Kidney Int 25:166, 1984.
130. Fairley KF, Adey FD, Ross IC, Kincaid-Smith P: Heparin treatment in severe pre-eclampsia and glomerulonephritis in pregnancy. In: Lindheimer MD, Katz AI, Zuspan FP (eds) Hypertension in pregnancy. New York: John Wiley and Sons, 1979, pp 103–112.
131. d'Apice AJF, Reti LL, Pepperell RJ, Fairley KF, Kincaid-Smith P: Treatment of severe pre-eclampsia by plasma exchange. Aust NZ J Obstet Gynaecol 20:231–235, 1980.
132. Becker GJ, Ihle B, Fairley K, d'Apice AJF, Kincaid-Smith P: Plasma exchange in pregnancy complicated by renal failure due to reflux nephropathy [abstr]. In: Proceedings of the 4th world congress, International Society for Study of Hypertension in Pregnancy, 1984, p 200.

10. ACUTE RENAL FAILURE IN PREGNANCY

NATHALIE PERTUISET, DOMINIQUE GANEVAL, and JEAN-PIERRE GRÜNFELD

1. INTRODUCTION

In the 1960s, obstetric acute renal failure (ARF) accounted for a substantial percentage of all cases of ARF, but there is compelling evidence that the incidence and the severity of pregnancy-related ARF have been declining steadily in industrialized countries during the last decade. This decline certainly reflects both the virtual disappearance of septic abortion and the improvement of prenatal care. In contrast, in nonindustrialized countries, both the incidence and the severity of ARF in pregnancy are still high. This chapter reviews the frequency of ARF in pregnancy, as well as clinical and pathophysiologic aspects of its causes and management, including the recently described, severe idiopathic postpartum renal failure, which is still poorly understood.

2. INCIDENCE

Estimates of the incidence of ARF in pregnancy in the 1960s were one case per 1400 [1] to 5000 deliveries [2]. At that time, ARF complicating pregnancy represented as much as 24%–40% of all cases of ARF [3, 4]. In recent years, a dramatic decrease in the incidence of ARF in pregnancy has been observed in industrialized countries. Pregnancy-related cases accounted for only 4.5% of all cases recorded in the last decade by Chapman and Legrain in France [4]. Similarly, Lindheimer et al. [5] reported that, in over 20,000 deliveries from 1973 to 1983, no patient has required dialysis. From their experience and that of others, they estimate that the current incidence of ARF in pregnancy is less than one case per 10,000 in Western countries [5]. Thus, the incidence of severe ARF requiring dialysis during pregnancy does not currently seem to be very different from that found in the general population, where it is estimated to be about 30 per million in Western European countries [6]. Gravidas should not be considered as a group more at risk for ARF than nonpregnant women. The marked decline of pregnancy-related ARF in most developed countries may be attributed to liberalized abortion laws and to better prenatal care. In developing countries, however, obstetric ARF still has a high incidence, reaching 22% in northern India [7].

The frequency distribution of ARF in relation to the duration of pregnancy is bimodal with two peaks at the end of the first and the third trimesters, respectively [8]. The former occurs at week 16 and is (or was) mainly due to septic abortion, whereas the latter, which occurs at week 38, has several causes, including primarily eclampsia and uterine bleeding. In the 1960s, Smith et al. [8], in their analysis of 70 obstetric patients with ARF, noted that the first trimestrial peak accounted for 60% of all obstetric ARF and the later for the remaining 40% [8]. In industrialized countries, however, these percentages have now changed: the number of cases of postabortum ARF have declined while those occurring in late pregnancy have risen. In addition, in last decade, attention has been focused on a third group of patients who suffer rare idiopathic postpartum renal failure one day to 12 weeks after delivery.

3. PROGNOSIS

The low mortality rate in pregnancy-related ARF as compared with nonobstetric ARF has been emphasized in most series. The average maternal mortality in 25 series published between 1950 and 1979 and reviewed by Finn [9] has been estimated as 16.8% with no difference between the first and the last decades of the study. Nevertheless, such mortality remains unacceptable if one considers the young age of this previously healthy population. In addition, the high risk of chronic renal failure due to the high incidence of bilateral renal cortical necrosis (BRCN) among the survivors must also be underlined. Recent data, however, from the National Maternity Hospital in Dublin showed a decline in the incidence of both abruptio placentae and BRCN during the past decade in pregnant women [10]. Acute cortical necrosis was observed in only one among 80,000 deliveries between 1971 and 1980 compared with 1 in 10,000 deliveries between 1961 and 1970 [10]. None of the patients died [10]. On the other hand, idiopathic postpartum renal failure, which often leads to irreversible renal failure, has been recognized by Robson et al. [11]. In obstetric ARF as a whole, the mortality rate is higher for the fetus than for the mother, with a high incidence of abortion and stillbirth. For example, among 52 cases of prepartum ARF referred to Necker Hospital in Paris from 1957 to 1979, there were 24 fetal deaths and six maternal deaths [12].

4. EFFECTS OF NORMAL GESTATION ON THE KIDNEY AND THE COAGULATION SYSTEM

Pregnancy is accompanied by morphologic and functional changes in the urinary system, by significant and complex alterations in volume homeostasis and by coagulation disorders. A substantial number of these changes should protect pregnant woman from ARF, whereas others may be predisposing. These alterations may influence the susceptibility to and the severity of acute renal failure in pregnancy and are of interest for our understanding of the pathogenesis and for the management of pregnancy-related ARF.

4.1. Renal morphologic and physiologic changes

The kidneys enlarge during pregnancy, probably due to increase in both vascular volume and interstitial space. Major morphologic changes involve the calices, renal pelves, and ureters. These structures undergo dilation and their peristaltic activity decreases as early as the third gestational month. Ureteral dilation has been attributed by some investigators to hormonal effects on smooth muscle while others regard mechanical obstruction as the major cause [13]. These alterations leading to urinary stasis may contribute to the propensity of pregnant women to develop upper urinary tract infection. Obstructive ARF secondary to enlarged uterus has also been reported in normal pregnancy. Renal hemodynamic changes begin shortly after conception. Both glomerular filtration rate (GFR) and renal blood flow increase from 30% to 50% above nonpregnant values [13]. These changes may protect gravidas against ARF. In certain experimental ARF, however, reduction of renal blood flow does not always appear as the primary event [14].

4.2. Volume homeostasis

In normal pregnancy, total body water increases from 6 to 8 liters. There is gradual accumulation of salt and water with expansion of both plasma and interstitial fluid volume. This "physiologic hypervolemia" may afford protection against ARF. Indeed, several investigators have shown that the severity of experimentally induced ARF in nonpregnant animals can be attenuated by the chronic ingestion of a high sodium chloride diet [14]. This protection, however, appears to be related to enhanced natriuresis rather than to chronic volume expansion. Bidani et al. [15], who examined the effects of volume expansion during pregnancy on the severity of glycerol-induced myoglobinuric ARF in rats, observed a decrease in the severity of ARF during the week 3 of gestation. In addition, earlier in pregnancy a greater protection against ARF was obtained by saline intake. These investigators suggested that protection resulting from saline intake may be independent of the degree of volume expansion, but may depend on the associated sustained natriuresis in the early stage of glycerol-induced myoglobinuric ARF [15]. These alterations in volume homeostasis during pregnancy are accompanied by a resetting of volume and osmolarity controls, and healthy pregnant women respond appropriately to volume manipulation.

Changes in various hormonal systems that influence renal hemodynamics and control salt and water balance have also been observed. Circulating levels of renin, angiotensin II, and aldosterone are elevated and vessels become refractory to the pressor action of angiotensin II. These alterations may affect the susceptibility of pregnant women to ARF. There are not, however, sufficient data to invoke a definite pathogenic role for the renin–angiotensin system in ARF. It has been suggested that renal vascular angiotensin-II receptors differ from systemic vascular angiotensin-II receptors. The results obtained by Sicinska et al. [16] are relevant in this regard. They have shown that angiotensin-II administration lowered GFR in late pregnant, but not in virgin rats. In addition, angiotensin II produced a smaller increase in blood pressure in pregnant than in virgin rats [16]. These results suggested a hyperreactivity of the glomerular vessels for angiotensin II during pregnancy. In addition, Collins and Baylis [17] have recently found that angiotensin II does not influence blood pressure and renal hemodynamics in unstressed pregnant rats, though in anesthetized pregnant rats angiotensin II exerts a net influence on renal hemodynamics [17]. There is also evidence that vasodilator prostaglandins increase during pregnancy, but their role in the pathophysiology of acute renal failure has not yet been evaluated clearly.

Water volume is disturbed in preeclamptic women who have a significant decrease in plasma volume compared with healthy pregnant women, and normal responses to volume and sodium manipulation are altered. Vascular sensitivity to angiotensin II is increased and there is a decrease of both plasma levels of angiotensin II and vasodilatator prostaglandins. These various alterations may predispose preeclamptic women to ARF.

4.3. Coagulation system disorders

Normal pregnancy is associated with an enhanced capacity to produce fibrin due to increased levels of factors VII, VIII, and X, and of plasma fibrinogen, whereas fibrinolytic activity is decreased until about 1 h after placental delivery. In addition, a decreased level of antithrombin III during pregnancy and parturition has been reported [18]. These coagulation disorders are observed especially in complicated pregnancy and may predispose pregnant women to ARF. Alterations in clotting factors consistent with disseminated intravascular coagulation (DIC) have been found in septic abortion, abruptio placentae, prolonged intrauterine death, and severe preeclampsia. Coagulation abnormalities may contribute to the propensity of pregnant women to develop BRCN in certain obstetric complications. In addition, the relationship of pregnancy to the experimental generalized Shwartzman reaction is of interest. It is well known that only one injection of endotoxin can produce a typical generalized Shwartzman reaction (with renal cortical necrosis) in pregnant rabbits and ten-day postpartum rats [19], whereas two properly spaced injections are required in nonpregnant animals. In most studies, however, DIC do not appear to be the primary event in pregnancy-related ARF. Conger et al. [19] have shown that, after a single endotoxin injection in ten-day postpartum rats, the decrease in single nephron glomerular filtration rate results from a decrease in both glomerular plasma flow and capillary pressure that precedes fibrin occlusion of vessels. Raij et al. [20] demonstrated that the initial event of BRCN during the Shwartzman reaction is a specific and local effect of endotoxin on the vascular endothelium. This finding supports the hypothesis of thrombi formation in areas of endothelium damage.

5. RENAL FAILURE IN SEPTIC ABORTION

The dramatic decrease in the incidence of obstetric ARF in industrialized countries mainly reflects the virtual disappearance of postabortum ARF. In France, septic abortion was a major cause of acute tubular necrosis (ATN) 20 years ago, but has declined since 1970. Kleinknecht et al. [21], in a series of 950 patients with ARF admitted to their unit, observed only one case of postabortum ARF, representing an incidence of 0.06%. No case of postabortum ARF has been observed at Necker Hospital since 1978. In contrast, in less developed countries, ARF due to septic abortion represents a substantial proportion of obstetric ARF. In their series in India, Chugh et al. [7] reported that, among 72 patients referred to their dialysis unit for obstetric ARF, 43 cases (59.7%) were related to septic abortion.

In most cases, abortion is deliberate. Initial symptoms (fever, vomiting, diarrhea, and generalized myalgias) appear suddenly a few hours to two days after the attempted abortion. They are rapidly accompanied by hypotension and signs of shock. Jaundice is often present. In severe cases, skin necrosis of the extremities has been described. Hemolytic anemia with indirect hyperbilirubinemia and hemoglobinuria, leukocytosis and thrombocytopenia, and clotting-test abnormalities suggestive of DIC are often found. Sepsis is primarily due to gram-negative bacteria such as *Escherichia coli.* Clostridial infection is now less common but, when present, usually leads to severe ARF. Bacterial identification may be difficult. Blood cultures are negative in about 80% of the cases and cultures from the uterus are positive in only half of the patients [5]. The oliguric or anuric phase of ARF generally persists for two or three weeks. The mortality rate in developed countries is approximately 10%. In nonindustrialized countries such as India, however, it remains as high as 47.5% [7]. Death usually occurs early in the course and appears to be primarily due to septic complications rather than to a direct result of ARF. In most patients who survive, renal function rapidly returns to normal. The incidence of BRCN in patients with postabortion ARF is low in most series. None of the 52 postabortum ARF patients reported from Hammersmith Hospital (London) had BRCN [8]; similarly, the incidence of BRCN during early pregnancy was only 1.5% at Necker Hospital [22]. In contrast, Chugh et al. [23] observed an incidence of BRCN as high as 39% among patients with postabortion ARF.

Septicemia and septic shock leading to postischemic ARF are the most common pathogenic factors in postabortum ARF. Intravascular hemolysis with hemoglobinuria and/or myonecrosis with myoglobinuria are often present in patients with clostridial infection. DIC is commonly found. The nephrotoxicity of abortifacient chemicals such as phenols and soaps often used in induced abortion has been emphasized. In addition, these substances may induce marked hemolysis.

Initial management should include intensive supportive therapy for shock, immediate use of antibiotics, and dialysis. Uterine evacuation may be necessary because of incomplete abortion. In the 1960s, many investigators advocated early abdominal hysterectomy [24]. More recently, Hawkins and colleagues [25] obtained a favorable outcome with normal renal function recovery in 17 out of 19 patients managed with intensive antibiotic therapy, peritoneal dialysis, and avoidance of surgical procedures. Indeed, modern antibiotic therapy usually eradicates infection from the uterus and prevents bacterial passage into the maternal circulation. Nevertheless, hysterectomy may be indicated in patients with necrotic uterine lesions that accompany abortion induced by chemicals and in the rare patients with uncontrolled uterine sepsis. There are no convincing data for the efficacy of exchange transfusions and hyperbaric oxygen therapy in clostridial infection.

6. RENAL FAILURE IN ACUTE PYELONEPHRITIS

Acute pyelonephritis is one of the most serious and common medical complications of pregnancy, affecting 1%–2% of all pregnant women [26, 27]. Several cases of ARF associated with acute pyelonephritis have been reported [12], and it is currently stated that pregnant women with such infection are more prone to develop ARF than are nongravid women. However, the frequency of severe ARF occurring in this setting seems low. Volume depression from vomiting and septicemia are probably the most important etiologic factors of ARF associated with pyelonephritis. In addition, acute pyelonephritis per se has an adverse effect on renal function in gravidas, whereas it does not alter renal function in nongravid patients. For instance, Whalley et al. [28], in an analysis of 130 gravidas with acute pyelonephritis, found a transient but marked decrease of glomerular filtration rate in about 20% of the cases. These authors postulated that the deleterious effect on renal function was related to an increased sensitivity of the renal vessels of gravidas to the vasoactive effect of bacterial endotoxins. Urinary stasis is probably another contributing factor to this detrimental effect.

Although acute pyelonephritis rarely leads to ARF in pregnancy, the severity of this complication with frequent fetal death has been underlined in the earlier literature. Hospitalization and prompt and vigorous treatment with antibiotics and intravenous fluids should particularly prevent volume depletion and septic shock. Subsequently, close surveillance for reinfection is recommended because of the frequent recurrence of infection. Finally, attention should be paid to the treatment of asymptomatic bacteriuria since, according to Whalley et al. [29], this may prevent 80% of antepartum pyelonephritis.

7. RENAL FAILURE DUE TO VOLUME CONTRACTION

7.1. Uterine hemorrhage

In late pregnancy, ARF frequently results from hemorrhagic complications. Ante- and postpartum hemorrhage were the major cause of ARF in late pregnancy in 16% of the cases in the series reported by Kennedy et al. [3], and in 7% of our own patients [12]. Severe uterine bleeding was noted as a precipitating factor in

59% of the cases in the study by Smith et al. [8]. Chugh et al. [7] considered blood loss as a contributing factor in 79% of their obstetric ARF cases. Diagnosis of antepartum hemorrhage may be difficult, and the severity of the bleeding may be underestimated since it is often not externally obvious. The propensity of toxemic women to develop hemorrhagic complications has long been emphasized. It has also been suggested that their renal sensitivity to blood loss is higher than that of normal gravidas. Thus, uterine hemorrhage may contribute to the development of ARF in such gravidas. For example, it was a precipitating factor of ARF in 68% of pregnant women with hypertension (or preeclamptic women) in one large series [8]. Both acute tubular necrosis and BRCN may complicate uterine hemorrhage. However, BRCN occurs primarily in preeclamptic women and in gravidas with abruptio placentae and severe coagulation disturbances. In such patients, early and adequate blood transfusion should prevent the renal functional shutdown.

7.2. Volume depletion secondary to sodium and water loss

Pernicious vomiting during pregnancy may lead to severe volume depletion and to either severe prerenal azotemia or acute tubular necrosis. In addition, consecutive potassium depletion resulting in vacuolar renal tubular changes may contribute to renal insufficiency in this syndrome, termed hyperemesis gravidarum. ARF associated with hyperemesis gravidarum may develop early or late in pregnancy. In one large series the onset of renal failure ranged from 14 to 32 weeks of gestation [30]. The etiology of this syndrome is still unclear. An organic cause for emesis can be found in some cases especially for late vomiting in pregnancy. Volume depletion may also contribute to the development of ARF in gravidas with acute pyelonephritis and in septic abortion. Early correction of water and electrolyte balance is the best prophylactic measure to prevent renal failure in these gravidas.

8. PREECLAMPSIA–ECLAMPSIA

Preeclampsia, a common complication of pregnancy, is characterized by hypertension plus proteinuria with or without overt edema. Severe preeclampsia is suspected when these abnormalities are severe and are associated with oliguria, overly elevated serum creatinine or upper quadrant abdominal pain, thrombocytopenia, and/or hepatocellular dysfunction. In neglected or fulminant cases of preeclampsia, a convulsive phase termed eclampsia may develop until 48 h postpartum. This disease affects primarily nulliparas and occurs rarely earlier than week 20 of gestation. Occasionally, however, preeclampsia occurs in multiparas, especially in women with vascular diseases including essential chronic hypertension, underlying renal disease, and multifetal pregnancy. It is generally accepted that ARF is a frequent complication of severe preeclampsia and eclampsia. The exact frequency of ARF complicating severe preeclampsia–eclampsia is, however, difficult to assess. The incidence of preeclampsia in retrospective studies dealing with obstetric ARF appears to be higher than that found in prospective studies on eclampsia. For example, in their retrospective study, Smith et al. [8] found evidence of preexisting hypertension or toxemia in 62% of pregnancy-related

ARF in late pregnancy and these symptoms were also noted by Kennedy et al. [3] in 33% of their cases. Similarly, in our own series, 12 out of 57 patients with ARF in late pregnancy had severe preeclampsia or eclampsia [12]. In contrast, in recent prospective studies, Lopez-Llera and Linares [31] found an incidence of ARF as low as 1% in 365 cases of eclampsia, and Pritchard and Pritchard [32] observed only one case of ARF among 154 eclamptic women. This discrepancy may be explained by several factors such as age, parity, presence or not of underlying renal disease, and/or treatment of preeclampsia–eclampsia. Indeed, in retrospective studies, most women were old gravidas, multiparas, and furthermore evidence of arteriolar and arterial changes (consecutive to underlying renal vascular disease) was found in several cases on histologic examination. In contrast, in prospective studies, women are younger and in most cases nulliparas, without underlying disease, and preeclampsia is better managed. These data suggest that: (a) ARF is more frequent in older gravidas and multiparas with "superimposed preeclampsia" than in "truly" preeclamptic women, and (b) earlier detection and better management of pregnancies complicated by preeclampsia–eclampsia should reduce the incidence of ARF in this setting.

The mechanisms whereby severe preeclampsia and eclampsia lead to ARF are not fully understood. It has been suggested that glomerular capillary obstruction resulting from glomerular endotheliosis leads to postglomerular ischemia and then to acute tubular necrosis, or occasionally to BRCN. There is no evidence, however, that glomerular changes are more severe and/or more diffuse in women with eclampsia-related ARF than in those without ARF. Tubular obstruction by intratubular hemoglobin casts due to intravascular hemolysis may also lead to ARF. Sheehan and Lynch [33] found intratubular hemoglobin casts in approximately 20% of fatal cases of eclampsia. Myoglobinuria due to repeated grand mal seizures may also be a contributing factor. It should be recalled, however, that the functional importance of tubular obstruction in acute pigment nephropathy remains questioned in humans. The presence of microangiopathic hemolytic anemia in ARF secondary to preeclampsia was first demonstrated by Brain et al. [34], who suggested that the causative mechanism was intravascular coagulation resulting in fibrin deposition in small vessels with secondary microangiopathic lesions [34]. Typical lesions of microangiopathy with intraluminal arteriolocapillary thrombosis and fibrinoid necrosis of the vascular walls have been documented in eclamptic women with ARF [34]. Reduced prostacyclin production in the umbilical artery, in amniotic fluid, and in plasma from patients with severe preeclampsia has been reported and could play a role [35]. As noted above, eclamptic women have an increased incidence of placental abruption and blood loss as well as volume depletion due to sodium and water loss. These are common precipitating factors of ARF in such women, whose intravascular volume is already decreased.

Preventive heparin therapy may be considered in preeclamptic multiparas in whom chronic vascular disease is often present and who are more susceptible to develop BRCN. A marked improvement in renal function has been reported with heparin therapy in some eclampsia-related ARF cases with thrombotic microangiopathy [34], but the efficiency of such treatment remains controversial. Fatal complications of heparin therapy have been observed.

9. ACUTE FATTY LIVER IN PREGNANCY

9.1. Clinical and laboratory features

Idiopathic acute fatty liver (AFLP) is the most serious hepatic disorder of pregnancy and is often complicated by ARF. This condition, recognized by Sheehan [36] in 1940 as a specific disease of pregnancy and characterized by jaundice, rapidly progressive hepatic failure, and fatty infiltration of liver, is rare. Since its first description by Stander and Cadden [37] in 1934, less than 100 cases have been reported in the literature [38–41]. Primagravidas are considered to be the group most at risk [42]. An association with toxemia has been reported in 20%–50% of cases [38, 40]. The illness usually starts during the third trimester of pregnancy or in early postpartum. Nausea, vomiting, and abdominal pain of sudden onset are the initial symptoms, which are rapidly followed by jaundice, fever, encephalopathy and, in severe cases, by coma due to hepatic failure. Complications such as severe hypoglycemia, gastrointestinal hemorrhage, pancreatitis, and postpartum bleeding are frequent. Hyperbilirubinemia associated with slightly elevated transaminase and alkaline phosphatase levels are characteristic laboratory findings. Leukocytosis is common and hyperuricemia is found in almost all the patients early in the course [41, 42]. Elevated levels of serum amylase and blood ammonia have been reported frequently. DIC have been documented by clotting tests in several patients [41, 43]. The incidence of ARF in this condition is high and was between 60%–90% in most series [40, 41]. Patients are frequently azotemic at the onset of the illness, but renal failure may occur later in the course. Renal failure is felt to be "functional" in most patients since urinary sodium levels are below 5 mmol/24 h [39, 40]. Nevertheless, some cases of acute tubular necrosis have been reported. Maternal death is due to hepatic failure itself, bleeding diathesis, or acute pancreatitis rather than to renal failure.

9.2. Pathology

The characteristic hepatic lesion consists of a diffuse cytoplasmic microdroplet fatty infiltration of hepatocytes sparing periportal liver cells. There is no disturbance of hepatic architecture. Cholestasis is often prominent. Necrosis and inflammatory changes are minimal or absent. Follow-up examination when obtained has always shown histologic recovery with progressive clearing of the fat, and return to normal liver structure [40, 42]. Mitochondrial ultrastructural changes including abundant crystalline inclusions and pleomorphism have been described [44].

The renal pathologic findings are variable. The most characteristic lesion is a fine fatty vacuolization of the proximal tubular cells that has been observed even in patients without ARF [45]. Less specific lesions have been described such as focal tubular necrosis and tubular regenerative changes [46]. Glomerular changes suggesting consumption coagulopathy such as fibrin deposition in glomerular capillaries have been rarely detected [47]. Finally, kidney structure may be normal in patients with ARF [38, 43].

Definite diagnosis of AFLP rests on hepatic biopsy. In the absence of histologic data, differential diagnosis includes severe preeclampsia with liver involvement, septicemia, viral hepatitis, and obstetric cholestasis. It should be stressed that jaundice is common in gravidas with ARF. In our own series, dealing with ARF in late pregnancy, the incidence of jaundice was 35% and AFLP was not diagnosed in any patients [12]. Estimation of fat liver content by computed tomography may sometimes be helpful in diagnosis [48].

9.3. Etiology and pathogenesis

The etiology of AFLP is still uncertain. The occurrence of a similar clinical syndrome with nearly the same histologic features following the intravenous administration of tetracycline to gravidas and to nonpregnant women has long been known. Since the first report by Kunelis et al. [49] of "tetracycline associated" fatty liver of pregnancy, at least 30 cases have been attributed to tetracycline toxicity [41]. Several cases of AFLP have been reported, however, since the cessation of tetracycline therapy in pregnant women. The clinical and histologic characteristics of AFLP have also been observed to have similarities with Reye syndrome. Furthermore, studies on hepatic mitochondrial urea-cycle enzyme activities revealed identical deficiencies such as ornithine transcarbamylase deficiency in the two syndromes [44]. Finally, many authors have suggested that nutritional factors may contribute to the development of the disease. Experimentally, diets deficient in methionine and choline can produce similar histologic lesions in female animals; in humans, Weber et al. [44] demonstrated that AFLP was associated with generalized hypoaminoacidemia. These data and the high incidence of twins (25%) noted by Burroughs et al. [40] in AFLP favor this latter hypothesis.

The pathogenesis of ARF in AFLP is not well understood. In any case, renal failure appears to be a secondary event. Renal involvement may be due to volume depletion or shock. Acute pancreatitis has been reported as a precipitating factor in some cases [38]. DIC may also be a contributing factor in the development of ARF, but histopathologic changes consistent with this hypothesis are scanty [47]. Finally, ARF may be related to renal hemodynamic alterations as in the so-called hepatorenal syndrome.

9.4. Prognosis and treatment

In the first reports of AFLP the mortality rate was estimated to be as high as 75%–85% for both the mother and the fetus [50]. In the last decade, a decline in maternal and fetal morbidities, probably due to earlier recognition of the disease and improved supportive therapy, has been reported [39–41]. Subsequent pregnancies reported in survivors had a favorable outcome and no recurrence of the disease was observed [40]. The treatment of AFLP is not specific and consists basically of vigorous supportive and corrective measures such as hemodynamic monitoring and correction of hypoglycemia and of clotting defects. Renal failure is rarely severe enough to require dialysis. For example, none of the three patients with AFLP managed at the University of Chicago Hospital required hemodialysis. Some authors claimed to have improved the outcome of AFLP with early delivery by cesarean section [40], but others found no evidence that delivery or termination of pregnancy affected the prognosis for the mother [41].

10. BILATERAL RENAL CORTICAL NECROSIS

Since the first report of postpartum renal cortical necrosis (BRCN) by Bradford and Lawrence in 1898 [51], the predominant association of this condition with pregnancy catastrophes has been well documented. Obstetric complications represent the main cause of BRCN in all published series, accounting for 50%–71% of overall cases [23, 52]. Thus, it is clear that gravidas with ARF are at a higher risk of BRCN than are nonpregnant women. Chugh et al. [7] in India have reported that 25% of all their obstetric renal failure cases had BRCN. In our own series, BRCN was diagnosed in 19 (33%) out of 57 gravidas with ARF in late pregnancy [12]. The incidence of BRCN in early pregnancy following spontaneous or induced septic abortion appears to be low in most series. In the study by Smith et al. [8], none of the 52 patients with postabortum ARF had BRCN. Similarly, in our institution, BRCN was observed in only 1.5% of postabortion renal failure, which is similar to the incidence observed in the nongravid population with with ARF [21].

Renal cortical necrosis is more likely associated with obstetric complications occurring during the third trimester or the postpartum period. In the study by Kleinknecht et al. [22], BRCN was present in 21% of patients with ARF in late pregnancy. Abruptio placentae with either concealed or overt hemorrhage is the most frequent presenting event and is responsible for 50%–70% of all cases of BRCN [30, 52]. Moreover, renal cortical necrosis is observed in about 50% of the gravidas with ARF complicating abruptio placentae [12, 53]. As noted above, however, recent data from Dublin indicate that the incidence of both abruptio placentae and renal cortical necrosis is declining [10]. Other obstetric complications associated with coagulation abnormalities such as prolonged intrauterine death, puerperal sepsis, postpartum hemorrhage, or amniotic fluid embolism are less likely to be the cause of BRCN. In contrast with earlier literature, the incidence of severe preeclampsia associated with BRCN appears to be low in recent publications. For example, in the series we reported [12], only one out of 12 toxemic gravidas had BRCN. Sheenhan and Lynch [53] noted that BRCN was present in only 2% of gravidas with preeclampsia. In their recent study, Chugh et al. [23] noted preeclampsia in only four of 35 patients with obstetric renal cortical necrosis. Furthermore, Kleinknecht et al. [22] noted that the incidence of toxemia was lower in gravidas with BRCN than in pregnant women with acute tubular necrosis. It should be stressed, however, that in the absence of a prior history of toxemia the exact frequency of preeclampsia may be difficult to assess if there is no accurate medical history, since blood pressure is usually low or normal at presentation.

Typically, renal cortical necrosis occurs primarily in multigravidas aged 30 years or older. The diagnosis should be suspected in gravidas with or without toxemia when ARF develops early in the third trimester of pregnancy, especially between weeks 26 and 30 [22]. Complete anuria is more common than in acute tubular necrosis and was present in 89.4% of patients with BRCN compared with only 11.5% of cases with acute tubular necrosis in one large series [7]. A long duration of anuria or severe oliguria lasting 15–20 days or more is also suggestive of BRCN. Involvement of organs other than the kidney in obstetric BRCN is uncommon, but a few cases with pituitary necrosis have been reported [12]. Disseminated intravascular coagulation has been demonstrated in many patients [54], but its incidence is not higher than in gravidas with ARF due to acute tubular necrosis. Definite diagnosis of renal cortical necrosis rests on histologic examination of renal biopsy and/or on selective renal angiography [22]. Both methods may also provide information on the extent of the lesion and therefore have prognostic value. Renal tissue, however, may be impossible to obtain in patients with severe coagulopathy. Diffuse renal cortical necrosis is characterized by a complete cortical destruction with only a thin rim of preserved subcapsular and juxtamedullary tissue; at light microscopy, most glomeruli are necrotic. The lack of cortical nephrogram on arteriogram is also diagnostic. In patchy necrosis, which is expected to imply the best prognosis, a lower percentage of glomeruli are destroyed and the cortical nephrogram appears heterogeneous, with a striated aspect. In this latter type of renal necrosis the diagnosis may be missed by renal biopsy due to the "patchy" nature of the lesion, and selective arteriography may be of great value. Cortical calcifications seen on x-rays are also suggestive, but they appear in only a few cases and, in addition, occur only after a few weeks. Finally, measures of mean renal blood flow by krypton or xenon washout techniques have been proposed to differentiate BRCN from acute tubular necrosis [22].

It has been stated frequently that renal cortical necrosis represents the clinical counterpart of the generalized Shwartzman reaction (see above). The initial event in the genesis of BRCN during the Shwartzman reaction is a specific and local effect of endotoxin on the vascular endothelium [20]. The propensity of pregnant women to develop BRCN has still not been elucidated. It is well known that only a single injection of endotoxin is required to elicit the Shwartzman reaction in pregnant animals. The severe clotting disorders observed in certain obstetric complications such as abruptio placentae or amniotic fluid embolism may play a role. These coagulation abnormalities are probably due to liberation of placental tissue thromboplastin. However, the incidence of BRCN in gravidas with ARF appears to be similar in women with or without DIC [54].

The prognosis is still poor, especially in diffuse renal cortical necrosis. In their recent study, Chugh et al. [23] noted maternal mortality as high as 82%. However, in other series from industrialized countries where supportive therapy with hemodialysis was provided over a long period, mortality of only 36% was found [12]. Partial recovery from renal failure occurs in a substantial number of patients after the acute episode and renal function may improve very slowly over a period of 1–3 years. Early recovery in the diffuse form is probably due to the recovery of juxtamedullary glomeruli and subsequent improvement to a functional adaptation of these juxtamedullary nephrons. Nevertheless, in a significant number of patients, subsequent deterioration in renal function may occur in the following years, leading to a requirement for regular hemodialysis [22]. Hyperfiltration in the surviving nephrons has been incriminated as a possible cause of this phenomenon [55].

Transplantation has been performed in patients with terminal renal failure. A high incidence of hyperacute graft rejection has been observed by some authors [56]. Subsequent successful pregnancy has been reported [57].

11. IDIOPATHIC POSTPARTUM RENAL FAILURE

11.1. Clinical and laboratory features

Idiopathic postpartum renal failure is a syndrome of acute, rapidly progressive renal failure occurring shortly after an uneventful pregnancy and delivery. This rare and often fatal syndrome was first described by Robson et al. [58] in 1968 as "irreversible postpartum renal failure," and several cases variously termed "malignant nephrosclerosis in women postpartum" [59], "postpartum intravascular coagulation with acute renal failure" [60], "postpartum renal failure with microangiopathic hemolytic anemia" [61], "the postpartum hemolytic uremic syndrome" [62], and "idiopathic postpartum renal failure" [63] have been reported in the literature. Although idiopathic postpartum renal failure appears to be a "new" syndrome, cases with similar features were described occasionally before the 1960s. The exact frequency of idiopathic postpartum renal failure is difficult to assess because many reports unfortunately include women with hypertensive disorders and/or delivery complications. Furthermore, idiopathic postpartum renal failure occurring later than three months after delivery has been reported [64, 65]. As uterine involution occurs by three months, it is not clear whether in such cases pregnancy was involved, especially in women using contraceptives.

This syndrome affects previously healthy women and may occur one day to several weeks after an apparently normal pregnancy and delivery. Patients usually present with an influenza-like illness followed by a rapidly progressive oliguric or often anuric renal failure. Blood pressure may be either normal or slightly elevated at presentation, but severe or malignant hypertension may appear during the course of the disease. An abnormal bleeding tendency with hematemesis, petechiae, hemoptysis, or vaginal bleeding is not uncommon. Symptoms of congestive heart failure are present in 30%–65% of patients [63, 66]. Generalized seizures occur in approximately 50% of patients [63].

Evidence of severe microangiopathic hemolytic anemia with anisocytosis and schizocytosis was noted in 70% of the cases reviewed by Segonds et al. [66]. Other indirect laboratory findings of hemolysis such as high reticulocyte count, indirect hyperbilirubinemia, and low serum haptoglobin level are common, but the Coomb test is always negative. In these cases with microangiopathic hemolytic anemia, the term "postpartum hemolytic uremic syndrome" is, therefore, appropriate. Thrombocytopenia and elevated serum levels of fibrinogen degradation products have been noted at the onset of the illness in almost all cases. Hypocompletemia has been found in a few patients [66].

11.2. Diagnosis

Diagnosis of idiopathic postpartum renal failure may be established after exclusion of other common causes of ARF such as abruptio placentae, postpartum hemorrhage, amniotic fluid emboli, and puerpueral sepsis.

Differentiation with thrombotic thrombocytopenic purpura (TTP) may be difficult. TTP may affect women either during pregnancy or in the late puerpuerium [67]. The absence of hypertension and renal failure is more typical of TTP, though renal function may be impaired. As in TTP, intravascular thrombosis or infarction of several organs has been found in several autopsies of postpartum renal failure [60, 63, 64]. It can also be difficult to differentiate postpartum hemolytic uremic syndrome from severe preeclampsia with microangiopathic hemolytic anemia and ARF. Clinically, however, toxemia is distinguished by severe hypertension and its occurrence no later than 48 h after delivery. Diagnosis of malignant hypertension may also be considered in cases of postpartum renal failure with severe hypertension occurring early in the course. Finally, hemolytic uremic syndrome (HUS) may develop in women during hormonal contraception. Hauglustaine et al. [68], in a review of 52 patients with hemolytic uremic postpartum syndrome, reported that five women were receiving oral contraception at the onset of the disease. It is unknown whether these latter cases should be attributed to current oral contraception or to recent pregnancy. Histopathologic changes observed in postpill syndrome were usually characteristic of thrombotic microangiopathy, but with more diffuse arteriolar changes [12].

11.3. Pathology

Heterogeneous renal histopathologic changes have been described in idiopathic postpartum renal failure. Two types of lesions may be seen: (a) glomerular capillaries and arteriolar changes typical of thrombotic microangiopathy and resembling those found in HUS in children, and (b) vascular lesions similar to those described in malignant nephrosclerosis or in scleroderma with renal involvement. In the former, characteristic lesions are thickening of capillary walls due to endothelial swelling and double-contoured appearance of basement membrane due to translucency of the subendothelial space. This subendothelial lucent space appears to contain a granular material on the electron micrograph. Capillary thrombi are found in 50% of the cases. Similar changes are detected in arterioles and small arteries, i.e., fibrin deposits, endothelial proliferation, fibrinoid necrosis, and intravascular thrombi. In the latter type, vascular changes are characterized by subendothelial mucoid intimal proliferation leading to narrowing of the vessel lumen and necrotizing arteritis. Involvement of interlobular arteries is more frequent than in thrombotic microangiopathy. Glomerular changes such as atrophy and sclerosis, wrinkled basement membranes, and interstitial edema and fibrosis are commonly seen and result from ischemia. It has been hypothesized that these two types of lesions may represent successive stages of this disease. However, anatomic data available in the literature do not provide sufficient information to confirm this hypothesis. The two types of glomerular lesions may coexist in the same biopsy specimen, and ischemic changes may be seen early in the course of the disease. Finally, an ischemic aspect is often prominent in idiopathic postpartum renal failure as it is in nonobstetric HUS in adults. Immunofluorescent studies usually show fibrin and C3 in mesangium, capillary wall, and arterioles [66, 69]. Infrequently, focal staining with anti-IgG and anti-IgM antisera is found [66, 70]. Kincaid-Smith [71] has suggested that a similar primary renal lesion is involved in preeclampsia and in postpartum renal failure. Several authors pointed out that vascular lesions are of great prognostic importance in idiopathic postpartum renal failure. Morel-Maroger et al. [69] have noted that patients with a favorable outcome had significantly less severe arterial intimal thickening compared with patients with a poor prognosis, whereas glomerular lesions have less prognostic value [69]. A higher incidence of severe postbiopsy hemorrhage in patients with HUS, compared with patients with other types of ARF, has been reported. These complications occur especially in patients in whom heparin therapy is instituted early after biopsy [69], and in those with hypertension even in the absence of heparin therapy [64, 65]. Renal biopsy is necessary in patients without unequivocal HUS. Conversely, in patients with clinical evidence of HUS, microangiopathic nephropathy can be anticipated, and renal biopsy must be discussed only with regard to its value in the therapeutic decision.

11.4. Etiology and pathogenesis

Various precipitating factors or etiologic agents have been implicated in the development of idiopathic postpartum renal failure. Oxytocic drugs and placental retention have been considered as possible etiologic factors in some cases. Symptoms consistent with viral infection as in HUS in childhood were noted in some patients. As in TTP, nonobstetric HUS, and postpill HUS, genetic and environmental factors have been implicated in a few kindreds [72]. In two HLA-identical sisters, postpartum HUS occurred in one, and the other developed postpill HUS [73].

The pathogenesis of idiopathic postpartum renal failure remains uncertain. Similarities with HUS, TTP, eclampsia with microangiopathic hemolytic anemia and, finally, experimental generalized Shwartzman reaction have been repeatedly underlined. In addition, Conger et al. [19] demonstrated that a single dose of endotoxin could induce the Shwartzman reaction in rats during the postpartum period. Injury to endothelial cells involving glomerular capillaries and extending to renal arterioles appeared to be the primary event. Various mechanisms initiating the endothelial damage, which leads to fibrin deposition, have been proposed. It has been suggested that circulating endotoxins may produce the endothelial damage. Such substances have rarely been detected in patients with HUS. There is likewise no evidence that DIC is the initial pathogenic event. Local renal intravascular coagulation is more likely to be involved in the pathogenesis of postpartum

HUS and may be triggered by the hypercoagulable state present in the early puerpuerium. A pathogenic role for immunologic factors has also been proposed due to the fact that immunoglobulins and C3 deposits in renal biopsy specimens as well as hypocomplementemia have been reported in some patients [66]. Evidence, however, of an immune complex disease has not yet been supported by convincing data [67]. Finally, low plasma activity of prostacyclin (PGI_2), a potent vasodilatator and inhibitor of platelet aggregation that appears important in the maintenance of vascular integrity, has been found in patients with HUS and TTP. A deficiency of plasma factor(s) stimulating vascular PGI_2 activity has been suggested [74]. This plasma defect might be determined genetically. Further experimentation is needed to delineate clearly the role of this deficiency in the pathogenic sequence of HUS.

11.5. Prognosis and treatment

In a review of 49 patients [66] with idiopathic postpartum renal failure, death occurred in 61%; among the survivors, terminal renal failure occurred in 12% and complete recovery of renal function in only 9.5%. Improvement of renal function usually occurs early, but may be delayed for as long as 1½ years [66]. Hypertension and proteinuria are common features in patients with residual impairment of renal function. Finally, recurrent postpartum HUS has been reported in rare cases [75].

A variety of treatments have been proposed. Their efficacy is difficult to evaluate because of the lack of controlled trials. Conservative management by peritoneal dialysis or hemodialysis and antihypertensive therapy is crucial and is probably an important factor in improving mortality. Bilateral nephrectomy has been performed in some patients with uncontrollable malignant hypertension [63, 66, 69]. Potent antihypertensive drugs such as angiotensin-converting enzyme inhibitors have limited the indication of bilateral nephrectomy to rare cases. A beneficial effect of captopril administration on both hypertension and renal function in a woman with postpill HUS has been observed [76]. The usefulness of anticoagulant therapy is disputed. Most reports indicate a beneficial effect of this treatment. For example, in a review of the literature yielding 52 cases, death occurred in 40.8% and partial or complete recovery of renal function in 44.4% of 27 anticoagulant-treated patients, whereas in 25 untreated patients, 19 (76%) died and only three (12%) had partial or complete renal function recovery [66]. It must be stressed, however, that most are isolated cases and uncontrolled studies. In addition, failure of heparin therapy has probably rarely been published. Most authors advocate that heparin must be administered as early as possible in the course of the disease [63, 69]. Morel-Maroger et al. [69] stressed the beneficial effect of anticoagulant therapy in patients with mild vascular lesions. In contrast, heparin therapy is not beneficial in hypertensive patients and/or in those with extensive and irreversible vascular and glomerular changes on biopsy specimen [69]. A beneficial effect of fibrinolytic therapy on renal function has not been proved. It should be recalled that several patients treated with heparin or a fibrinolytic agent had severe hemorrhagic complications [63, 69]. Antiplatelet therapy alone or combined with heparin has also been tried and a beneficial effect has been reported. Complete recovery of renal function after infusion of antithrombin-III concentrate in an antithrombin-III-deficient women with postpartum HUS has been reported [77]. Fresh frozen plasma infusion and plasmapheresis have been advocated in TTP and HUS by Misiani et al. [78]. Webster et al. [79] also observed a beneficial effect of intravenous infusion of prostacyclin and of fresh frozen plasma on renal function in one case of postpartum HUS. Successful renal transplantation has been performed in patients with postpartum HUS. No recurrence of HUS in the transplant was observed in several patients [12, 63, 69].

12. MISCELLANEOUS CAUSES OF ACUTE RENAL FAILURE

Occasionally, obstructive ARF may occur in gravidas with polyhydramios [80], incarcerated gravide uterus, or even in women with uncomplicated gestation [81].

Amniotic fluid embolism, which occurs primarily in multiparas after prolonged labor, may also induce ARF. Pregnant women with underlying renal disease are more prone to develop acute tubular necrosis even in the absence of chronic renal insufficiency, especially when increased blood pressure or superimposed preeclampsia is present [5].

Finally, ARF in gravidas may be caused by coincidental factors such as acute glomerulonephritis, drug nephrotoxicity, incompatible blood transfusions, or bacterial endocarditis. These pregnancy-unrelated cases of ARF represent only about 5% of all obstetric ARF.

13. MANAGEMENT OF ACUTE RENAL FAILURE IN PREGNANCY

Management of ARF in gravidas is the same as that in nonpregnant patients. The vital importance of blood replacement and even "overtransfusion" in those women with frequent and severe uterine hemorrhage must be recalled. Dialysis should be undertaken early in order to maintain urea nitrogen around 30 mg/dl. Both peritoneal dialysis and hemodialysis may be used in gravidas with ARF [5, 82]. The advantages of these two techniques are disputed. Smith et al. [8] considered peritoneal dialysis as the best method and stressed that "neither pelvic peritonitis nor enlarged uterus are contraindications." The catheter must be inserted under direct vision through a small incision and high in the abdomen. Nevertheless, hemodialysis has been used with success in several patients [12]. Preservation of a good uteroplacental perfusion requires a careful monitoring of fluid balance during dialysis. Close attention to the possibility of hemorrhagic complications due to heparinization is necessary. Fetal survival in gravidas undergoing hemodialysis has been reported [83].

REFERENCES

1. Knapp RC, Hellman LH: Acute renal failure in pregnancy. Am J Obstet Gynecol 78:570–577, 1959.
2. Kerr DNS, Elliot W: Renal disease in pregnancy. Practitioner 190:459–467, 1967.
3. Kennedy AC, Burton JA, Luke RG, Briggs JD, Linsay RM, Allison MEM, Edward N, Dargie HJ: Factors affecting the prognosis in acute renal failure. Q J Med 42:73–86, 1973.

4. Chapman A, Legrain M: Acute tubular necrosis and interstitial nephritis. In: Hamburger J, Crosnier J, Grunfeld JP (eds) Nephrology. New York: John Wiley and Sons, 1979, pp 383–410.
5. Lindheimer MD, Katz AI, Ganeval D, Grunfeld JP: Acute renal failure in pregnancy. In: Brenner BM, Lazarus JM (eds) Acute renal failure. Philadelphia: WB Saunders, 1983, pp 510–526.
6. Chapman A: Etiologie et pronostic actuel de l'insuffisance renale aigue en France: Resultats d'une enquete. In: Cartier F (ed) L'insuffisance renale aigue. Paris: L'Expansion scientifique francaise, 1978, pp 37–54.
7. Chugh KS, Singhal PC, Sharma BK, Yash PAL, Thomas Mathew M, Kamla Dhall, Datta BN: Acute renal failure of obstetric origin. Obstet Gynecol 48:642–646, 1976.
8. Smith K, Browne JCM, Schackman R, Wrong OM: Acute renal failure of obstetric origin: an analysis of 70 patients. Lancet 2:351–354, 1965.
9. Finn WF: Recovery from acute renal failure. In: Brenner BM, Lazarus JM (eds) Acute renal failure. Philadelphia: WB Saunders, 1983, pp 252–268.
10. Donohoe JF: Acute bilateral cortical necrosis. In: Brenner BM, Lazarus JM (eds) Acute renal failure. Philadelphia: WB Saunders, 1983, pp 252–268.
11. Robson JS, Martin AM, Ruckley VA, MacDonald MK: Irreversible post-partum renal failure. Q J Med 37:423–435, 1968.
12. Grunfeld JP, Ganeval D, Bournerias F: Acute renal failure in pregnancy. Kidney Int 18:179–191, 1980.
13. Lindheimer MD, Katz AI: Kidney function and disease in pregnancy. Philadelphia: Lea and Febiger, 1977.
14. Stein JH, Lifschitz MD, Barnes LD: Current concepts on the pathophysiology of acute renal failure. Am J Physiol 234:F171–F181, 1978.
15. Bidani A, Churchill PC, McDonald FD, Fleishmann L: Glycerol-induced myohemoglobinuric acute renal failure in the pregnant rat. Nephron 26:35–40, 1980.
16. Sicinska J, Bailie MD, Rector FC Jr: Effects of angiotensin on blood pressure and renal function in pregnant and nonpregnant rats. Nephron 8:375–381, 1981.
17. Collins R, Baylis C: Effects on angiotensin II (AII) inhibition on blood pressure (AP) and renal hemodynamics in late pregnant (P) rat. Clin Res 32:444A, 1984.
18. Bonnar J: Acute and chronic coagulation problems in pregnancy. In: Poller (ed) Recent advances in blood coagulation. Edinburgh: Churchill Livingstone, 1977, pp 363–378.
19. Conger JD, Falk SA, Guggenheim SJ: Glomerular dynamics and morphologic changes in the generalized Shwartzman reaction in postpartum rats. J Clin Invest 67:1334–1346, 1981.
20. Raij L, Keane WF, Michael AF: Unilateral Shwartzman reaction: cortical necrosis in one kidney following in vivo perfusion with endotoxin. Kidney Int 12:91–95, 1977.
21. Kleinknecht D, Bochereau G, Chauveau P: Y a-t-il encore des accidents graves de l'avortement provoque? Nouv Presse Med 9:460, 1980.
22. Kleinknecht D, Grunfeld JP, Cia Gomez P, Moreau JF, Garcia-Torres R: Diagnostic procedures and long-term prognosis in bilateral renal cortical necrosis. Kidney Int 4:390–400, 1973.
23. Chugh KS, Singhal PC, Kher VK, Gupta VK, Malik GH, Narayan G, Datta BN: Spectrum of acute cortical necrosis in Indian patients. Am J Med Sci 286:10–20, 1983.
24. Bartlett RH, Yahia C: Management of septic chemical abortion with renal failure: report of five consecutive cases with five survivors. N Engl J Med 281:747–753, 1969.
25. Hawkins DF, Sevitt LH, Fairbrother PF, Tothill AU: Management of septic chemical abortion with renal failure: use of a conservative regimen. N Engl J Med 292:722–725, 1975.
26. Kincaid-Smith P: Bacteriuria and urinary infection in pregnancy. Clin Obstet Gynecol 2:533, 1968.
27. Gilstrap LC, Cunningham FG, Whalley PJ: Acute pyelonephritis during pregnancy: an anterospective study. Obstet Gynecol 57:409–413, 1981.
28. Whalley PJ, Cunningham FG, Martin F: Transient renal dysfunction associated with acute pyelonephritis of pregnancy. Obstet Gynecol 46:174–177, 1975.
29. Whalley PJ: Bacteriuria of pregnancy. Am J Obstet Gynecol 97:723, 1967.
30. Ober WE, Reid DE, Romney SL, Merrill JP: Renal lesions and acute renal failure in pregnancy. Am J Med 21:781–810, 1956.
31. Lopez-Llera M, Linares GR: Factors that influence maternal mortality in eclampsia. In: Lindheimer MD, Katz AI, Zuspan FP (eds), Hypertension in pregnancy. New York: John Wiley and Sons, 1976, p 41.

32. Pritchard JA, Pritchard SA: Standardized treatment of 154 consecutive cases of eclampsia. Am J Obstet Gynecol 123:543–549, 1975.
33. Sheehan HL, Lynch JB: Pathology of toxaemia of pregnancy. Edinburgh: Churchill Livingstone, 1973, p 220.
34. Brain MC, Kuah KB, Dixon HG: Heparin treatment of haemolysis and thrombocytopenia in preeclampsia. J Obstet Gynaecol Br Common 74:702–711, 1967.
35. De Gaetano G, Livio M, Donati MB, Remuzzi G.: Platelet and vascular prostaglandins in uraemia, thrombotic microangiopathy and preeclampsia. Philos Trans R Soc Lond [B] 294:-339–342, 1981.
36. Sheehan H: The pathology of acute yellow atrophy and delayed chloroform poisoning. J Obstet Gynaecol Br Commonw 47:49–62, 1940.
37. Stander HJ, Cadden JF: Blood chemistry in preeclampsia and eclampsia. Am J Obstet Gynecol 28:856–871, 1934.
38. Bletry O, Roche-Sicot J, Rueff B, Degott C: Steatose hepatique aigue gravidique. Nouv Presse Med 8:1835–1838, 1979.
39. Davies MH, Wilkinson SP, Hanid MA, Portmann B, Brudenell JM, Newton JR, Williams R: Acute liver disease with encephalopathy and renal failure in late pregnancy and the early puerpuerium: a study of fourteen patients. Br J Obstet Gynaecol 87:1005–1014, 1980.
40. Burroughs AK, Seong NGH, Dojcinov DM, Sheuer PJ, Sherlock SVP: Idiopathic acute fatty liver of pregnancy in 12 patients. Q J Med 204:481–497, 1982.
41. Pockros PJ, Peters RL, Reynolds TB: Idiopathic fatty liver of pregnancy: findings in ten cases. Medicine (Baltimore) 63:1–11, 1984.
42. Koff RS: Case records of Mass. Gen. Hosp. N Engl J Med 304:216–224, 1981.
43. Cano RI, Delman MR, Pitchumoni CS, Lev R, Rosenthal WS: Acute fatty liver of pregnancy: complicated by intravascular coagulation. JAMA 231:159–161, 1975.
44. Weber FL, Snodgrass PJ, Powell DE, Rao P, Huffman SL, Brady PG: Abnormalities of urea-cycle enzyme activities hepatic ultrastructure in acute fatty liver of pregnancy. J Lab Clin Med 94:27–41, 1979.
45. Ober WB, Lecompte PM: Acute fatty metamorphosis of the liver associated with pregnancy. Am J Med 19:743–758, 1955.
46. Recant L, Lacy P: Fulminating liver disease in a pregnant woman at term. Am J Med 35:231–240, 1963.
47. Kahil ME, Fred HL, Brown H, David JS: Acute fatty liver of pregnancy. Arch Intern Med 113:63–69, 1964.
48. Bydder GM, Kreel L, Chapman RWG, Harry D, Scherlock S: Accuracy of computed tomography in diagnosis of fatty liver. Br Med J 281:1042, 1980.
49. Kunelis CT, Peters JL, Edmonson HA: Fatty liver of pregnancy and its relationship to tetracycline therapy. Am J Med 38:359–377, 1965.
50. Varner M, Rinderknecht N: Acute fatty metamorphosis of pregnancy: a maternal mortality and literature review. J Reprod Med 24:177–180, 1980.
51. Bradford JR, Lawrence TWP: Endarteritis of the renal arteries causing necrosis of both kidneys. J Pathol Bacteriol 5:195, 1898.
52. Sheehan HL, Moore HC: Renal cortical necrosis and the kidney of concealed hemorrhage. Springfield IL: Charles C Thomas, 1953.
53. Sheehan HL, Lynch JB: Pathology of toxaemia of pregnancy. Edinburgh: Churchill Livingstone, 1973, p 287.
54. Kleinknecht D, Kanfer A, Josso F: Intravascular coagulation and heparin therapy in acute renal failure: a reappraisal. Eur J Clin Biol Res 17:695–700, 1972.
55. Brenner BM, Meyer TW, Hostetter TH: Hemodynamically mediated glomerular injury and the progressive nature of kidney disease. Kidney Int 23:647–655, 1983.
56. Gelfand MC, Friedman Ea, Knepshield JH, Karpatkin S: Detection of antiplatelet antibody in patients with renal cortical necrosis. Kidney Int 6:426–430, 1974.
57. Effersoe P, Raaschou F, Thomsen AC: Bilateral renal cortical necrosis: a patient follow-up over 8 years. Am J Med 33:455–458, 1962.
58. Robson JS, Martin AM, Ruckley VA, MacDonald MK: Irreversible postpartum renal failure: a new syndrome. Q J Med 37:423–435, 1968.
59. Sheer RL, Jones DB: Malignant nephrosclerosis in women post-partum: a note on microangiopathic hemolytic anemia. JAMA 201:106–110, 1967.

60. Rosenmann E, Kanter A, Bacani RA, Pirani CL, Pollak VE: Fatal late postpartum intravascular coagulation with acute renal failure. Am J Med Sci 257:259–273, 1969.
61. Luke RG, Siegel RR, Talbert W, Holland N: Heparin treatment for postpartum renal failure with microangiopathic hemolytic anemia. Lancet 2:750–752, 1970.
62. Eisinger AJ: The postpartum hemolytic uremic syndrome. J Obstet Gynaecol Br Commonw 79:139–143, 1972.
63. Sun NCJ, Johnson WJ, Sung DTW, Woods JE: Idiopathic postpartum renal failure: review and case report of a successful renal transplantation. Mayo Clin Proc 50:395–401, 1975.
64. Churg J, Koffler D, Paronetto F, Rorat E, Barnett RN: Hemolytic uremic syndrome as a cause of postpartum renal failure. Am J Obstet Gynecol 108:253–261, 1970.
65. Ponticelli C, Imbasciati A, Tarantino G, Graziani G, Redaelli B: Post-partum renal failure with microangiopathic haemolytic anaemia. Nephron 9:27–41, 1972.
66. Segonds A, Louradour N, Suc JM, Orfila C: Postpartum hemolytic uremic syndrome: a study of 3 cases with a review of the literature. Clin Nephrol 12:229–242, 1979.
67. Neame PB: Immunologic and other factors in thrombotic thrombocytopenic purpura (TTP). Semin Thromb Hemost 6:416–429, 1980.
68. Hauglustaine D, Vandamme B, Vanrenterghem Y, Michielsen P: Recurrent hemolytic uremic syndrome during oral contraception. Clin Nephrol 15:147–153, 1981.
69. Morel-Maroger L, Kanfer A, Solez K, Sraer JD, Richet G:Prognostic importance of vascular lesions in acute renal failure with microangiopathic hemolytic anemia (hemolytic–uremic syndrome): clinicopathologic study in 20 adults. Kidney Int 15:548–558, 1979.
70. Schoolwerth AC, Sandler RS, Klahr S, Kissane JM: Nephrosclerosis postpartum and in women taking oral contraceptives. Arch Intern Med 136:178–185, 1976.
71. Kincaid-Smith P: The similarity of lesions and underlying mechanism in preeclamptic toxemia and postpartum renal failure: studies in the acute stage and during follow up. In: Kincaid-Smith P, Mathew TH, Becker EL (eds) Glomerulonephritis, morphology, natural history, and treatment. II. New York: John Wiley and Sons, 1973, p 1013.
72. Grottum KA, Flatmark A, Myhre E, Jansen H, Teisberg P, Oystese B, Husby G, Hovig T: Immunological hereditary nephropathy. Acta Med Scand [Suppl] 197:571, 1975.
73. Modesto A, Durand D, Orfila C, Suc JM: Syndrome hemolytique uremique chez deux germains HLA identiques. Nephrologie 5:47, 1984.
74. Remuzzi G, Misiani R, Marchesi D, Livio M, Mecca G, De Gaetano G, Donati MB:Haemolytic–uraemic syndrome: deficiency of plasma factor(s) regulating prostacyclin activity. Lancet 2:-871–872, 1978.
75. Gomperts ED, Sessel L, Du Plessis V, Hersch C: Recurrent post-partum haemolytic uraemic syndrome. Lancet 1:48, 1978.
76. Hoorntje SJ, Prins EJL, Smit AJ, Donker AB JM: Reversal of long-standing renal insufficiency by captopril in a patient with relapsing hemolytic uremic syndrome due to an oral contraceptive. Ann Intern Med 94:355–357, 1981.
77. Brandt P, Jespersen J, Gregersen G: Postpartum haemolytic–uraemic syndrome treated with antihrombin-III. Nephron 27:15–18, 1981.
78. Misiani R, Appiani A, Edefonti A, Gotti E, Betinelli A, Giani M, Rossi E, Remuzzi G, Mecca G: Haemolytic uraemic syndrome: therapeutic aspect of plasma infusion. Br Med J 285:1304–1306, 1982.
79. Webster J, Rees AJ, Lewis PJ, Hensby CN: Prostacyclin deficiency in haemolytic–uraemic syndrome. Br Med J 281:271, 1980.
80. Quigley MM, Cruikshank DP: Polyhydramnios and acute renal failure. J Reprod Med 19:92, 1977.
81. Bennett AH, Adler S: Bilateral ureteral obstruction causing anuria secondary to pregnancy. Urology 20:631–633, 1982.
82. Kelleher S, Berl T: Acute renal failure in pregnancy. Semin Nephrol 1:61–68, 1981.
83. Cole EH, Bear RA, Steinberg W: Acute renal failure at 24 weeks of pregnancy: a case report. Can Med Assoc J 122:1161–1162, 1980.

11. SUCCESSFUL PREGNANCIES IN WOMEN ON REGULAR DIALYSIS TREATMENT AND WOMEN WITH A FUNCTIONING TRANSPLANT

SABRI CHALLAH, ANTONY J. WING, MICHEL BROYER, and GIANFRANCO RIZZONI

1. INTRODUCTION

The first child born to a patient on renal replacement therapy was delivered by cesarean section on 10 March 1958 [1]. The mother was the recipient of a renal graft from an identical twin and was not on immunosuppressive drugs. Eight years later, in April and September 1966, two normal children were born by spontaneous vaginal delivery to recipients of related living donor transplants, both of whom were being treated with azathioprine and prednisone [2–4]. In the following year, the first successful pregnancy after transplantation of a cadaver kidney occurred [5]. Since then, individual patients in Europe have been documented in detail [6–9] and a few small series described [10–14]. Experience of centers reporting to the Human Kidney Transplant Registry was reviewed by Goldby [15]; Nolan et al. [16] added two of their own patients to published information on 23 others and, in 1975, Rifle and Traeger [17] presented an international survey of 103 pregnancies in women who had been transplanted. In 1979, Rudolph et al. [18] published the results of a questionnaire survey of pregnancy in grafted patients that involved most of the renal transplant centers in North America. The 440 pregnancies they collected, including 40 from the literature, had resulted in 221 term and 54 premature births. Davison [19] reviewed 1068 pregnancies in 717 patients, but there may have been some overlap among the series he aggregated. It has been estimated that one out of every 50 women of childbearing age with a functioning renal transplant becomes pregnant [20].

The first description of pregnancy and successful delivery in a patient on chronic hemodialysis was by Confortini et al. [21], and subsequently further individual case reports have been published [22–24]. More recently, successful pregnancy in a woman on CAPD has been reported [25].

The Registry of the EDTA–ERA (European Dialysis and Transplant Association–European Renal Association) collects information on patients being treated by dialysis and transplantation in 32 countries, and annual reports have given a summary of reported live births and abortions [26]. Returns are made to the Registry by means of both a center and individual patient questionnaires. Since 1978, successful pregnancies have been recorded on the center questionnaire, and each notification followed up with a request for further information. The data required include sex of child, birth weight, duration of pregnancy, feeding practice, presence of congenital abnormalities and, from 1982 onward, body length, head circumference, and immunosuppressive regimen used during gestation. A detailed survey of pregnancies reported before 31 December 1978 has been carried out, and the results on 125 births published [27]. Between 1979 and the end of 1982, a further 185 successful pregnancies were reported to the Registry. Results on a total of 310 pregnancies are presented in this chapter; only babies whose date of birth was given are included.

2. NUMBER OF LIVE BIRTHS

Table 11-1 shows the number of live births reported to the EDTA–ERA Registry up to the close of 1982. Births prior to 1979 are aggregated and results are shown separately according to treatment status of the mother. There were 275 successful pregnancies in grafted patients compared with only 35 recorded on dialysis. The 310 pregnancies resulted in 317 live births with a slight preponderance of females in the ratio 1.1:1 (table 11-2).

Table 11-3 shows pregnancies reported to the Registry by country of birth; the prominence of the United Kingdom with a total of 116 successful pregnancies is undoubtedly related to its active transplant program.

Multiple pregnancies appear to have occurred with increased frequency in patients with transplants [28]. Sciarra et al. [13] included one pair of twins in their series of 17 pregnancies in transplant recipients, and Lower et al. [29] reported

Table 11-1. Successful pregnancies reported to the EDTA–ERA Registry up to the end of 1982, shown according to treatment status of mother.

	Number of successful pregnancies					
Mode of treatment	Up to end 1978	1979	1980	1981	1982	Total
Transplanted patients	109	30	48	44	44	275
Dialyzed patients	16	5	2	8	4	35
Total	125	35	50	52	48	310

Table 11-2. Number and sex of children born alive to mothers on the EDTA–ERA Registry, up to the end of 1982.

	Number of children born alive					
Sex of child	Up to end 1978	1979	1980	1981	1982	Total
Male	54	17	31	17	23	142
Female	63	18	19	33	26	159
Not recorded	14	0	0	2	0	16
Total	131	35	50	52	49	317

Table 11-3. Successful pregnancies notified to the EDTA–ERA Registry up to the end of 1982, shown according to country of treatment of the mother.

	Number of successful pregnancies					
Country	Up to end 1978	1979	1980	1981	1982	Total
Austria	1	1	0	1	0	3
Belgium	5	1	4	0	1	11
Czechoslovakia	3	2	0	2	0	7
Denmark	4	0	3	1	2	10
Fed Rep Germany	3	4	1	3	2	13
Finland	9	1	0	1	1	12
France	14	5	7	7	9	42
German Dem Rep	2	0	0	0	4	6
Greece	2	0	3	1	3	9
Ireland	3	0	0	0	0	3
Israel	2	0	0	0	0	2
Italy	7	2	3	3	2	17
Netherlands	1	1	2	3	2	9
Norway	1	0	1	0	2	4
Poland	0	0	0	0	1	1
Spain	4	5	1	4	4	18
Sweden	9	0	0	6	0	15
Switzerland	4	0	1	1	0	6
United Kingdom	47	12	23	19	15	116
Yugoslavia	4	1	1	0	0	6

premature twins who died. There was one set of twins among 86 births collected by Rifle and Traeger [17] and four in the series reported by Rudolph et al. [18]. The Registry has records of seven multiple births, six sets of twins and one set of triplets, and 12 second or subsequent babies.

Although in the past, the Registry has recorded information on 57 therapeutic and 16 spontaneous abortions in women with transplants, and 45 therapeutic and 16 spontaneous abortions in women on dialysis [26], data are no longer collected on incomplete pregnancies. Between 25% and 28% of all pregnancies in grafted patients end in therapeutic abortion; reasons include unstable renal function prior to pregnancy, deteriorating renal function during pregnancy, severe hypertension, ureteric or ileal conduit compression, emotional instability, hereditary renal disease, uncertainity about maternal long-term survival, and unwanted childbirth [18, 19]. Rates of spontaneous abortion, stillbirth, and ruptured ectopic pregnancy are similar in transplanted patients to those in the normal population [18]. It has been estimated that 42% of all conceptions in grafted patients do not go beyond the first trimester [19].

3. COURSE OF PREGNANCY AND ITS IMPACT ON RENAL FUNCTION

The youngest mother identified to the Registry was 19 and the oldest was a 42-year-old dialysis patient. The interval between first renal replacement therapy and delivery varied greatly from nine months to over ten years, and pregnancy was reported more commonly among living donor than cadaveric recipients [27].

Information on clinical problems during pregnancy was collected in the 1978 EDTA–ERA survey. A quarter of the mothers took antihypertensive drugs and the management of hypertension appeared to be particularly difficult in patients on dialysis. Most patients took extra hematinics, and supportive blood transfusions were usually required for patients on dialysis. Preeclampsia is reported in about 30% of cases in the literature compared with only 8% of healthy subjects [18]. In the larger series, respiratory and urinary infections are reported as common occurrences [13, 30].

Rejection episodes do not appear to be a major problem in mothers who have been transplanted [18]. Among the 44 pregnancies in grafted patients reported to the EDTA–ERA Registry in 1982, 39 mothers were on steroids plus azathioprine throughout pregnancy, and one was on steroids alone; in four cases, no information on immunosuppressive regimen was given. In five patients the dose of azathioprine was reduced in the last six months of the pregnancy, and in one case the dose of prednisolone was lowered. The dose of azathioprine used in combination varied from 50 to 150 mg daily.

Of great concern are changes in transplant function associated with the pregnancy. Of the 125 mothers identified to the Registry before 1979, 17% had evidence of damage to the transplant during the pregnancy. This seems most likely to occur both toward the end of pregnancy and also postpartum [31]. The increase in glomerular filtration rate characteristic of early pregnancy is also evident in transplant recipients [32] and it is conceivable that this may mask deterioration of graft function; some authors describe a reduction in glomerular filtration rate in the third trimester, with return to normal after delivery, while others have found no change in transplant function [3, 4]. Permanent impairment of renal function has been noted previously during pregnancy [7] and this has been progressive in at least three reported patients [5, 13, 33].

Of the 35 children born to women on dialysis in the EDTA–ERA series, 15 were conceived before first renal replacement therapy. Although conception and successful pregnancy can occur without significant residual glomerular filtration rate [23], most of the patients in this group have some residual renal function [17,

24]. Careful blood pressure control, maintenance of good nutrition, and limitation of predialysis blood urea levels necessitate increased hours and frequency of dialysis [22, 23], but the duration and frequency of treatments recorded by our correspondents did not appear excessively burdensome [27].

4. DELIVERY

Preterm delivery (i.e., before week 37 of gestation) occurred in 52% of our series, and this is consistent with other reports in the literature [19]. Of births recorded by the Registry, 66% were premature (i.e., less than 37 weeks of gestation and yielding an infant of less than 2500 g). Intervention for obstetric reasons is common in this group of patients, but also premature labor has been attributed to poor renal function, and this may be a contributory factor in some patients [34]. Other maternal complications may have some influence upon the maturity of the infant, including preeclampsia, which was seen in 32.4% of premature deliveries and 26.8% of term deliveries reported by Rudolph et al. [18]. Premature delivery in the general population is seen twice as often in patients with chronic hypertension or with preeclampsia.

The mean duration of pregnancy recorded by the Registry was 35.7 weeks for patients who underwent transplantation and 33.2 weeks for patients who underwent dialysis. Table 11-4 shows that gestation is invariably shorter in the dialysis than the transplant group.

The incidence of cesarean section is high in mothers on renal replacement therapy, and has been reported as 25% [19]; in the 1978 Registry survey, 47% of recorded deliveries were by this route.

The transplanted kidney does not usually produce mechanical problems during delivery, but Rudolph et al. [18] reported six cases out of 440 pregnancies where labor was obstructed by the graft.

5. THE INFANTS

5.1. Birth weight

The mean birth weight of children born to transplanted and dialyzed mothers in the Registry's series is shown in table 11-5. For grafted mothers, the average birth weight is consistently above 2500 g, for dialyzed mothers consistently below.

Table 11-4. Mean duration of pregnancy in weeks for births reported to the EDTA–ERA Registry up to the end of 1982, shown according to treatment status of the mother.

	Mean duration of pregnancy (weeks)					
Treatment status	Up to 31.12.78	1979	1980	1981	1982	All years
Transplanted (*n*)	35.0 (105)	36.4 (28)	36.0 (46)	36.0 (44)	36.3 (42)	35.7 (265)
Dialyzed (*n*)	33.3 (14)	34.3 (4)	34.0 (2)	31.9 (8)	34.3 (8)	33.2 (32)

Table 11-5. Mean birth weight, in kilograms, of children born to mothers on the EDTA–ERA Registry, shown according to treatment status of the mother.

Treatment status	Mean birth weight (kg)					
	Up to 31.12.78	1979	1980	1981	1982	All years
Transplanted (*n*)	2.5 (103)	2.6 (28)	2.6 (43)	2.6 (43)	2.6 (43)	2.6 (265)
Dialyzed (*n*)	1.9 (12)	1.8 (4)	1.6 (2)	1.7 (8)	1.8 (4)	1.8 (30)

Rudolph et al. [18] studied the relationship between birth weight and the interval between transplantation and delivery; they showed that the percentage of term deliveries with normal weight (i.e., 37 weeks and weighing over 2500 g) was greatest in those who gave birth two years or more after transplantation. In this group, over 80% of term infants had birth weights over 2500 g, compared with 73% of those born 1–2 years after transplantation, and only 46% born within a year of grafting. This finding is not substantiated in the Registry's results: 78% (80 of 102) of term infants born two or more years after transplantation had normal birth weight compared with 76% (16 of 21) of those born within two years of grafting. Both full-term infants born within a year of transplantation weighed in excess of 2500 g.

The mean body length and mean head circumference of the infants, which were recorded for the first time in 1982, were 47.9 and 32.5 cm, respectively.

5.2. Chromosomal and genetic abnormalities

Regular information about chromosomal studies was requested by the Registry for the first time in 1982. In only two cases had studies been performed; in one child there was a translocation abnormality, found also in the mother. In the 1978 survey, 16 children had undergone chromosomal analysis and chromatid breaks were discovered in two. Out of 16 children studied elsewhere, 11 were found to have structural chromosome abnormalities [6, 35, 36], which had usually disappeared by one year of age.

The congenital abnormalities reported to the Registry are shown separately for transplanted and dialyzed mothers in tables 11-6 and 11-7. In total, 14 abnormalities in 12 children were recorded. Pulmonary artery stenosis and ureterovesical stenosis have been reported elsewhere in the literature [18]. Congenital abnormalities do not appear to occur with increased frequency in the children born to mothers on renal replacement therapy compared with the general population.

In large doses, azathioprine is teratogenic in mice and rabbits [37] but not rats [38], so that the risk of modest doses taken by patients with stable renal function (about 2 mg/kg daily) may not be excessive. Transplant patients studied in 1978 who gave birth to children with congenital abnormalities were found to be taking a significantly higher daily dose of azathioprine than those who had normal children [27]. Although congenital abnormalities result from very large doses of

Table 11-6. Congenital abnormalities described in children born to transplanted mothers on the EDTA–ERA Registry.

Congenital abnormalities (transplanted mothers)
Plagiocephaly with neurologic damage
Congenital heart disease
Bilateral pes equinovarus
Cerebral palsy (frontal hemangioma)
Hypospadias
Anal atresia
Agenesis of the thumb
Pigeon chest
Strabismus
Hydrocephalus
Medullary cystic disease
Ureterovesical stenosis

Table 11-7. Congenital abnormalities described in children born to dialyzed mothers on the EDTA–ERA Registry.

Congenital abnormalities (dialyzed mothers)
Malformation of the nasopharynx
Pulmonary artery stenosis

steroids in experimental animals, the consensus is that the risk to the fetus from the doses used after transplantation is small [9, 10, 39]. There is only one report of a pregnancy in a transplant patient taking cyclosporin [40].

The effects of maternal immunosuppression on the fetal immune system include lymphoid and adrenal hypoplasia [29], thymic aplasia, and adrenal insufficiency [11]. Congenital cytomegalovirus infection recorded in one of our patients has been reported elsewhere in the literature [41]; the virus has been implicated as a cause of later mental retardation [42]. Hepatitis-B antigenemia may be a hazard in pregnancies of transplant recipients [43]. If the patient is an asymptomatic carrier, the risk of the baby becoming antigen positive is very low compared with 75% in the presence of acute hepatitis in late pregnancy or within a few months after delivery [44]. Hepatitis-B immunoglobulin given prophylactically to neonates immediately after birth has been shown to prevent the carrier state in 75% of newborns [45].

5.3. Breast feeding

Of the children reported to the Registry, 29 were breast fed. In 1981, 23% of the mothers breast fed their infants, compared with only 8.2% in 1982, and around 16% in 1979 and 1980. The concentration of azathioprine and its metabolites in breast milk is low [46], but there is no information on the long-term effect of breast feeding in these patients on which to base sound advice.

5.4. Subsequent course

The only enquiry that the Registry has so far made about the subsequent history of children born to patients on renal replacement therapy has been about survival at four weeks. Of 157 children on whom we have this information, five were dead at four weeks; the deaths all occurred prior to 1982, when cause of death was first requested. In the survey carried out by Rudolph et al. [18], 216 out of 217 children who survived the neonatal period were alive and well in 1979, the oldest aged ten years. It is the hope of the Registry to follow up its records of children born to transplanted and dialyzed patients, and already a cooperative study is being planned to look at the incidence of malignancy in this very special group of people.

6. CONTRACEPTIVE ADVICE

In 1979, the Registry enquired about the provision of contraceptive advice to women on renal replacement therapy. Among 752 centers in Europe treating women of child-bearing age, only 11% gave contraceptive advice to all women; a further 46% counseled some of their patients. The most popular stated method of contraception was the oral contraceptive pill, followed by intrauterine devices, and the condom. In view of the real danger of unwanted pregnancy in transplanted women, with the attendant risks to the graft, it is surprising that so few units offer contraceptive advice routinely. It should clearly be policy to do so. In the same way, transplanted patients who want children must be counseled about the risk they take upon themselves and upon their unborn children. That pregnancy is possible with a graft demonstrates the high quality of life achieved on renal replacement therapy.

REFERENCES

1. Murray JE, Reid DE, Harrison JH, Merrill JP: Successful pregnancies after human renal transplantation. N Engl J Med 269:341–343, 1963.
2. Hume DM, Lee HM, Williams GM, White HJO, Ferré J, Wolf JS, Prout GR, Slapak M, O'Brien J, Kilpatrick SJ, Kauffman HM, Cleveland KJ: Comparative results of cadaver and related donor renal homograft in man and immunologic implications of the outcome of second and paired transplants. Ann Surg 164:352–392, 1966.
3. Board JA, Lee HM, Draper DA, Hume DM: Pregnancy following kidney transplantation from a non-twin. Obstet Gynecol 29:318–323, 1967.
4. Kaufman JJ, Dignam W, Goodwin WE, Martin DC, Goldman R, Maxwell MH: Successful normal childbirth after kidney homotransplantation. JAMA 200:162–165, 1967.
5. Caplan RM, Dossetor JB, Maughan GB: Pregnancy following cadaver kidney homotransplantation. Am J Obstet Gynecol 106:644–648, 1970.
6. Gevers RH, Hintzen AHJ, Kalff MW, Ruys JH, Dooren LJ, Van Rood JJ, Van Went JJ, Schaberg A: Pregnancy following kidney transplantation. Eur J Obstet Gynaecol 1:147–157, 1971.
7. Horbach J, Van Liebergen F, Mastboom J, Wijdeveld P: Pregnancy in a patient after cadaveric renal transplantation. Acta Med Scand 194:237–240, 1973.
8. Robertson JG, Cockburn F, Woodruff M: Successful pregnancy after cadaveric renal transplantation. J Obstet Gynaecol Br Commonw 81:777–780, 1974.

9. Jacob ET, Grunstein S, Shapira Z, et al.: Successful pregnancy in a recipient of a cadaver kidney allograft. Isr J Med Sci 10:206–212, 1974.
10. Merkatz IR, Schwartz GII, David DS, Stenzel KH, Riggio RR, Whitsell JC: Resumption of female reproductive function following renal transplantation. JAMA 216:1749–1754, 1971.
11. Penn I, Makowski E, Droegemueller W, Halgrimson CG, Starzl TE: Parenthood in renal homograft recipients. JAMA 216:1755–1761, 1971.
12. Merrill LK, Board JA, Lee HM: Complications of pregnancy after renal transplantation including a report of spontaneous uterine rupture. Obstet Gynecol 41:270–274, 1973.
13. Sciarra JJ, Toledo-Pereyra LH, Bendel RP, Simmons RL: Pregnancy following renal transplantation. Am J Obstet Gynecol 123:411–425, 1975.
14. Von D Scholz P, Hengst H, Schilling G, May G, Schmitt E, Mebel M: Schwangerschaft nach nierentransplantation: ein bericht über 6 erfolgreiche verläufe bei multiplen riskofactoren. Z Urol Nephrol 76:175–189, 1983.
15. Goldby M: Fertility after renal transplantation. Transplantation 10:201–207, 1970.
16. Nolan GH, Sweet RL, Laros RK, Roure CA: Renal cadaver transplantation followed by successful pregnancies. Obstet Gynecol 43:732–739, 1974.
17. Rifle G, Traeger J: Pregnancy after renal transplantation: an international survey. Transplant Proc [Suppl 1] 7:723–728, 1975.
18. Rudolph JE, Schweizer RT, Bartus SA: Pregnancy in renal transplant patients. Transplantation 27:26–29, 1979.
19. Davison JM: Pregnancy in renal transplant recipients: clinical perspectives. Contrib Nephrol 37:170–178, 1984.
20. Editorial: Pregnancy after renal transplantation. Br Med J 1:733–734, 1976.
21. Confortini P, Galanti G, Ancona G, Giongo A, Bruschi E, Lorenzini E: Full term pregnancy and successful delivery in a patient on chronic haemodialysis. Proc Eur Dial Transplant Assoc 8:74–78, 1971.
22. Unzelman RF, Alderfer GR, Chojnacki RE: Pregnancy and chronic haemodialysis. Trans Am Soc Artif Intern Organs 19:144–149, 1973.
23. Ackrill P, Goodwin FJ, Marsh FP, Stratton D, Wagman H: Successful pregnancy in patients on regular dialysis. Br Med J 2:172–174, 1975.
24. Rigenbach M, Renger B, Beavais P, Imbs JF, Eschbach J, Frey G: Grossesse et accouchement d'un enfant vivant chez une patiente traitéé par haemodialyse iterative. J Urol Nephrol (Paris) 84:360–366, 1978.
25. Cattran DC, Benzie RJ: Pregnancy in a continuous ambulatory peritoneal dialysis patient. Peritoneal Dial Bull 3:13–14, 1983.
26. Wing AJ, Brunner FP, Brynger H, Chantler C, Donckerwolcke RA, Gurland HJ, Hathway RA, Jacobs C, Selwood NH: Combined report on regular dialysis and transplantation in Europe. Proc Eur Dial Transplant Assoc 7:4–76, 1978.
27. Registration Committee of the European Dialysis and Transplant Association: Successful pregnancies in women treated by dialysis and kidney transplantation. Br J Obstet Gynaecol 87:-839–845, 1980.
28. MacLean AB, Briggs JD, Sharp F, Macpherson SG: Successful triplet pregnancy in renal transplant recipient. Scott Med J X:320–322, 1980.
29. Lower GD, Stevens LE, Najarian JS, Reemtsma K: Problems from immunosuppressives during pregnancy. Am J Obstet Gynecol 111:1120–1121, 1971.
30. Salant DJ, Marcus RG, Milne FJ, Meyers AM, Botha JR, Myburgh JA: Pregnancy in renal transplant recipients. S Afr Med J 50:1288–1290, 1976.
31. Legrain M: Transplantation rénale et grossesse. Gynecologie 27:535–538, 1976.
32. Davison JM, Elliott RW, Kerr DNS, Proud G, Taylor RMR, Ward MK, Wilkinson R: Effect of pregnancy on renal function in kidney transplant recipients. Clin Exp Hypertens 81:322, 1982.
33. Moore TC, Hume DM: The period and nature of hazard in clinical renal transplantation. Ann Surg 170:12–24, 1969.
34. Felding CF: Obstetric aspects in women with histories of renal disease. Acta Obstet Gynecol Scand 48:2–43, 1969.
35. Price HV, Salamen JR, Laurence KM, Langmaid H: Immunosuppressive drugs and the foetus. Transplantation 21:294–298, 1976.
36. Leb DE, Weisskopf B, Kawovitz BS: Chromosome aberrations in the child of a kidney transplant recipient. Arch Intern Med 128:441–444, 1971.

37. Githens JH, Rosenkrantz JG, Tunnock SM: Teratogenic effects of azathioprine (Imuran). J Pediatr 66:959–961, 1965.
38. Rosenkrantz JG, Githens JH, Cox SM, Kellum DL: Azathioprine (Imuran) and pregnancy. Am J Obstet Gynecol 97:387–394, 1967.
39. Bongiovanni AM, McPadden AJ: Steroids during pregnancy and possible fetal consequences. Fertil Steril 11:181–185, 1960.
40. Lewis GJ, Lamont CAR, Lee HA, Slapak M: Successful pregnancy in a renal transplant recipient taking cyclosporin A. Br Med J 286:603, 1983.
41. Evans TJ, McCollum JPK, Valdimarsson H: Congenital cytomegalovirus infection after maternal renal transplantation. Lancet 1:1358–1360, 1975.
42. Hurley R: Antenatal infection associated with fetal malformation. In: Scrimgeour JB (ed) Towards the prevention of fetal malformation. Edinburgh: Edinburgh University, 1978, pp 101–119.
43. Skinhoj P, Cohn J, Bradburne AF: Transmission of hepatitis type B from healthy HBs Ag-positive mothers. Br Med J 1:10–11, 1975.
44. Dalquist E, Nordenfelt E: Neonatal hepatitis type B: a three year follow-up. Scand J Infect Dis 6:305–308, 1974.
45. Immunization Practices Advisory Committee: Immunoglobulins for protection against viral hepatitis. Ann Intern Med 96:193–197, 1982.
46. Verco CJ, Hawkins DF: Pregnancy after renal transplantation. Br J Obstet Gynaecol 3:29–33, 1982.

12. PREGNANCY FOLLOWING RENAL TRANSPLANTATION

ISRAEL PENN

1. INTRODUCTION

As the results of kidney transplantation continue to improve, greater numbers of patients with chronic renal failure are being rehabilitated. An important aspect of this process is restoration of sexual function and the opportunity to become a parent should one so desire. In this chapter, we discuss sexual function before and after transplantation and the risks of pregnancy to the mother and the fetus. This study is based on one of the largest series in the world of pregnancies produced by male and female kidney transplant recipients followed at a single institution, the University of Colorado Medical Center (Denver), by the author and his colleagues [1–5]. Where necessary, these data are supplemented by additional information obtained from the published literature.

2. SEXUAL FUNCTION BEFORE AND AFTER TRANSPLANTATION

2.1. Males

Chronic renal failure is frequently associated with sexual dysfunction [5, 6]. Loss of libido and impotence occurred in 48% of men in one large series studied [7]. During maintenance dialysis therapy, only 8% had improvement in sexual function. In some patients, sexual function improves after restoration of satisfactory renal function by transplantation but, in others, sexual dysfunction may persist or even develop de novo [6]. In several series, impotence was present in 22%–43%

of transplant patients [3, 7–9]. Organic causes of impotence that have been blamed include operative interference with penile blood flow or nerve supply, decreased plasma zinc levels, decreased serum hormone levels, poor allograft function, and side effects of corticosteroid and antihypertensive drugs [6]. Psychogenic factors may also play an important role [6]. Depression and anxiety decrease sexual activity, as does the poor self-image of the patient whose body has been drastically changed by surgery and corticosteroid therapy. Chronically ill men who adopt roles they consider to be feminine may feel unable to resume male sexual roles. Occasionally, a man who has received a woman's kidney feels that he is part woman inside and can no longer function as a man. Some patients may feel that transplantation is a form of castration, while others fear that intercourse will damage the transplanted kidney (which is placed low down in the iliac fossa). Whatever the cause, impotence is a source of great distress to the patient, and a number of marriages have terminated as a result of it. Occasionally it is possible to improve potency through a reduction in dosage of corticosteroid or antihypertensive drugs or by the administration of testosterone. Rare patients have improved marital relations after the surgical insertion of a permanent indwelling penile prosthesis. Sexual dysfunction therapy, on the other hand, is still underutilized.

Another problem has prevented parenthood in a small number of male patients. In the early years of transplantation it was routine practice in many medical centers to divide the spermatic cord when obtaining exposure in the iliac fossa for insertion of the kidney allograft. When this was done bilaterally, as in patients who needed two or more transplants, the patient was left sterile. This was not a problem in the early years of transplantation when patient survival was a few weeks or months. As long-term survivals were attained and parenthood became a possibility, we recommended that every effort be made to preserve the spermatic cord [10]. This procedure is now widely practiced.

2.2. Females

Sexual dysfunction occurs in 26% of females with chronic renal failure [7]. They experience loss of libido, anovulatory vaginal bleeding, or amenorrhea. During maintenance dialysis therapy, only 6% experience improvement in sexual function. As a result, pregnancy only occurs in about one of 200 women of childbearing age having dialysis therapy [11]. By 1981, conception and successful completion of pregnancy by a woman on hemodialysis had been reported on only eight occasions [12]. A unique case has been reported of a pregnant dialysis patient who underwent renal transplantation during the second trimester with a successful outcome for mother, child, and the allografted kidney [13].

Many dialysis patients have improved sexual function after successful renal transplantation and, in addition, their fertility increases. Thus, patients have the opportunity to become parents if they so desire [1–5] and about one of every 50 women of childbearing age, having a functioning renal transplant, becomes pregnant [11]. A high-risk group of patients, in whom the results of renal transplantation have been progressively improving, are those with renal failure caused by juvenile-onset diabetes mellitus. To date, at least three successful pregnancies have been described in such patients [14–16].

3. MENSTRUATION AND CONTRACEPTION FOLLOWING RENAL TRANSPLANTATION

Before transplantation, female patients are either amenorrheic or have infrequent episodes of vaginal bleeding that occur at intervals ranging from three to six months. On the average, menstruation reappears an average of six months after transplantation (range, 3–12 months) [1].

Because of the uncertain life expectancy following renal transplantation, both male and female patients must be counseled on family planning. Those desiring parenthood must be warned that they may not live long enough to rear their children to adulthood and may leave their spouses with the problem of raising their children [1–5]. The importance of this is borne out by the fact that five of the 39 mothers and two of the 50 fathers in the author's series at the University of Colorado died after becoming parents [5]. All patients who have completed their families or have no desire to have children should be offered sterilization either at the time of transplantation or at some time thereafter. Those wishing to become parents should be advised to practice contraception for at least 18 months after transplantation [1–5]. In a few instances, however, pregnancies have occurred at an early period after transplantation in individuals who were under the mistaken impression that they were incapable of having children and, therefore, did not take any contraceptive precautions [1].

As thromboembolism and hypertension are common in renal transplant patients, we are disinclined to use oral contraceptive agents because they may increase the incidence of these complications [3]. In the normal female population, there have been reports of serious and even fatal infections following the insertion of intrauterine devices. Theoretically this complication is more likely to occur in immunosuppressed renal transplant patients. Although this has not been our experience thus far, we recommend less risky forms of contraception such as the diaphragm, condom, and contraceptive foams and creams [3].

4. RISKS OF PREGNANCY FOLLOWING RENAL TRANSPLANTATION

Pregnant patients should consult their obstetricians as soon as pregnancy is suspected. They should then be followed in a high-risk obstetric clinic, in conjunction with a member of the transplant team or a nephrologist, at biweekly intervals until week 36 of gestation and then weekly until the onset of labor [1–5]. The patient's blood pressure and weight are measured. Standard renal function tests, including determination of blood urea nitrogen levels, serum creatinine levels, and creatinine clearance should be performed at regular intervals. The urine should be analyzed for specific gravity, 24-h protein content, glucose, and electrolyte levels. In addition, microscopic examinations should be performed and cultures obtained.

Most pregnancies have occurred in patients receiving conventional immunosuppressive therapy with azathioprine, corticosteroids and, in some cases, antilymphocyte globulin [1–5]. At present, at least two successful pregnancies have occurred following the use of the new immunosuppressive agent, cyclosporine [17, 18].

A major concern is for the function of the kidney during and after gestation [1–5]. Many immunologists regard pregnancy as an immunologically privileged state, which protects the mother from rejecting the fetus, and which may also protect the allograft. On theoretical grounds, rejection might not be expected to occur during gestation. In fact, some women have had substantial reductions or even cessation of immunosuppressive therapy during pregnancy without deterioration of renal function [19]. In the author's experience (see below), most recipients with satisfactory pregestational renal function experience no significant change during pregnancy and delivery, although transient deterioration of function may occur during pregnancy. However, one patient did develop permanent renal functional impairment. In addition, several authors have reported patients in whom renal functional impairment developed during pregnancy and persisted following delivery [20–26].

The overall incidence of permanently impaired renal function in the author's series was 7% [5]. Most occurred in patients with allograft problems that were present before pregnancy. Because of the greatly increased risks involved, one must strongly advise those with impaired function not to become pregnant. If they do, however, the pregnancy should be terminated if any further functional deterioration occurs, because of the danger that such damage may become permanent [3–5]. The cause of the functional deterioration is not known. Presumably, it results from an ongoing process of chronic rejection [3].

Theoretically, the termination of pregnancy and its naturally occurring immunosuppressed state should be followed by an increased risk of rejection. On occasions, some workers have augmented the dose of corticosteroids during or after delivery, for periods ranging from five days to three months after termination of pregnancy [19]. The author has found that increased dosage of corticosteroid therapy was unnecessary except for 100-mg doses of hydrocortisone given every 8 h for 24 h, commencing with the onset of parturition to protect the patient from the stress of labor [2].

In the author's series there were 58 pregnancies in 39 female transplant recipients [1–5]: 25 patients had single pregnancies, ten had two, three had three, and one had four pregnancies. Of 39 pregnancies that occurred in patients, who were normotensive or had normal renal function before transplantation, 84% had no difficulties. The major problems were preeclampsia, which occurred in five pregnancies (14%), and deterioration of renal function, which occurred in one pregnancy (3%). In contrast, of 21 pregnancies that occurred in patients who had hypertension and/or impaired renal function before transplantation, only six (29%) were uneventful. Ten (48%) were complicated by preeclampsia, five (24%) ended in therapeutic abortions for medical as well as emotional reasons, and three (14%) were complicated by deterioration of renal function during pregnancy or postpartum. One pregnancy was also complicated by severe gestational diabetes. The overall incidence of preeclampsia in the 58 pregnancies was 26%. This is approximately four times greater than that seen in the general population [3]. No patients developed eclampsia. To the author's knowledge, only one case of eclampsia has been reported in a renal transplant recipient [27]. We regard all increases in proteinuria with suspicion, although some authors state that proteinuria frequently increases during the third trimester, but that it has no negative significance, even though there may be a transitory decrease in glomerular filtration rate near term [19].

The transplanted kidney does not cause mechanical dystocia during labor as it is usually situated in the false pelvis and vaginal delivery is possible in most pregnancies [1–5]. Cesarean section is indicated purely for obstetric reasons, mainly fetal distress and cephalopelvic disproportion. Tubal ligation at the time of cesarean section may be advisable in patients who do not wish to have any additional children, or in patients where further pregnancies may be high-risk procedures because of hypertension or impaired allograft function. The renal allograft blood vessels and ureter may be subjected to compression during labor, but we have not observed any harmful consequences as a result of this [3]. If there is any question of allograft compression or of obstruction of labor by the transplanted kidney, some workers recommend simultaneous intravenous pyelography and x-ray pelvimetry [19, 27, 28].

Some authors have described an increased incidence of infections in transplant patients during pregnancy [25], and they should be carefully monitored particularly for urinary tract infections. Because of the risk of infection, we cannot overemphasize the importance of aseptic technique during examination and delivery. Because of this hazard, labor is induced with oxytocin in patients who present with premature rupture of the membranes. The ever-present danger of infection is emphasized by the only pregnancy-related death that occurred in the author's series [5]. The patient, who had preexisting hypertension, developed preeclampsia and gestational diabetes. Fetal distress and a breech presentation necessitated a cesarean section. Postoperatively the patient developed wound infection and a tuboovarian abscess that required emergency subtotal hysterectomy and bilateral salpingo-oophorectomy. She died of sepsis several weeks later.

Abortions occurred in nine of 58 pregnancies in the author's series [5]. One occurred spontaneously. Most of the eight therapeutic abortions were performed at the patients' request since they did not desire to be parents. In addition, five of them had impaired renal function and/or hypertension, factors that helped in making the decision in favor of therapeutic abortion, and two recipients also had emotional instability.

During pregnancy, urinary levels of estrogen are low. Some authors believe that administered corticosteroids cross the placenta, suppress fetal corticotropin and, therefore, suppress the precursors that are necessary for estrogen synthesis [29]. However, low urinary estriol levels have been observed in a patient immunosuppressed with cyclosporine only, without additional steroids. Presumably another explanation for low urinary estriol excretion in pregnant renal transplant recipients is a relatively lower glomerular filtration rate [17].

5. FOLLOW-UP OF WOMEN WITH TRANSPLANTED KIDNEYS FOLLOWING PREGNANCY

Patients should be followed indefinitely particularly as regards to long-term function of the allograft, and for complications that may occur in any organ transplant recipient, such as side effects of individual immunosuppressive agents, infections, and cancers [30]. Certain cancers of the female genital tract are particularly common among organ transplant recipients. Up to September 1984, the Cincinnati Transplant Tumor Registry (CTTR) had received data on 2211 types of cancer that had occurred in 2070 organ transplant recipients [31]. Of these, 736 patients were women. In transplant patients, in situ carcinomas of the uterus are increased 14-fold as compared with age-matched controls [30, 31]. In the CTTR, 133 (18%) of the 736 women had carcinomas of the cervix. In situ lesions made up at least 80% of the cases. Carcinomas of the body of the uterus were uncommon (only 14 cases). Perhaps this is because most transplant patients are young whereas these neoplasms occur mainly in postmenopausal women.

Carcinomas of the vulva, perianal skin, and anus were much more common than in the nontransplant population and occurred at an earlier age. They were found in 45 women patients. Compared with the general population, the recipients were surprisingly young, their average age at the time of transplantation being 30 (range, 15–55) years. The tumors appeared at an average of 92 (range, 9–215) months. In some patients there was a "field effect" with involvement by cancer of the vulva and vagina and/or cervix of the uterus. A history of condyloma acuminatum or herpes genitalis suggests an etiologic role by oncogenic viruses in these immunosuppressed patients.

Other tumors of the female sex organs were carcinomas of the breast (67 cases), carcinomas of the ovary (23 cases), carcinomas of the vagina (five cases), and a carcinoma of an endometrial implant in the rectovaginal septum (one case). These various malignancies were not increased in incidence compared with controls. The frequency of genital malignancies, however, particularly of the uterine cervix and vulva, emphasizes the need for all postadolescent female transplant patients to undergo regular examinations of the breast and pelvic organs and to have routine cervical smears performed [30, 31].

6. RISKS TO THE FETUS

6.1. Offspring of male transplant patients

The only concern is that the children may be born with congenital malformations [1–5]. Studies in humans have shown that azathioprine may cause chromosome aberrations [32] and it is theoretically possible that the sperm could be affected. In the author's experience, 50 men patients were responsible for 67 pregnancies, which resulted in 60 live births and two spontaneous abortions [5]. Two children were born with multiple congenital anomalies and one of them died at birth.

Among the abnormalities in the other was a myelomeningocele, but there was also a family history of spina bifida.

6.2. Offspring of female transplant patients

Theoretically the immunosuppressive agents and other drugs given to the mother during pregnancy, or metabolites of these drugs, may cross the placenta or be excreted in the colostrum or breast milk and cause immunosuppressive or other side effects on the fetus. Our own studies showed no detectable levels of 6-mercaptopurine (the major metabolite of azathioprine) in cord blood, maternal blood, colostrum, or milk [1]. In contrast, corticosteroids readily cross the human placenta [29] and may cause transient adrenal insufficiency in the neonate [1]. In one study cyclosporine was not found in the infant's cord blood [18] but, in another, significant levels were found in the cord blood and in breast milk [17]. The authors recommended that mothers treated with cyclosporine should avoid breast feeding [17]. Neither infant manifested side effects of cyclosporine [17, 18].

Of 58 pregnancies in the author's series, 48 resulted in live births, including one set of twins [1–5]. The major problem was prematurity (birth before week 37 of gestation), which occurred in 23 infants (48%). Premature labor is quite common in nontransplant patients with poor renal function. Some of the premature deliveries in the author's series may have resulted from this cause, but in the remaining cases there is no obvious explanation for the premature onset of labor. One of the complications of prematurity is respiratory distress syndrome. Some physicians believe that steroid therapy given to the mother before delivery may prevent this disorder in the premature infant [33]. Despite the fact that the mothers in the author's series received corticosteroid therapy, however, four premature infants did in fact develop respiratory distress syndrome.

In the author's series, 34 (71%) of the 48 infants had an uncomplicated neonatal course. The remaining 14 (29%) had one or more complications. The most common were five (10%) with congenital anomalies, four (8%) with respiratory distress syndrome, two (4%) with adrenocortical insufficiency, two (4%) with septicemia, and two (4%) with hyperviscosity. There were two deaths in the neonatal period, one from sepsis and the other from respiratory distress syndrome. The congenital anomalies included two infants with pulmonary artery stenosis, of whom one also had an intraarticular hemangioma, one with bilateral inguinal hernias, one with a deformed hand, and one with a patent ductus arteriosus. It is uncertain whether these were coincidental developments or were caused by the immunosuppressive therapy given to the mothers. Experiments in animals have shown that both of the commonly used agents, azathioprine and corticosteroids, may be teratogenic [34–36]. However, other workers have reported a low incidence of congenital defects in infants born to mothers with renal transplants [19, 25, 37].

As mentioned above, infants born to chronically immunosuppressed mothers may themselves suffer side effects of the immunosuppressive therapy [1–5]. Two newborns in the author's series developed serious infections that caused the death of one of them. Two others had adrenocortical insufficiency with signs of peripheral vascular collapse including lethargy, mottled skin, and hypotension. Any infant showing deterioration during the first few days of life should have an urgent workup for these complications. If indicated, treatment with hydrocortisone, intravenous electrolyte solutions, antibiotics, and gamma globulin should be started. The children in the University of Colorado series have now been followed from 11 months to 15 years [38]. Unusual childhood infections or malignant tumors were not observed. All children appear to be growing and developing without problems specifically attributable to their mothers' kidney transplant.

There are several other theoretical long-term risks to these infants. Experiments in female mice, given low doses of 6-mercaptopurine during pregnancy, indicate that many of the female offspring may be sterile or, if they become pregnant, they have smaller litters and more dead fetuses than the offspring of mothers that have not received the drug [39]. Long-term follow-up of the children of transplant patients will provide an answer as to whether similar problems may occur in humans.

Chromosome aberrations have been observed in the lymphocytes of several infants born to renal transplant mothers [40, 41]. Although these disappeared within 32 months, there are two theoretical risks. Abnormalities may have persisted in tissues not studied, including the primordial ova, and these may give rise to abnormalities in the next generation. Another possibility is that chromosome abnormalities may precede the development of cancers in the affected offspring. Thus far, none have been reported.

7. CONCLUSIONS

The improving long-term results of renal transplantation make it likely that greater numbers of transplant recipients will desire to become parents. As pregnancy has risks to the female transplant patient and to the fetus, transplant recipients must be counseled regarding family planning. The option of sterilization should be offered if the patient desires it. If female patients have impaired renal function prior to conception and there is further deterioration during pregnancy, termination of the gestation should be recommended. If the pregnancy continues, there is a risk of permanent impairment of renal function. In patients with satisfactory renal function before pregnancy, there may be transient deterioration of function during gestation, but usually this returns to preexisting levels in the postpartum period. Renal transplant patients have a 26% risk of developing preeclampsia during pregnancy. Usually the transplanted kidney does not produce any mechanical dystocia during labor. During vaginal delivery, there is no apparent mechanical injury to the transplanted kidney. Since there is a 14-fold increase in the incidence of in situ carcinoma of the cervix, and an increased incidence of carcinoma of the vulva, in female transplant recipients it is essential that these patients have pelvic examinations and vaginal cytology prior to transplantation and at regular intervals afterward.

The risk to the offspring of male transplant patients is small. There is a substantial hazard, however, to the newborn of female recipients: 48% of the newborns were delivered prior to week 37 of gestation, and 29% had one or more complications during the neonatal period; these included respiratory distress syndrome, congenital anomalies, lymphopenia and adrenocortical insufficiency, infection, and hyperviscosity.

REFERENCES

1. Penn I, Makowski E, Droegemueller W, Halgrimson C, Starzl TE: Parenthood in renal homograft recipients. JAMA 216:1755–1761, 1971.
2. Makowski EL, Penn I: Parenthood following renal transplantation. In: De Alvarez RR (ed) The kidney in pregnancy. New York: John Wiley, 1976, pp 215–227.
3. Penn I, Makowski EL, Harris P: Parenthood following renal transplantation. Kidney Int 18:-221–233, 1980.
4. Penn I, Makowski EL, Harris P: Parenthood following renal and hepatic transplantation. Transplantation 30:397–400, 1980.
5. Penn I, Makowski EL: Parenthood in kidney and liver transplant recipients. Transplant Proc 13:36–39, 1981.
6. Dubovsky SL, Penn I: Psychiatric considerations in renal transplant surgery. Psychosomatics 21:481–491, 1980.
7. Levy NB: Sexual adjustment to maintenance hemodialysis and renal transplantation: national survey by questionnaire, preliminary report. Trans Am Soc Artif Intern Organs 19:138–143, 1973.
8. Abram HS, Hester LR, Sheridan WF, Epstein GM: Sexual function in patients with chronic renal failure. J Nerv Ment Dis 160:220–226, 1975.
9. Salvatierra O Jr, Fortman JL, Belzer FO: Sexual function in males before and after renal transplantation. Urology 5:64–66, 1975.
10. Penn I, Mackie G, Halgrimson C, Starzl TE: Testicular complications following renal transplantation. Ann Surg 176:697–699, 1972.
11. Editorial: Pregnancy after renal transplantation. Br Med J 1:733–734, 1976.
12. Kobayashi H, Matsumato Y, Otsubo O, Otsubo K, Naito T: Successful pregnancy in a patient undergoing chronic hemodialysis. Obstet Gynecol 57:382–386, 1981.
13. Burleson RL, Sunderji SG, Aubry RH, Clark DA, Marbarger P, Cohen RS, Scruggs BF, Lagraff S: Renal allotransplantation during pregnancy. Successful outcome for mother, child and kidney. Transplantation 36:334–335, 1983.
14. Tagatz GE, Arnold NI, Goetz FC, Najarian JS, Simmons RL: Pregnancy in a juvenile diabetic after renal transplantation (class T diabetes mellitus). Diabetes 24:497–501, 1975.
15. Kitzmiller JL, Aiello LM, Kaldany A, Younger MD: Diabetic vascular disease complicating pregnancy. Clin Obstet Gynecol 24:107–123, 1981.
16. Levine MG, Miodovnik M, Siddiqi TA, First MR, Knowles HC: A successful pregnancy in a juvenile diabetic with a renal transplant complicated by pre-eclampsia. Transplantation 35:-498–499, 1983.
17. Lewis GJ, Lamont CAR, Lee HA, Slapak M: Successful pregnancy in a renal transplant recipient taking cyclosporin A. Br Med J 286:603, 1983.
18. Klintmalm G, Althoff P, Appleby G, Segerbrandt E: Renal function in a newborn baby delivered of a renal transplant patient taking cyclosporine. Transplantation 38:198–199, 1984.
19. Rifle G, Traeger J: Pregnancy after renal transplantation: an international survey. Transplant Proc 7:723–728, 1975.
20. Board JA, Lee HM, Draper DA, Hume DM: Pregnancy following kidney homotransplantation from a non-twin. Obstet Gynecol 29:318–323, 1967.
21. Caplan RM, Dossetor JB, Maughan GB: Pregnancy following cadaver kidney homotransplantation. Am J Obstet Gynecol 106:644–648, 1970.
22. Gevers RH, Hintzen AHJ, Kalff MW, Ruys JH, Dooren LJ, Van Rood JJ, Van Went JJ, Schaberg A: Pregnancy following kidney transplantation. Eur J Obstet Gynaecol 1:147–157, 1971.
23. Merrill LK, Board JA, Lee HM: Complications of pregnancy after renal transplantation including a report of spontaneous rupture. Obstet Gynecol 41:270–274, 1973.

24. Moore TC, Hume DM: The period and nature of hazard in clinical renal transplantation. II. The hazard to transplant kidney function. Ann Surg 170:12–24, 1969.
25. Rudolph JE, Schweitzer RT, Bartus SA: Pregnancy in renal transplant patients: a review. Transplantation 27:26–29, 1979.
26. Sciarra JJ, Toledo-Pereyra LH, Bendel RP, Simmons RL: Pregnancy following renal transplantation. Am J Obstet Gynecol 125:411–425, 1975.
27. Williams PF, Jelen J: Eclampsia in a patient who had had a renal transplant. Br Med J 2:972, 1979.
28. Corry RJ, Thompson J: Renal transplantation case studies. Garden City NY: Medical Examination Publication Company, 1977, p 83.
29. Coulam CB, Zincke H, Sterioff S: Pregnancy after renal transplantation: estrogen secretion. Transplantation 33:556–558, 1982.
30. Penn I: The price of immunotherapy. Curr Probl Surg 18:681–751, 1981.
31. Penn I: Mechanisms of malignant development after transplantation. In: Proceedings of the 20th annual meeting of the Japan Transplantation Society, Tokyo, Japan, September 1984 (In press.)
32. Jensen MK: Chromosome studies in patients treated with azathioprine and Amethopterin. Acta Med Scand 182:445–455, 1967.
33. Liggins GC, Howie RN: A controlled trial of antepartum glucocorticoid treatment for prevention of the respiratory distress syndrome in premature infants. Pediatrics 50:515–525, 1972.
34. Githens JH, Rosenkrantz JG, Tunnock SM: Teratogenic effects of azathioprine. J Pediatr 66:-959–961, 1965.
35. Rosenkrantz JG, Githens JH, Cox SM, Kellum DL: Azathioprine and pregnancy. Am J Obstet Gynecol 97:387–394, 1967.
36. Bongiovanni AM, McPadden AJ: Steroids during pregnancy and possible fetal consequences. Fertil Steril 11:181–186, 1960.
37. Merkatz IR, Schwartz GH, David DS, Stenzel KH, Riggio RR, Whitsell JS: Resumption of female reproductive function following renal transplantation. JAMA 216:1749–1754, 1971.
38. Weil R III, Barfield N, Schroter GPJ, Bauling PC: Children of mothers with kidney transplants. Transplantation Proc, 1985 (in press).
39. Reimers TJ, Sluss PM: 6-Mercaptopurine treatment of pregnant mice: effects on second and third generations. Science 201:65–67, 1978.
40. Leb DF, Weisskopf B, Kanovitz BS: Chromosome aberrations in the child of a kidney transplant recipient. Arch Intern Med 128:441–444, 1971.
41. Price HV, Salaman JR, Laurence KM, Langmaid H: Immunosuppressive drugs and the fetus. Transplantation 21:294–298, 1976.

13. URINARY TRACT INFECTION IN PREGNANCY

IAIN R. McFADYEN

1. INTRODUCTION

The normal urinary tract is sterile from bladder neck to kidney. Urinary tract infection (UTI) is the presence of microorganisms in the urinary tract. Bacteriuria is the presence of bacteria in the bladder urine: this may be restricted to the bladder (cystitis) or also involve the ureteric urine and kidney (pyelonephritis). Either kind of UTI may be accompanied by symptoms and signs (overt infection), or none may be present despite the active proliferation of organisms (covert infection). The urethra also is part of the urinary tract. It may be the seat of some symptoms because of infection within itself or because infected urine is passing through it. Also, bacteria may travel from the introitus along the urethra into the bladder urine and produce UTI. The intrinsic lesions of urethritis have recently been well reviewed elsewhere [1] so here the urethra will be considered only as it is relevant to UTI.

Urinary tract infection is one of the most common complications of pregnancy, but its diagnosis frequently is difficult or imprecise. It may be mimicked by other lesions, some of which are trivial and some life-threatening. To clarify this review of the problems and significance of UTI in pregnancy, diagnosis is discussed first.

2. DIAGNOSIS OF UTI

Diagnosis depends on accurate determination of whether or not organisms are present in the urinary tract and, if any are present, on recognition of their species.

This can be done only by examination of the urine or of a renal biopsy. Interpretation of the bacterial content of a specimen of urine requires knowledge of how that urine was obtained, since it could be contaminated by organisms in the urethra or on the vulva [2, 3]. Only 2% of women who had sterile bladder urine passed a midstream specimen (MSU) that was free of all organisms, 17% of the MSUs contained 10–100 organisms/ml, 40% 100–1000/ml, 24% 1000–10,000/ml, 11% 10,000–100,000/ml, and 7% of these women with sterile urine passed an MSU containing more than 100,000 organisms/ml: half of the organisms grown from these urines were Gram-negative bacilli [4]. Some degree of contamination in midstream specimens appears to be almost inevitable. It is identification of what is contamination and what is not that makes interpretation of an MSU difficult. Kass [2] recognized this when he proposed that more than 100,000 ($>10^5$) bacteria/ml urine was a "significant" growth, indicating infection of the urine with 80% certainty. The value of $>10^5$/ml was selected because it was the bacterial count present in the urine of 95% of patients with dysuria, flank pain, and pyrexia: it was also the concentration of bacteria present in 6% of outpatients who had no symptoms of infection, but of whom more than half gave a history of urinary infection and who showed a 95% reproducibility between MSU and catheter specimens (CSU), while those with lower bacterial counts had little correlation between MSU and CSU (the organisms were usually saprophytes of skin and urethra) and only 15% gave a history of infection [2, 5]; also, urine obtained by percutaneous puncture of the bladder usually showed either no growth or $>10^5$ organisms/ml [6, 7]. This critical level of "significance" is valid only with thorough cleansing of the periurethral urea: contamination rates as high as 50% may occur, suggesting that vulval preparation was not satisfactory [8–10].

Assuming that vulval preparation was satisfactory so that a bacterial count of $>10^5$/ml had only a 1 in 5 chance of being due to contamination of a urine that was truly sterile, Kass [2] proposed that two consecutive MSUs that contained $>10^5$ organisms/ml gave a 96% probability of correctly indicating infection of the bladder urine, since the first had an 80% probability of being correct and the second would by being sterile reveal that four-fifths of the original 20% (i.e., 16%) contained $>10^5$ bacteria/ml as a consequence of contamination. This would be true if contamination were random, but it is not [9]: those who contaminate once tend to do so recurrently, and this is likely to occur with the physiologic and pathologic discharges of pregnancy and the puerperium. Thus, a single MSU in pregnancy that contains $>10^5$ organisms/ml has at least a 10%–20% chance of that bacterial growth being due to contamination, and possibly of the chance of contamination being greater, while two consecutive MSUs from that patient containing $>10^5$/ml increase the chance of accurate diagnosis, but even this is not certain. An MSU that is sterile or that contains only a few organism is likely to be accurate, when the various caveats discussed later are taken into account, and so is a reasonable indication of the absence of infection. Further research has, however, increased the uncertainty of diagnosis of UTI from midstream urines.

Of asymptomatic women with $>10^5$ Gram-negative bacteria in an MSU, 92%

had the same organism in a later percutaneous suprapubic aspiration specimen (SPA) while only 70% of those with Gram-positive organisms in MSU had the same in SPA [11]. So, in interpreting the significance of growth in an MSU, the species of organism is relevant. Lower bacterial counts of 10^4–10^5/ml are not necessarily due to contamination: 5% are bacteriuric [5]; 74% of those with Gram-negative organisms and 30% with Gram-positive organisms in such concentrations in an MSU had the same organisms in SPA [11]. Certain organisms such as *Staphylococcus saprophyticus* may be multiplying in the urine, but rarely reach bacterial counts $> 10^5$/ml [12]. The patients' symptoms may also be relevant to interpretation: among 187 dysuric women, the optimal sensitivity and specificity for bacterial counts of *Coliform* organisms in MSU was found to be $> 10^2$/ml [13].

Mixtures of organisms in an MSU cannot be disregarded or taken to mean that the bacterial count is due to contamination: 1%–3% of infections are due to more than one organism, or urine infected by one organism may be contaminated by another during collection and produce a mixed growth on culture [4, 11, 13–15]. Mixed infection suggests underlying pathology such as stone, tuberculosis, or diverticula.

White cell content of an MSU may also be potentially misleading. Pyuria is present in only 50% of those with an infected urine whether the bacterial content is greater or less than 10^5/ml [11, 13, 16–18], so 50% of those with infection have no pyuria: thus the presence or absence of pyuria cannot be used to determine whether or not a specimen of urine should be cultured. Pyuria may be present when the bladder urine is sterile because of urethritis, vulval contamination, infection that has been inadequately treated and is going to reappear, or with chronic infections such as tuberculosis. Microscopy may also reveal characteristic clumps of *Staphylococcus saprophyticus* [12] casts and other relevant abnormalities.

Midstream urines may be useful in excluding infection, but the value of an MSU in making a positive diagnosis of UTI is reduced by the inherent uncertainty of a single specimen. Two more accurate methods of obtaining urine for culture are available: catheter specimens (CSU) and suprapubic aspiration (SPA). Catheter specimens containing $> 10^5$/ml have at least a 95% confidence level [5], and counts of 1000/ml or more of a single organism or 3000/ml or more of a mixed organism probably accurately reflect the content of the bladder urine since these are the numbers expected from urethral contamination [4, 19]. With a satisfactory technique, catheterization rarely introduces infection, and instillation of antiseptic into the bladder at the end of the procedure almost eliminates the risk in a single catheterization [20]. Furthermore, since a CSU frequently will be obtained for accurate diagnosis when there is clinical suspicion of UTI, it is likely that antibacterial treatment will be started immediately, which will also prevent the establishment of infection should the CSU be sterile. Catheter specimens have considerable advantages in accuracy as pregnancy advances, since the abdominal distension, vaginal laxity, and discharge discourage satisfactory MSU samples. In the puerperium, a CSU is even more indicated because of the potential for contamination from the lochial discharge, particularly if there are perineal or abdominal wounds.

Diagnostic catheterization does not increase the number of puerperal urinary infections [20].

Suprapubic aspiration is the most certain method of diagnosing UTI. Any bacteria found in the urine indicates infection: bacterial counts are potentially misleading (as well as being unnecessary) because of the dilution of the urine required for SPA. It is better than 99% accurate and is safe in pregnancy up to 32–34 weeks: after this, the pregnant uterus compresses the bladder so that it can be penetrated and the uterus entered [4, 15]. Provided that the bladder is full, SPA is no more uncomfortable than venepuncture.

2.1. Falsely high bacterial counts

Whatever the method of collection of urine, bacterial numbers may be increased by delays in culturing the specimen. Since bacteria may divide every 20–30 min, organisms that originally were present in small numbers (as the result of urethral or vulval contamination) can reach "significant" levels rapidly if there is delay in transporting the specimen to the laboratory or in setting up the culture; or contaminant organisms may overgrow true infection. Keeping the urine specimen at 4°C does not alter colony counts significantly for at least 48 h [19]. Another method of avoiding such fallacious results is to use slides coated with culture medium ("dip slides") that are dipped into freshly passed urine and incubated immediately; 18–24 h later, growth on the slide accurately reflects the bacterial content of the original urine specimen, but the result is as likely to be a consequence of urethral or vulval contamination as in any other MSU, may be in as many as 40% of "positive" dipslides [21].

2.2. Falsely low bacterial counts

Reduced or no bacterial growth may be obtained from an infected urinary tract if the urine contains a bacteriostatic agent. A single 500-mg dose of ampicillin may reduce the concentration from 10^9/ml to less than 10^5/ml for 3–4 days before the concentration again rises above 10^5/ml [22]. If the laboratory knows that the urine contains an antibiotic, penicillinase or other relevant agents can be placed in the culture medium to aid maximum appropriate bacterial growth: in one series, however, 21% of specimens contained antibiotics of which the laboratory were not informed when the request for examination was made, and 21% of urines from patients who were thought to be taking antibiotics did not contain any antibiotic [23]. Chlorhexidine or other antiseptics used for cleaning the vulva before an MSU is obtained may get into the specimen and effectively sterilize it [24], so preparative cleaning is best done with saline or water. Metabolic products excreted in the urine may also be bacteriostatic [25]. Diuresis or increased frequency of micturition may dilute the urinary concentration of bacteria or not allow sufficient time for bacterial multiplication to occur so that only low bacterial counts are found: the anxious patient who has a cup of coffee before she arrives at the clinic and is then asked by the nurse to produce a specimen of urine just before she is seen by the doctor is not likely immediately to produce an MSU, or any other specimen of urine, suitable for accurate diagnosis: better that she return later with a full bladder. Organisms that grow slowly or have special requirements for culture may also produce false-negative results: they are discussed later.

3. CLINICAL DIAGNOSIS OF UTI

Symptoms associated with UTI are of little help in its diagnosis. Such symptoms are present in only 50% of whose who are infected; only 30%–50% of those with these symptoms have infected urine and almost half of those with upper urinary tract infection have no symptoms [15, 16, 26–31]. This lack of correlation between infection and symptoms is true both for the initial presentation of infection and for recurrence after treatment [15]. "Urinary" symptoms may be minimal or absent in UTI or they may be mimicked by many other conditions. Iliac fossa pain indistinguishable from that of UTI may be produced by appendicitis or other intestinal disorders, by ovarian cysts that rotate or bleed, by round or broad ligament structures, or by abdominal wall or retroperitoneal tissues. Increased frequency of micturition is normal in pregnancy, as is nocturia that may occur as often as four times a night in a normal uninfected pregnancy [15]. Stress incontinence may be due to UTI [32], but it is also a consequence of the relaxation of the support of the bladder that occurs during pregnancy [33]. Burning dysuria can be due to urethritis [1], viruria [34], chlamydial infection of the urine [35], acid urine [25], or to vulvitis. The last is commonly monilial, secondary to treatment with broad spectrum antibiotics that may have been prescribed for a UTI, so that the vulvitis produces symptoms suggestive of persistence or recurrence of the infection. Loin pain may have orthopedic or other origins but, even if it is present in a patient with UTI, it does not help to localize the site of infection, since a fifth of those whose infection is localized to the bladder, without ureteric or renal involvement, have loin pain [36]. Hematuria, however, is usually a consequence of infection [15], and renal angle pain with pyrexia is likely to be due to UTI. Acute retention of urine or persistent vomiting that does not respond to treatment also may be due to UTI.

The patient's previous history sometimes is relevant. Urinary problems in the past are more common in bacteriurics than in others, but the association is not strong. One study revealed that urinary symptoms had been experienced previously by 91% of bacteriurics, but also by 63% of uninfected controls: if the history was restricted to the previous year, the relationship was stronger, 69% of bacteriurics having had urinary symptoms during that time but only 18% of controls [37]. In another group of patients, 38% of those with bacteriuria had a proven urinary tract infection in the past, but this was true of only 15% of those who were currently free of infection [38]. Women who had pyelonephritis in childhood have an increased incidence of pyelonephritis in pregnancy [39, 40], and pyelonephritis in one pregnancy increases the chances of symptomatic infection in later pregnancies [41]. Although history alone is not helpful in diagnosing asymptomatic bacteriuria, it may aid the identification of a group at risk for developing symptomatic infection during pregnancy [42].

4. CLINICAL EXAMINATION

Clinical examination may suggest the possibility of UTI, but rarely produces a conclusive diagnosis. Too many conditions can produce abdominal tenderness or other symptoms: even renal angle tenderness can be due to orthopedic or other problems. UTI is a condition that is dependent on laboratory studies of diagnosis.

5. CHANGES IN THE URINARY TRACT

During pregnancy there is a gradually progressive dilatation of the ureters above the pelvic brim [43–45]. This starts earlier in multiparous patients than in primigravidas and may appear as early as six weeks. After delivery it recedes and in most women it has disappeared within two months, but in some there is permanent residual dilatation. The dilatation is a result of a combination of hormonal relaxation of the smooth muscle of the ureters [46] and physical obstruction by the pregnant uterus rising out of the pelvis such as is seen with large gynecologic tumors rising out of the pelvis [45]. Because the uterus tends to be dextrorotated, the dilatation is usually greater on the right than the left. As the capacity of the ureters increases due to the dilatation, flow down them slows in the majority of women: ureteric emptying time may be 4–5 times as long as in the nonpregnant. In women with bacteriuria, this slowing of urine flow may be increased by the antiperistaltic effect of *Escherichia coli* endotoxin [47].

Ureteric reflux is uncommon in normal pregnancy, occurring in only 0–3% [48–50]. It is prevented by proliferation of the Waldeyer sheath around the ureter in the bladder wall, which produces an even more effective valvular effect than in the nonpregnant [44, 45]. Infected urine may, however, render this valve ineffective [51], but reflux due to this may be abolished by cure of the infection [52, 53], although it does persist in some cases [54].

Bladder tone decreases during pregnancy, paralleling the ureteric changes. The urethra elongates and the supports of the bladder also relax [33]. Bladder capacity increases with the loss of tone: starting from the third month of gestation it may reach 1300 ml by the eighth month, but there is no residual urine [55]. After delivery, tone decreases and capacity increases further, and residual volumes are sometimes present for a few days [55–58], which increases the probability of any bacteria that enter the bladder proliferating there [59, 60]. Like the ureteric changes, bladder tone and capacity return to normal in the next eight weeks in almost every case. In the puerperium, the vaginal epithelium thins, a relative atrophy due to the physiologic hormonal changes [61]. Bladder epithelial changes tend to mimic those of the vagina so, if there is some atrophy of the bladder epithelium, the intrinsic defenses of the bladder may be less effective. During pregnancy the urethra elongates, except in those who develop stress incontinence [62].

6. SITE OF INFECTION

The site of infection in UTI can be detected by cystoscopy with catheterization of the ureters. Infection present in the ureteric urine shows involvement of the upper urinary tract, and the patient is often said to have pyelonephritis, although this technique cannot prove renal involvement. The site of infection can also be deduced from "washout" tests in which the bladder is cleared of bacteria by the instillation of antiseptic followed by copious lavage: urine then collected from the catheter in the empty bladder is considered to be purely ureteric so infection in that urine indicates upper urinary tract involvement. Reduction of renal concentrating ability and increased excretion of β_2 microglobulin [63] suggest tubular dysfunction secondary to renal involvement by the infection. The presence of antibody-coated bacteria (ACB) in the urine was shown to be related to upper tract involvement [64], but they are also found with cystitis and urethritis, and may be absent in upper UTI, so the sensitivity of this investigation is only 83% and specificity 77% [63, 65].

Ureteric catheterization of patients who were not pregnant [4] showed upper urinary tract involvement in 60%: unilateral in 28% and bilateral in 32%. Similar studies in pregnancy have shown a similar distribution [66]: 50% had ureteric involvement, bilateral in half of these. "Washout" tests [31, 67] and reduction in renal concentrating ability [68, 69] confirm this distribution of infection. About 10% of those who have only cystitis at the beginning of pregnancy have infected ureteric urine by delivery [70]: since this was found in "washout" tests as well as catheterization studies, it is not an artifact.

7. INFECTING ORGANISMS

7.1. *Escherichia coli*

Escherichia coli is the infecting organism in 75%–90% of UTI in pregnancy (table 13-1). It is so the world over, and has remained so for decades. Since the infecting route for almost all UTI is from the fecal reservoir to urethra and bladder via the periurethral area [71–73], common fecal commensal organisms tend to be the common urinary pathogens; *E. coli* and group-B streptococci are both in that category [74]. Pregnancy alters the balance of organisms on the periurethral area

Table 13-1. Percentages of organisms isolated from specimens of urine obtained in three ways

	MSU [38]	CSU [135]	SPA [15]
Escherichia coli	78	68	76.5
Klebsiella–enterobacter	14.5	4.5	2.5
Citrobacter	—	4.5	—
Streptococcus faecalis	—	—	6.1
Coag. neg. staphylococci	2.1	14	8.3
Proteus spp.	3.5	—	4.5
Pseudomonas	0.7	—	—
β-Haem. streptococci	—	—	4.5

Bacterial counts included are MSU > 10^5/ml, CSU > 10^4/ml (this series also had 12% with growth 10^3–10^4/ml, but the organisms were not stated), and SPA any growth. Mixed growth was found in 2% SPA and 9% of CSU.

(as do menstruation and oral contraceptives) so that *E. coli,* group-B streptococci, and *Strepococcus faecalis* become more common [75, 76]. The same serotypes of *E. coli* are found in the patient's urine as are in her feces, except in covert infection where they may be different [77], presumably because the fecal serotype has changed since the urinary infection was established. Some serotypes of *E. coli* are more common than others in UTI because they are more common in the population rather than because they are more virulent [78]. *Escherichia coli* is not, however, the most common organism in the feces, but there are several factors that make it more likely than other organisms to establish infection. It is the balance between these factors and maternal defenses that determine whether or not infection is established.

7.2. Factors favoring *Escherichia coli*

Those *E. coli* likely to produce UTI are more resistant to low vaginal pH than others [79]. *Escherichia coli* grows more quickly in urine than most other organisms [80]. The endotoxin of *E. coli* reduces ureteric peristalsis, which encourages persistence of infection [47]. The K antigen of *E. coli* destroys complement and inhibits phagocytosis [81], and the strains rich in K antigen are most frequently found in renal infection [82, 83]. All of these favor *E. coli,* as does another property that it shares with other urinary pathogens, that of adherence to cells.

Escherichia coli have flagellae (for movement), but they also have shorter hair-like projections called pili, which allow the bacteria to adhere to epithelial cells. Urinary strains of *E. coli* are more piliated than are fecal strains [84]. The more virulent the *E. coli,* the better they adhere: strains producing acute pyelonephritis adhere more efficiently than those that produce covert infection [85, 86]. Bacteria in the stationary phase adhere better than those in the logarithmic growth phase [87]. Adherence depends also on receptors on the cells. There are more receptors on the uroepithelial and vulval cells of women prone to UTI than on those of healthy women; even though an individual's cell receptivity for bacteria may change from day to day, this difference persists consistently [86, 88, 89]. Treatment with antibiotics reduces adherence, but it remains above healthy control levels [89]. The epithelial cells to which adhesion is important are the vaginal introital and uroepithelial cells, but adhesion to them correlates well with adhesion to buccal epithelial cells [89]. The cells of amniotic membrane are also potential sites for adhesion [90].

The *E. coli* that produce covert infection differ from those in overt UTI by characteristics in addition to serotype and adhesiveness. Those in covert infections have fewer virulence factors such as the O and K antigens [91] and these are less antigenic [92]. They are more sensitive to the effects of normal human serum [93]. The strains of the covert organisms tend to be rough rather than smooth [92, 94]. A maternal adaptation may account for part of the difference between overt and covert infection and that is development of tolerance to the bacterial endotoxin [95].

7.3. Other organisms

Some other organisms do have factors in their favor and produce UTI (table 13-1). Some staphylococci are more adherent than *E. coli* [12]. The proteus species are very motile and adherent. Their pili, however, are not wholly to their advantage since these make them more susceptible to phagocytosis: perhaps because of this, they appear to be able to change their state of piliation in vivo and proteus without pili are more nephrotoxic than the piliated [96].

Anaerobic, microaerophilic, and slow-growing organisms are found in urine, but their significance has not yet been determined. Anaerobic growth may be discouraged by the high $p0_2$ in urine [80], but the presence of aerobes or facultative anaerobes might encourage growth of anaerobes [97]. Such organisms that cannot be grown with the usual overnight incubation in air but require 48–72 h in 7% CO_2 or other special environments have been obtained from SPA specimens [98]. *Gardnerella vaginalis, Lactobacillus* species, *Streptococcus* species, *Corynebacterium* species and other vaginal or perineal skin commensals have all been found. Appropriate antibacterial treatment eliminates them [99] but, even in pregnancy, they may disappear spontaneously [15]: persistence may be more likely with underlying renal pathology. Other fastidious organisms such as *Chlamydia trachomatis, Ureaplasma, Urealyticum,* and *Mycoplasma hominis* certainly are involved in urethritis and vaginitis, but whether or not they are significant in bacteriuria or to the pregnancy has yet to be decided [1, 100].

Viruses do not appear to be a common cause of UTI [101], but they may produce symptoms [34]. Whether this is while they are multiplying in the urinary tract or just passing through it is not certain.

8. MATERNAL DEFENSE MECHANISMS

Both local and general defenses are important in the prevention of invasion of the urinary tract, and in controlling infection once it has occurred.

Healthy women rarely have *E. coli* or other Gram-negative rods on their periurethral tissues, although they may appear there transiently during menstruation: 30% of women prone to UTI persistently carry *E. coli* or other Gram-negative organisms such as *Streptococcus faecalis* on their introitus for long periods even when the urine is free from infection [73, 102]. The remaining 70% who are prone to UTI are intermittently colonized at the introitus, but have long periods of apparently normal flora there: generally, however, those prone to infection have pathogens on the vulvovaginal epithelium in larger numbers and for longer than those who are not prone to infection [102]. Antibody to the 0 antigen of the prominent fecal strain of *E. coli* is present on the vulvovaginal epithelial of 77% of healthy women, but only on 26% of those prone to UTI, although it may appear transiently in these patients during an episode of infection [103]. Since bacterial infection of the bladder occurs from the rectum via the periurethral area and urethra [72], these antibodies that reduce colonization of the introitus help to prevent infection. Antibiotics given for UTI alter the fecal flora, but not that of the introitus, the one exception being trimethoprim, which crosses the vaginal mucosa and does affect the vulvovaginal flora [102]. The antibodies that appear on the introitus are not an inflammatory exudate from the serum, but a secretion from the vagina [103]. These periurethral defenses protect also against streptococci and other organisms.

If invasion of the bladder does occur, one of the primary defenses is flushing by frequent emptying. Large numbers of *E. coli* introduced into a healthy bladder disappear within 72 h and do not return [104], but the rate of disappearance is more rapid than would be expected from simple flushing [105], so reduction of bacterial numbers is also due to other defense mechanisms. Women who delay emptying for several hours after they first feel the urge to micturate tend to have recurrent UTI [60, 106]: delayed emptying allows more time for bacterial multiplication, stretches the bladder wall, and reduces blood flow through it and, by increasing the volume of infected urine per square centimeter of bladder wall, reduces the effectiveness of its intrinsic defenses. Production of secretory IgA (SIgA) by the bladder mucosa and urethra is an important part of these defenses [107]. SIgA is increased in the urine of adults with UTI [108] and may prevent bacterial attachment to the bladder mucosa directly [109] or by transforming the organisms from smooth capsulated to rough forms that are less virulent [91]. It has also been postulated that infection with *E. coli* that adhere poorly may protect against infection with more virulent strains [110].

General maternal defenses alter during pregnancy so that infection is less likely to be controlled. Leukocyte activity against *E. coli* is less effective in women with bacteriuria [111]. Immune mechanisms also are less effective against bacterial infection during pregnancy [112, 113], but, despite these many advantages that the bacteria enjoy, the majority of infections are cured without difficulty. The balance is not tipped too far against the mother.

9. PREVALENCE OF UTI

Bacteriuria is a complication, but not a consequence, of pregnancy. Within a geographic area, the prevalence of bacteriuria is very similar in those who are pregnant and those who are not: 8% of infertile women and 6.6% of pregnant women from the same area were bacteriuric [114] and, in another city, 5%–6% of married women who never had been pregnant and 6.8% of those who were had bacteriuria [115]. Sexual intercourse is the major factor in determining the incidence and prevalence of bacteriuria in women: transient bacteriuria frequently follows intercourse (probably due to bacteria entering the bladder from the urethra) and occasionally it persists [116, 117]. Among nuns and five- to 14-year-old schoolgirls, the prevalence is about 1% [118, 119]. In 15–19 year olds, the prevalence rises to 3.5% and, in most pregnant populations, it is 4%–7%. These and other studies of the nonpregnant were carried out before oral contraception was widely used: since this encourages persistence of bacteriuria [120], the current prevalence may be slightly higher. Contrariwise, screening and treatment of bacteriuria may have reduced its prevalence [121].

Many groups have been screened for bacteriuria by MSU, CSU, and SPA. While prevalence is generally 4%–7%, the reported range is 2%–18.5%. Ethnic differences account for a small part of this: although the very high rate of 18.5% was found in a Moari population [122], such differences can usually be explained by underlying pathology or by differences in social class. Bacteriuria is twice as common in Negroes with sickle cell trait [123] and sickle cell disease [124]. Social class differences, however, consistently have the closest association with prevalence: the higher the social class, the lower the prevalence, from 2% in the affluent [125] to 9.9% in the indigent [126], possibly because treatment for relatively minor symptoms is more readily available for, and more quickly sought by, the upper social classes [127]. Bacteriuria tends to be more common in those under 20 [15, 128], and then remains steady for the remainder of the childbearing years. The relevance of parity is not agreed: some have found no relationship between bacteriuria and parity and some have found that bacteriuria increased; perhaps the parous are more likely to produce contaminated urines. Diabetes probably has an association with bacteriuria. Diabetic schoolgirls have 1.6%–2% bacteriuria [129], but older diabetic women who are not hospital patients had an 18.8% prevalence compared with a 7.9% in nondiabetic women [130]. There may be an increased incidence of abnormal glucose tolerance among bacteriuric pregnant women [131]. Most reviews of prevalence are of hospital populations, frequently those that attract "high risk" patients [126]. Examination of all pregnant women in the Cardiff area delivered at home or in hospital revealed a prevalence of 3.8% [128], but this was only "asymptomatic" bacteriuria, so the prevalence of all bacteriuria was likely to be about twice this, and so in the same range as for hospital populations.

That the prevalence of bacteriuria discovered in MSU, CSU, and SPA specimens is so close is unexpected in view of the different possibilities of error of diagnosis with each of these. As SPA includes all bacteriuria discovered, this may be partly balanced by the false positives on MSU. Catheter specimens might be expected to be intermediate, since they would be certain about the 10^3–10^5 bacteria/ml specimens, but almost all CSU series included as bacteriuria only those counts greater than 10^5/ml. The one series that included all bacterial counts had a prevalence of 10%, but included only "normal" obstetric patients without defining normality [132]. The consistency of results the world over, however, does suggest that the prevalence of bacteriuria is usually in the 4%–7% range.

10. NATURAL HISTORY OF UTI

While the prevalence of bacteriuria is constant, the individuals who are affected change. In any year, between one-quarter and one-third of women with bacteriuria lose it spontaneously and a similar number acquire the infection. Spontaneous cure is more likely with staphylococci [133] and fastidious organisms [15] than with *E. coli.* During the six months that pregnant women are under medical supervision, 0.5%–1% of those who are not bacteriuric early in pregnancy will develop it [15, 131]. Spontaneous cure during pregnancy is, however, not common: instead of one-quarter to one-third of bacteriurics clearing without treatment, the spontaneous cure rate is 0–3% [15, 38, 124, 134]. The differences in pregnancy that discourage disappearance of bacteriuria are not only the alterations in defense mechanisms, the slowing of urine flow, and the fall in vaginal pH that encourages pathogenic *E. coli.* The urine of pregnant women contains large quantities of glucose, amino acids, and other nutrients that encourage bacterial growth [135], as does its reduced pH in pregnancy [57, 136]. Perhaps because of this, 30% of pregnant women with untreated bacteriuria develop severe symptoms [15, 131].

The puerperium is a period of increased bacteriuria. Bacteria enter the bladder at delivery: the more traumatic the delivery, the more likely are bacteria to appear [137], although simple forceps does not produce an increase over spontaneous delivery [19]. Because residual urine also appears in the puerperium, the conditions favor bacterial growth [55]. Spontaneous clearance does occur in 70% during the next six weeks, but it tends to persist in the remainder [19, 138, 139]. Bacteriuria that was not treated during pregnancy continues after delivery [138, 139]. Even if it was treated, it recurs after delivery in about 30% of women and, in many, persists over the next ten years [134, 140, 141]. In a small but significant proportion, this persistence is accompanied by deterioration in renal function [141] (see chapter 9).

10.1. Subsequent pregnancies

Since bacteriuria persists in the years following delivery in 25%–40%, and (depending on how long after the pregnancy they are reviewed) appears in 1%–5% [15, 140], those mothers who conceive again have a prevalence that is considerably greater than normal. If they are not treated prophylactically, they again have a 30% incidence of acute UTI [41].

11. EFFECTS ON THE FETUS

The fetus of the mother with bacteriuria has an increased risk of midtrimester abortion [134], and has a perinatal mortality rate twice that of those without the infection [131, 142], the mortality excess tending to be in those in whom the urinary tract infection was discovered within 15 days of delivery, the highest rate occurring in those who have maternal hypertension coexisting with bacteriuria. The commonest causes of death are pulmonary hyaline membrane disease and congenital malformation. A marked increase in perinatal mortality has been found among diabetic women with asymptomatic bacteriuria [143]: the rate of perinatal death was 50% in bacteriuric women with microvascular disease and 15% in those with microvascular disease but no urinary infection.

As with many renal diseases there is an increased risk of intrauterine growth retardation if the infection involves the kidney [144], and also of placental growth retardation [142]. The underlying mechanism that determines the growth retardation is not certain. Possibly *E. coli* endotoxin affects the vessels of the placental bed [145, 146], or it could be related to suppression of immunologic mechanisms. Infections such as malaria and laparotomous leprosy, which depress immunologic mechanisms [147, 148], are associated with reduction in the rate of fetal growth.

Immunosuppression with drugs retards fetal growth in rats and humans because of reduction of the number of cells in the fetus [149]. Experimental pyelonephritis in rats depresses their immune response as could occur in human bacteriuria and retards fetal growth [150].

Premature labor is more common in acute pyelonephritis. Baird [137] found in a deprived community in the UK that 27% of mothers with pyelonephritis had babies weighing less than 5 ½ lb if the infection was unilateral, and 42% of it was bilateral; if it was the mother's first pregnancy, 55% of birth weights were below 5 ½ lb. More recently in the USA, symptomatic UTI has been associated with a doubling of the incidence of low birth weight [151, 152]. Certainly it is a common clinical experience that some women who present with preterm labor have an active UTI. Whether or not all covert UTI is associated with an increased incidence of preterm labor is still undecided. Certainly it is with polyhydramnios, abruptio placentae, and infection of the amniotic fluid [142], all common causes of premature labor. Also the presence of group-B streptococci in a pregnant woman's urine has been linked to an increased incidence of both premature rupture of the membranes and premature delivery, both being about twice as common as in the uninfected [153]. There are a number of reasons for the uncertainty and confusion about the relationship of all bacteriuria to prematurity: (a) Almost every published series has defined prematurity as a birth weight of 2.5 kg or less, but few differentiated between the preterm fetus and one born light-for-dates. (b) Associated conditions have been found with the prematurity, but not all are agreed about this: some have found that prematurity is increased in hypertensive women with bacteriuria [152, 154], while others have found the prematurity is increased, but unrelated either to preeclampsia or to twins [134]. (c) The number of cases analyzed. For statistically reliable conclusions to be reached, 1500–2000 bacteriuric women would need to be investigated if the incidence of premature labor was 5% [131]. This would require screening of 30,000–40,000 pregnant women. The collaboration of several centers would be required for such an investigation to be completed in a reasonable time, and it is likely that there would be problems in establishing uniform policy, diagnosis, and treatment. Also, since women suffering from symptomatic infection are more likely to have premature babies than those suffering from asymptomatic bacteriuria and since the high incidence of symptomatic infection among asymptomatic women who are not treated is accepted, it would be difficult to withhold treatment from any woman with covert bacteriuria.

1.2. EFFECTS OF UTI ON THE MOTHER

Apart from the development of "acute pyelonephritis," in one-third of mothers, if bacteriuria is not treated, the most significant maternal effects are on renal function. UTI may, however, also affect the cardiovascular and hemopoietic systems.

12.1. Effects of bacteriuria in childhood

Bacteriuria before the age of 4 may lead to scarred kidneys and reduction of the GFR by up to 50% as these girls mature [155]. Renal concentrating ability reduces with increasing age, and this is accelerated by childhood UTI [156]. If bacteriuria in childhood is not treated with antibiotics, or is followed by renal scarring, these girls when aged 18 show no renal dysfunction apart from reduced fractional reabsorption of glucose [157]. Should they become pregnant, however, they have less than physiologic increases in GFR, and greater than normal amounts of glycosuria due to the reduced fractional reabsorption of glucose: the additional demands of pregnancy may unmask otherwise unrecognizable renal damage.

12.2. Effect of infection during pregnancy on renal function

GFR is reduced by bacteriuria in acute pyelonephritis, the creatinine clearance being less than 80 ml/min in 25% of patients, and less than 60 ml/min in 10% (normal, 125–200 ml/min), but this is reversed by treatment [134, 158, 159].

Renal concentrating ability in normal pregnancy is 750–1250 mOsm/liter, whereas in bacteriuria this is reduced to below 700 mOsm/liter maximum [158, 160]. The effect is produced by infection ascending to the kidneys and not by infection confined to the bladder; the reduction is greater in bilateral than unilateral pyelonephritis [158, 161]. It occurs with organisms other than *E. coli* [133]. The concentrating ability returns toward normal with effective treatment of the infection [158, 161, 162], but the more the concentrating ability is reduced, the more difficult it is to treat the infection satisfactorily [128]. The impaired concentrating ability does not correlate with creatinine clearance, and those with impaired concentration are more likely to become clinically ill [163]. These effects are also seen in women who are not pregnant. Recently it has been shown in the nonpregnant that excretion of β_2-microglobulin, which reflects proximal tubular dysfunction such as may occur in pyelonephritis, also improves with treatment [63]. Rarely, pyelonephritis in pregnancy precipitates renal failure (see chapter 10).

Anemia has been found to be more common in some populations of bacteriurics, being most marked in those who have symptomatic UTI: the more severe the infection and the more treatment it required, the more anemic the patient [15, 164]. This could be due to deficient erythropoietin excretion by diseased kidneys, to hemoglobinopathy since it is more likely that bacteriuric patients will have sickle cell trait or disease, but the mechanism appears frequently to be increased destruction of red blood cells and reduced production [164].

Preeclampsia and hypertension in pregnancy frequently are due to underlying renal pathology. Thus, it would be anticipated that both of these maternal complications would be more common with bacteriuria, but there is no clear view on this. Restrictions and exclusions in the patients considered may have obscured differences. Some reviewed only those who had a blood pressure of 140/90 mm Hg or more with generalized edema and proteinuria [134, 165]; others excluded those with a history of hypertension or with a diastolic blood pressure of 85 mm Hg or more at their first visit to the clinic (without stating when this was) and required that the diastolic pressure rise to 100 mm Hg for inclusion as hypertensive [154]. Diuretics were given in one series and only if the mothers then failed to lose weight and required admission to hospital for hypertension were they included

[131]. Others failed to differentiate between transient and persistent hypertension. While many have not found any increase in preeclampsia or hypertension in bacteriuric pregnancies [131, 132, 165], others have [134, 154], particularly in those whose infection was resistant to treatment [15].

1.3. TREATMENT

Urinary infection may be cured by treatment, or it may relapse, it may recur, or it may persist. Cure rates tend to be lower in pregnancy than at other times, not only because of the factors that encourage bacterial growth, but also because the duration of follow-up is longer. A sterile urine 1–2 weeks after the completion of treatment frequently is the criterion of cure in the nonpregnant whereas, during pregnancy, surveillance may easily continue for a further 28 weeks until delivery, and into the puerperium, which allows greater opportunities for reappearance of bacteriuria. A possible fallacy of "cure" is that contamination of the urine may be diagnosed as infection and this vulvovaginal contamination be eliminated by the antibacterial therapy so that subsequent urines are not contaminated and thus are apparently "cured." On the other hand, a broad-spectrum antibiotic may produce a profuse vulvovaginitis that not only is accompanied by dysuria, but may contaminate the urine and suggest that it remains infected.

Relapse is the reappearance in the urine of the same organism as produced the original infection: reinfection is the appearance of a different organism, which includes a different serotype of *E. coli.* Relapse is more likely with infection that involves the ureteral urine, and reinfection with bladder bacteriuria [166]. Relapse is usually associated with recolonization of the introitus, rarely to persistence of infection in the kidney unless there is an anatomic abnormality of the urinary tract or infected stones [102]. Relapse may occur within 72 h of the end of treatment, or it may take 1–2 or more weeks [15, 166]. Failure of treatment frequently is due to the appearance of resistant organisms in the feces and periurethral area [167]. Reappearance of infection or difficulty in eradicating it is not necessarily related to abnormality in the urinary tract or to renal infection [15, 168].

Some antibacterial drugs are better avoided during pregnancy because of their effects on the fetus or mother. Tetracycline can cause staining of the permanent dentition [169] or slowing of growth of long bones [170]. Sulfonamides (particularly the long-acting variety) can cross the placenta and compete for bilirubin-carrying capacity, which may produce jaundice in the neonate, so they are better avoided if delivery is likely [171]. Chloramphenicol may affect hematopoiesis or produce the grey syndrome in the neonate [172]. Trimethoprim is used in the treatment of UTI either alone or in combination with a sulfonamide (cotrimoxazole): it is better avoided during pregnancy as it is a folic acid antagonist [173]. Nitrofurantoin produces gastrointerstinal upset and may not be taken by the patients for whom it is prescribed [157], so if it is the only drug to which an organism is sensitive it should be prescribed to be taken with meals.

Bacteriuria should be treated whenever it is found, as treatment reduces the incidence of symptomatic UTI from 30%–40%, to less than 5%, and it also reduces the other ill-effects of UTI on the mother and fetus [15, 131, 134]. The drug used should be the one to which the infecting organism is most sensitive.

Duration of treatment required depends on the presentation of the UTI: whether it is covert or accompanied by a few symptoms, or an acute UTI possibly with some previous history, or a chronic infection known to exist before pregnancy that requires continuing control during the pregnancy.

13.1. Covert UTI or UTI with few symptoms or minimal previous history

Treatment is not required immediately, so bacterial sensitivity can be awaited. Renal function studies are not required. First-choice treatment is one or two 3-g doses of cephalexin or amoxycillin. This is as effective as conventional five- to ten-day course both in the nonpregnant [80, 127, 174] and in the pregnant [21, 175]. The advantages of this regimen are that patient compliance is not a problem and that side effects are minimized: after a ten-day course of ampicillin or amoxycillin, 25% of nonpregnant women were found to have vaginal candidiasis, but this appeared in only 2% after a single-dose treatment [127]; and seven days of amoxycillin produced resistance in 26% of fecal Enterobacteriaceae that in some cases persisted for weeks, whereas single-dose treatment had no such effect [80, 174], so drug resistance is unlikely to occur. It is also cheaper.

Single-dose or double-dose treatment cures 65%–70% of pregnant women for 6–23 weeks [21, 175], which is very similar to the 62%–75% achieved by conventional five- to ten-day courses [15]. One group did find that seven days of amoxycillin was better than two large doses, but follow-up of these patients was only for 2–7 days [176]. The majority of organisms are sensitive to either cephalexin or ampicillin, but, if they are not, a single dose of 100 mg nitrofurantoin [177] or 2 g of a sulfonamide [178] might be considered. Whatever drug is used, the patients must be followed closely for the remainder of the pregnancy, and into the puerperium, because those who will be cured cannot be predicted by the renal concentrating ability [21] or other criteria. Urine should be cultured two weeks after treatment and thereafter monthly until delivery. If infection reappears, then the patient should be treated as described in section 13.2.

13.2. Acute UTI, or recurrence after single dose or history of UTI

The drug used should be the one indicated by bacterial sensitivity testing but, if the patient is so ill that this cannot be awaited, the drug of first choice is cephalexin, to which few organisms are resistant and which has few side effects; or the antibacterial to which most organisms are sensitive in the patients' locality. If the patient is severely unwell or is vomiting, the initial doses may be given intravenously or intramuscularly, but usually oral treatment is sufficient. It may be necessary to review renal function, particularly if the patient has a previous history of UTI. The drugs should be given for 5–10 days, but the initial drug may need to be changed if the patient's pyrexia is not falling, her localizing symptoms are not improving, or bacterial sensitivity shows that another drug would be better. If, however, the patient's clinical condition is not improving, the diagnosis should be reviewed in case some other lesion such as appendicitis is the basis of the patient's pyrexia and other symptoms. If there is suspicion of a blocked ureter, an ultrasound examination of the kidneys to exclude an obstructed ureter on one side, or a single-shot IVP, may be required to clarify the diagnosis so that any block present can be relieved.

Treatment for 5–10 days will produce cure for the rest of the pregnancy in 50%–65% of pregnant women [15, 168, 179, 180]. Continuous treatment will produce slightly better rates of cure, but may well produce antibacterial resistance in organisms that would produce problems with treatment in the puerperium or of the neonate. Five to seven days of treatment produces as satisfactory a result as 10–14 days.

Following this treatment, an MSU should be obtained 10–14 days after its end, and thereafter monthly until delivery. The urine should also be cultured in the early puerperium and six weeks after delivery. It is likely that half of those treated in this way will have no recurrence for the rest of that pregnancy [15]. Those that recur should be treated as described in section 13.3.

13.3. Previous chronic urinary tract infection on continuous therapy, or relapse or reinfection following 5–10 days of treatment

These patients' renal function should be reviewed at least once after treatment has been started. Treatment should be continuous and under close supervision. The drug should be one to which the organisms are sensitive. Methenamine should not be used, as it is ineffective [181]. With such continuous therapy, relapse or reinfection will be very much less common, but it will not be totally prevented [179, 182–184]. The treatment should be continued through labor and certainly for the first few days of the puerperium.

Patients in whom bacteriuria is not cleared by treatment must be thoroughly investigated to ensure that there is no underlying pathology. The possibilities for such investigation are reduced during pregnancy, as is definitive treatment, so each case should be reviewed individually.

After delivery, patients who have been treated may well have a recrudescence of infection producing a puerperal pyrexia. Covert bacteriuria should then be sought.

Full urologic investigation is not worthwhile in every patient who was bacteriuric during pregnancy, abnormal IVP being found in only 14%: it is, however, worthwhile if the patient's infection required repeated treatment during the pregnancy, if it has been resistant to infection, if unusual organisms such as *Streptococcus viridans* produced the infection, if renal function has been significantly affected, or if she was hypertensive during pregnancy, had a light-for-dates baby, or a significant previous history.

14. SCREENING FOR BACTERIURIA IN PREGNANCY

UTI (covert or overt) is one of the most common complications of pregnancy. It has affects on both mother and fetus. Treatment of covert infection prevents the mother developing clinical UTI, and in many cases improves her renal function. Single-dose treatment is effective in the majority and has few side effects. Although some patients do develop bacteriuria for the first time during pregnancy, the numbers are not large: a unit that delivers 3000 patients each year with an incidence of 5% of bacteriuria at booking will (with the precautions described earlier) reveal 150 women with bacteriuria that is either covert or overt. Assuming that these mothers book at 12 weeks, it is likely that 0.5%–1.0% of the remainder will develop bacteriuria during the rest of pregnancy, which will amount to 14–28 mothers. Thus, although the latter group will not be detected by screening at booking, the majority of patients with bacteriuria will be and the potential ill-effects can then be prevented by treatment. Over 20 years, such a policy in one unit reduced the incidence of acute antepartum pyelonephritis by 75% [185]. Effective screening can, however, be carried out only from urine specimens obtained from well-prepared women and interpreted in the knowledge of their origin. History and clinical examination are of little value. A pregnant woman with burning dysuria who has to get up three times during the night to pass urine is as likely to have a sterile urine as she is to be bacteriuric [186].

REFERENCES

1. Wong ES, Stamm WE: Urethral infections in men and women. Annu Rev Med 34:337–358, 1983.
2. Kass EH: Chemotherapeutic and antibiotic drugs in the management of infections of the urinary tract. Am J Med 18:764–781, 1955.
3. Guze LB, Beeson PB: Observations of the reliability and safety of bladder catheterization for bacteriologic study of the urine. N Engl J Med 255:474–475, 1956.
4. Stamey RA, Govan DE, Palmer JM: The localization and treatment of urinary tract infections: the role of bactericidal urine levels as opposed to serum levels. Medicine (Baltimore) 44:1–36, 1965.
5. Kass EH: Asymptomatic infections of the urinary tract. Trans Assoc Am Physicians 69:56–64, 1956.
6. MacDonald RA, Levitin H, Mallory GK, Kass EH: Relation between pyelonephritis and bacterial counts in the urine: an autopsy study. N Engl J Med 256:915–918, 1957.
7. Monzon OT, Ory EM, Dobson HL, Carter E, Yow EM: A comparison of bacterial counts of urine obtained by needle aspiration of the bladder, catheterization and midstream-voided methods. N Engl J Med 259:764–767, 1958.
8. Kaitz AL, Hodder EW: Bacteriuria and pyelonephritis of pregnancy: a prospective study of 616 pregnant women. N Eng J Med 265:667–672, 1961.
9. Cohen SN, Kass EH: A simple quantitative urine culture. N Engl J Med 277:176–180, 1967.
10. Norden CW, Kass EH: Bacteriuria of pregnancy: a critical appraisal. Annu Rev Med 19:-431–470, 1968.
11. Little PJ, Peddie BA, Sincock AR: Significance of bacterial and white cell counts in midstream urines. J Clin Pathol 33:58–60, 1980.
12. Hovelius B, Mardh P-A, Bygren P: Urinary tract infections caused by *Staphylococcus saprophyticus:* recurrences and complications. J Urol 122:645–647, 1979.
13. Stamm WE, Counts GW, Running KR, Fih S, Turck M, Holmes KK: Diagnosis of coliform infection in acutely dysuric women. N Engl J Med 307:463–467, 1982.
14. Nanra RJ, Friedman A, O'Keefe C, Hubbard M, Fairley KF: Response to treatment of renal and bladder infections. In: Kincaid-Smith P, Fairley KF (2ds) Renal infections and renal scarring. Melbourne: Mercedes, 1971, pp 175–179.

15. McFadyen IR, Eykyn SJ, Gardner NHN, Vanier TM, Bennett AE, Mayo ME, Lloyd-Davies RW: Bacteriuria in pregnancy. J Obstet Gynaecol Br Commonw 80:385–405, 1973.
16. Kass EH: Bacteriuria and the diagnosis of infections of the urinary tract. Arch Intern Med 100:709–714, 1957.
17. Little PJ: Prevention of pyelonephritis of pregnancy. Lancet 1:566–569, 1965.
18. Thysell H: Evaluation of chemical and microscopical methods for mass detection of bacteriuria. Acta Med Scand 185:393–400, 1969.
19. McFadyen IR, Hicks L: Catheterization, delivery and puerperal bacteriuria. Am J Obstet Gynecol 105:916–924, 1969.
20. McFadyen IR, Simmons SC: Prevention of urinary infection following major vaginal surgery. J Obstet Gynaecol Br Commonw 75:871–875, 1968.
21. Campbell-Brown M, McFadyen IR: Bacteriuria in pregnancy treated with a single dose of cephalexin. Br J Obstet Gynaecol 90:1054–1059, 1983.
22. Cattell WR, Sardeson JM, Sutcliffe MB, O'Grady F: Kinetics of urinary bacterial response to antibacterial agents. In: O'Grady F, Brumfitt W (eds) Urinary tract infection. London: Oxford University Press, 1968, pp 212–226.
23. Cruickshank JG, Gawler AHL, Hart RJC: Costs of unnecessary tests: nonsense urines. Br Med J 280:1355–1356, 1980.
24. Bollgren I, Vaclavenkova V, Hurvell B, Bergqvist G: Periurethral aerobic microflora of pregnant and non-pregnant women. Br Med J 1:1314–1317, 1978.
25. Bodel PT, Cotran R, Kass EH: Cranberry juice and the antibacterial action of hippuric acid. J Lab Clin Med 54:881–888, 1959.
26. Gallagher DJA, Montgomerie JZ, North JDK: Acute infections of the urinary tract and the urethral syndrome in general practice. Br Med J 1:622–626, 1965.
27. Mond NC, Percival A, Williams JD, Brumfitt W: Presentation, diagnosis and treatment of urinary-tract infections in general practice. Lancet 1:514–516, 1965.
28. Mestitz P, McIntosh WG, Sleigh JD: Laboratory evaluation of the significance of urinary symptoms. Practitioner 195:328–334, 1965.
29. Gruneberg RN, Brumfitt W: Single-dose treatment of acute urinary tract infection: a controlled trial. Br Med J 3:649–651, 1967.
30. MacNaughtan G, Laurence AR, Knox JDE: Urinary-tract infections in general practice: self-help in diagnosis. Practitioner 189:416–420, 1967.
31. Boutros P, Mourtada N, Ronald AR: Urinary infection localization. Am J Obstet Gynecol 112:379–381, 1972.
32. Warrell DW, Russell CS: Investigation and treatment of over 200 complicated cases of urinary incontinence. J Obstet Gynaecol Br Commonw 72:564–574, 1965.
33. Francis WJA: The onset of stress incontinence. J Obstet Gynaecol Br Commonw 67:899–903, 1960.
34. Davies JG, Taylor CM, White RHR, George RH, Purdham Dr: Cytomegalovirus infection associated with lower urinary tract symptoms. Br Med J 1:1120, 1979.
35. Burney P, Marson WS, Evans M, Forsey T: Chlamydia trachomatis and lower urinary tract symptoms among women in one general practice. Br Med J 286:1549, 1983.
36. Fairley KF: The routine determination of the site of infection in the investigation of patients with urinary tract infection. In: Kincaid-Smith P, Fairley KF (eds) Renal infection and renal scarring. Melbourne: Mercedes, 1971, pp 107–116.
37. Sussman A, Asscher AW, Waters WE, Evans JAS, Campbell H, Evans KT, Williams JE: Asymptomatic significant bacteriuria in the non-pregnant woman. I. Description of a population. Br Med J 1:799–803, 1969.
38. Elder HA, Santamarina BAG, Smith S, Kass EH: The natural history of asymptomatic bacteriuria during pregnancy: the effect of tetracycline on the clinical course and the outcome of pregnancy. Am J Obstet Gynecol 111:441–462, 1971.
39. Wharton LR, Gray LA, Guild HG: The late effects of acute pyelitis in girls. JAMA 109:-1597–1602, 1937.
40. Davison JM, Sprott MS, Selkon JB: The effect of covert bacteriuria in schoolgirls on renal function at 18 years and during pregnancy. Lancet 2:651–655, 1984.
41. Gilstrap LC, Cunningham FG, Whalley PJ: Acute pyelonephritis in pregnancy: an anterospective study. Obstet Gynecol 57:409–413, 1981.

42. Chng PK, Hall MH: Antenatal prediction of urinary tract infection in pregnancy. Br J Obstet Gynaecol 89:8–11, 1982.
43. Duncan JW, Seng MI: Factors disposing to pyelitis in pregnancy. Am J Obstet Gynecol 16:557–578, 1982.
44. Baird D: The upper urinary tract in pregnancy and puerperium, with special reference to pyelitis of pregnancy. J Obstet Gynaecol Br Emp 42:733–774, 1936.
45. Hundley JM, Walton JM, Hibbitts JT, Siegel IA, Black CB: Physiologic changes occurring in the urinary tract during pregnancy. Am J Obstet Gynecol 30:625–649, 1935.
46. Van Wagenen G, Jenkins RH: Pyeloureteral dilatation of pregnancy after death of the fetus: an experimental study. Am J Obstet Gynecol 56:1146–1151, 1948.
47. Teague N, Boyarsky S: Further effects of coliform bacteria on ureteral peristalsis. J Urol 99:720–723, 1968.
48. Bunge RG: Further observations with delayed cystograms. J Urol 71:427–434, 1954.
49. Heidrick WP, Mattingly RF, Amberg JR: Vesicoureteral reflux in pregnancy. Am J Obstet Gynecol 29:571–578, 1967.
50. Mattingly RF, Brokowf HI: Clinical implications of ureteric reflux in pregnancy. Clin Obstet Gynecol 21:863–873, 1978.
51. Bumpus HC: Urinary reflux. J Urol 12:341–346, 1924.
52. Hanley HG: Transient stasis and reflux in the lower ureter. Br J Urol 34:283–285, 1962.
53. Hutch JA, Ayres RD, Noll LE: Vesicoureteral reflux as cause of pyelonephritis of pregnancy. Am J Obstet Gynecol 87:478–485, 1963.
54. Williams JD, Reeves DS, Condie AP, Franklin ISN, Leigh DA, Brumfitt W: The treatment of bacteriuria in pregnancy. In: O'Grady F, Brumfitt W (eds) Urinary tract infection. London: Oxford University Press, 1968, pp 160–169.
55. Muellner SR: Physiological bladder changes during pregnancy and the puerperium. J Urol 41:691–695, 1939.
56. Slotnick IJ, Prystowsky H: Microbiology of the female genital tract. I. The infectious hazard of prophylactic catheterization of the urinary bladder prior to delivery. Am J Obstet Gynecol 93:1102–1111, 1963.
57. Roberts AP, Beard RW: Some factors affecting bacterial invasion of the bladder during pregnancy. Lancet 1:1133–1136, 1965.
58. Burkhart FL, Porges RF, Gibbs CE: Bladder capacity post partum and catheterization. Obstet Gynecol 26:176–179, 1965.
59. Shand DG, O'Grady F, Nimmon CC, Cattell WR: Relation between residual urine volume and response to treatment of urinary infection. Lancet 1:1305–1306, 1970.
60. Adatto K, Dobbie KG, Galland L, Granowetter L: Behavioural factors and urinary tract infection. JAMA 241:2525–2526, 1979.
61. Hytten FE, Lind T: Diagnostic indices in pregnancy. Basle: Ciba-Geigy, 1973, pp 22–24.
62. Iosif S, Uemsten U: Comparative urodynamic studies of continent and stress incontinent women in pregnancy and in the puerperium. Am J Obstet Gynecol 140:645–650, 1981.
63. Schardijn HGC, Statius van Eps LW, Pauw W, Hoefnagel C, Nooyen WJ: Comparison of reliability of tests to distinguish upper from lower urinary tract infection. Br Med J 289:-284–287, 1984.
64. Thomas V, Shelokov A, Forland M: Antibody-coated bacteria in the urine and the site of urinary-tract infection. N Engl J Med 290:588–590, 1974.
65. Mundt JA, Polk BF: Identification of site of urinary-tract infections by antibody-coated bacteria assay. Lancet 2:1172–1175, 1979.
66. Fairley KF, Bond AG, Adey FD, Habersberger P, McCredie M: The site of infection in pregnancy bacteriuria. Lancet 1:939–941, 1966.
67. Fairley KF, Bond AG, Brown RB, Habersberger P: Simple test to determine the site of urinary-tract infection. Lancet 2:427–428, 1967.
68. Kaitz AL: Urinary concentrating ability in pregnant women with asymptomatic bacteriuria. J Clin Invest 40:1331–1338, 1961.
69. Clark H, Ronald AR, Cutler RE, Turck M: The correlation between site of infection and maximal concentrating ability in bacteriuria. J Infect Dis 120:47–53, 1969.
70. Fairley KF, Radford NJ, Whitworth JA: Spontaneous ascent of infection from bladder to kidney in pregnancy. Med J Aust 2:1116–1118, 1972.

71. Gruneberg RN, Leigh DA, Brumfitt W: Relationship of bacteriuria in pregnancy to acute pyelonephritis, prematurity, and fetal mortality. Lancet 1:1–3, 1969.
72. Stamey TA, Timothy M, Millar M, Mihara G: Recurrent urinary infections in adult woman: the role of introital enterobacteria. Calif Med 115:1–19, 1971.
73. Bollgren I, Wingberg J: The periurethral aerobic flora in girls highly susceptible to urinary infections. Acta Paediatr Scand 65:81–87, 1976.
74. Badri MS, Zawaneh S, Cruz AC, Mantilla G, Baer H, Spellacy WN, Ayoub EM: Rectal colonisation with group B *Streptococcus:* relation to vaginal colonisation of pregnant women. J Infect Dis 135:308–312, 1977.
75. Bollgren I, Vaclavenkova V, Hurvell B, Bergqvist G: Periurethral aerobic microflora of pregnant and non-pregnant women. Br Med J 1:1314–1317, 1978.
76. Ross JM, Needham JR: Genital flora during pregnancy and colonization of the newborn. J R Soc Med 73:105–110, 1980.
77. Roberts AP, Linton JD, Waterman AM, Gower PE, Koutsaimanis KG: Urinary and faecal *Escherichia coli* O-serogroups in symptomatic urinary-tract infection and asymptomatic bacteriuria. J Med Microbiol 8:311–318, 1975.
78. Gruneberg RN, Leigh DA, Brumfitt W: *Escherichia coli* serotypes in urinary tract infection: studies in domiciliary, ante-natal and hospital practice. In: O'Grady F, Brumfitt W (eds) Urinary tract infection. London: Oxford University Press, 1968, pp 68–97.
79. Stamey TA, Kaufman MF: Studies of introital colonization in women with recurrent urinary infections. II. Comparison of growth in normal vaginal fluid of common versus uncommon serogroups of *Escherichia coli.* J Urol 114:264–267, 1975.
80. Anderson JD, Eftekhar F, Aird MY, Hammond J: Role of bacterial growth rates in the epidemiology and pathogenesis of urinary infections in women. J Clin Microbiol 10:766–771, 1979.
81. Glynn AA, Brumfitt W, Howard CJ: K Antigens of *Escherichia coli* and renal involvement in urinary-tract infections. Lancet 1:514–516, 1971.
82. Mabek CE, Orskov F, Orskov I: *Escherichia coli* stereotypes and renal involvement in urinary-tract infection. Lancet 1:1312–1314, 1971.
83. Kaijser B: Immunology of *Escherichia coli:* K antigen and its relationship to urinary-tract infection. J Infect Dis 127:670–677, 1973.
84. Gerstl F, Semenitz E: Zur morphologie der gesseln und fimbrien von *Escherichia*-Stammen. Zentrabl Bakteriol 232:48–54, 1975.
85. Svanborg Eden C, Hanson LA, Jodal U, Lindberg U, Sohl Akerlund A: Variable adherence to normal human urinary tract epithelial cells of *Escherichia coli* strains associated with various forms of urinary tract infection. Lancet 2:490–492, 1976.
86. Fowler JE, Stamey TA: Studies of introital colonization in women with recurrent urinary infections. VII. The role of bacterial adherence. J Urol 117:472–476, 1977.
87. Svanborg Eden C, Eriksson B, Hanson LA: Adhesion of *Escherichia coli* to human uroepithelial cells in vitro. Infect Immun 18:767–774, 1977.
88. Kallenius G, Winberg J: Bacterial adherence to periurethral epithelial cells in girls prone to urinary tract infections. Lancet 2:540–543, 1978.
89. Schaeffer AJ, Jones JM, Dunn JK: Association of in vitro *Escherichia coli* adherence to vaginal and buccal epithelial cells with susceptibility of women to recurrent urinary tract infections. N Engl J Med 304:1062–1066, 1981.
90. Galask RP, Varner MW, Petzold R, Wilbur SL: Bacterial attachment to the chorioamniotic membranes. Am J Obstet Gynecol 148:915–926, 1984.
91. Hanson LA, Ahlstedt S, Fasth U, Jodal B, Kaijser P, Larsson U, Lindberg S, Olling A, Sohl Akerlund A, Svanborg Eden C: *E. coli* antigens, human immune response, and the pathogenesis of urinary tract infections. J Infect Dis [Suppl] 136:S144–149, 1977.
92. Lindberg U, Hanson LA, Jodal U, Lidin-Janson G, Lincoln K, Olling S: Asymptomatic bacteriuria in school girls. II. Differences in *Escherichia coli* causing asymptomatic and symptomatic bacteriuria. Acta Paediatr Scand 64:432–436, 1975.
93. Olling S, Hanson LA, Holmgren J, et al.: The bactericidal effect of normal human serum on *E. coli* strains from normals and from patients with urinary tract infections. Infection 1:24–28, 1973.
94. Hanson LA, Ahlstedt S, Jodal U, Kaijser B, Larson P, Lidin-Janson F, Lincoln K, Lindberg U,

Mattsby I, Olling S, Peterson H, Sohl A: The host–parasite relationship in urinary tract infections. Kidney Int 8:S28–34, 1975.
95. McCabe WR: Endotoxin tolerance. II. Its occurrence in patients with pyelonephritis. J Clin Invest 42:618–625, 1963.
96. Silverblatt FJ, Ofek I: Effects of pili on susceptibility of *Proteus mirabilis* to phagocystosis and on adherence to bladder cells. In: Kass EH, Brumfitt W (eds) Infections of the urinary tract. Chicago: University of Chicago Press, 1975, pp 49–59.
97. Meijer-Severs GJ, Aarnoudse JG, Mensink WFA, Dankert J: The presence of antibody-coated anaerobic bacteria in asymptomatic bacteriuria during pregnancy. J Infect Dis 140:653–658, 1979.
98. McFadyen IR, Eykyn SJ: Suprapubic aspiration of urine in pregnancy. Lancet 1:1112–1114, 1968.
99. Maskell R, Pead L, Allen J: The puzzle of "urethral syndrome": a possible answer? Lancet 1:1088–1089, 1979.
100. Brumfitt W, Hamilton-Miller JMT, Ludlam H, Gooding A: Lactobacilli do not cause frequency and dysuria syndrome. Lancet 2:393–396, 1981.
101. Israel MS, Joekes AM: Renal biopsy virus tissue cultures: a negative report and comparison with bacterial cultures from renal biopsy. In: O'Grady, Brumfitt W (eds) Urinary tract infection. London: Oxford University Press, 1968, pp 49–52.
102. Schaeffer AJ, Stamey TA: Pathogenicity of Enterobacteriaceae isolated from the vaginal vestibule. In: Kass EH, Brumfitt W (eds) Infections of the urinary tract. Chicago: University of Chicago Press, 1978, pp 60–68.
103. Stamey TA, Wehner N, Mihara G, Condy M: The immunologic basis of recurrent bacteriuria: role of cervicovaginal antibody in enterobacterial colonization of the introital mucosa. Medicine (Baltimore) 57:47–56, 1978.
104. Cox CE, Hinman F: Factors in resistance to infection in the bladder. I. The eradication of bacteria by vesical emptying and intrinsic defense mechanisms. In: Kass EH (ed) Progress in pyelonephritis. Philadelphia: FA Davis, 1965, pp 563–570.
105. O'Grady F, Gauci CL, Watson BW, Hammond B: In vitro models simulating conditions of bacterial growth in the urinary tract. In: O'Grady F, Brumfitt W (eds) Urinary tract infection. London: Oxford University Press, 1968, pp 80–90.
106. Lapides J, Costello RT, Zierdt DK, Stone TE: Primary cause and treatment of recurrent urinary infection in women: preliminary report. J Urol 100:552–555, 1968.
107. Marsh FP, Banerjee R, Panchamia P: The relationship between urinary infection, cystoscopic appearance, and pathology of the bladder in man. J Clin Pathol 27:297–307, 1974.
108. Uehling DT, Steihm ER: Elevated urinary secretory IgA in children with urinary tract infection. Pediatrics 47:40–46, 1971.
109. Fubara ES, Freter R: Protection against enteric bacterial infection by secretory IgA antibodies. J Immunol 111:395–403, 1973.
110. Miller TE, Creaghe E: Bacterial interference as a factor in renal infection. J Lab Clin Med 87:792–803, 1976.
111. Mitchell GW, Jacobs AA, Haddad V, Paul BB, Strauss RR, Sbarra AJ: The role of the phagocyte in host–parasite interactions. XXV. Metabolic and bactericidal activities of leukocytes from pregnant women. Am J Obstet Gynecol 108:804–813, 1970.
112. Ledger WJ: Bacterial infections complicating pregnancy. Clin Obstet Gynecol 21:455–475, 1978.
113. Harkness RA: Oestrogens and host resistance. J R Soc Med 73:161–164, 1980.
114. Sleigh JD, Robertston JD, Isdale MH: Asymptomatic bacteriuria in pregnancy. J Obstet Gynaecol Br Commonw 71:74–81, 1964.
115. Chalmers GC: Bacilluria in pregnancy. Excerpta Med Int Congr Ser 67:25, 1963.
116. Bran JL, Levison HE, Kaye D: Entrance of bacteria into the female urinary bladder. N Engl J Med 286:626–629, 1972.
117. Buckley RH, McGluckin H, MacGregor RR: Urine bacterial counts after sexual intercourse. N Engl J Med 298:321–324, 1978.
118. Kunin CM, Deutscher R, Paquin A: Urinary tract infection in school children: an epidemiologic, clinical and laboratory study. Medicine (Baltimore) 43:91–130, 1964.
119. Kunin CH, McCormack RC: An epidemiologic study of bacteriuria and blood pressure among nuns and working women. N Engl J Med 278:636–642, 1968.

120. Evans DA, Liao L, Hennekens Ch, Kass EH: Clearance of bacteriuria on discontinuing oral contraception. Br Med J 1:152, 1980.
121. Laughlin LW, Williams DN, Kass EH, Taylor JO, Donner A: Favourable effect of treatment on bacteriuria. In: Kass EH, Brumfitt W (eds) Infections of the urinary tract. Chicago: University of Chicago Press, 1978, pp 151–152.
122. Bailey RR: Urinary infection in pregnancy. NZ Med J 71:216–220, 1970.
123. Whalley PJ, Martin FG, Peters PC: Significance of asymptomatic bacteriuria detected during pregnancy. JAMA 193:879–881, 1965.
124. Pathak UN, Tang K, Williams LL, Stuart KL: Bacteriuria of pregnancy: results of treatment. J Infect Dis 120:91–103, 1969.
125. Turck M, Goffe B, Petersdorf RG: Bacteriuria of pregnancy: relation to socioeconomic factors. N Engl J Med 266:857–860, 1962.
126. Henderson M, Entwhistle G, Tayback M: Bacteriuria and pregnancy outcome: preliminary findings. Am J Public Health 52:1887–1893, 1962.
127. Rubin RH, Fang LST, Jones ST, Munford RS, Slepack JM, Varga PA, Onheiber L, Hall Cl, Tolkoff-Rubin NE: Single-dose amoxycillin therapy for urinary tract infection: multicentre trial using antibody-coated bacteria localization technique. JAMA 244:561–564, 1980.
128. Williams GL, Campbell H, Davies KJ: The influence of age, parity and social class on the incidence of asymptomatic bacteriuria in pregnancy. J Obstet Gynaecol Br Commonw 76:-229–239, 1969.
129. Pometta D, Rees SB, Younger D, Kass EH: Asymptomatic bacteriuria in diabetes mellitus. N Engl J Med 276:1118–1121, 1967.
130. Vejlsgaard R: Bacteriuria in patients with diabetus mellitus (a controlled study). In: Kass EH (ed) Progress in pyelonephritis. Philadelphia: FA Davis, 1965, pp 478–491.
131. Savage WE, Hajj SN, Kass EH: Demographic and prognostic characteristics of bacteriuria in pregnancy. Medicine (Baltimore) 46:385–407, 1967.
132. Low JA, Johnston EE, McBride RL, Tuffnell P: The significance of asymptomatic bacteriuria in the normal obstetric patient. Am J Obstet Gynecol 90:897–906, 1964.
133. Mabeck CE: Studies in urinary tract infections. II. Urinary tract infection due to coagulase-negative staphylococci. Acta Med Scand 186:39–45, 1969.
134. Kincaid-Smith P, Bullen M: Bacteriuria in pregnancy. Lancet 1:395–399, 1965.
135. Gruneberg RN, Brumfitt W: Single-dose treatment of acute urinary tract infection: a controlled trial. Br Med J 3:649–651, 1967.
136. Asscher AW, Sussman M, Waters WE, Evans JAS, Campbell H, Evans KT, Williams JE: Asymptomatic significant bacteriuria in the non-pregnant woman. II. Response to treatment and follow-up. Br Med J 1:804–806, 1969.
137. Baird D: Infection of the urinary tract in the puerperium. J Obstet Gynaecol Br Emp 43:-435–452, 1936.
138. Kass EH: The role of asymptomatic bacteriuria in the pathogenesis of pyelonephritis. In: Quinn EL, Kass EH (eds) Biology of pyelonephritis. London: Churchill, 1960, pp 399–412.
139. Cobbs CG, Strickler JC, McGovern JH, Kaye D: The post partum renal status of women with untreated asymptomatic bacteriuria during pregnancy. Am J Obstet Gynecol 99:221–227, 1967.
140. Zinner SH, Kass EH: Long-term (10–14 years) follow-up of bacteriuria in pregnancy. N Engl J Med 285:820–824, 1971.
141. Kaijser B, Hanson LA, Jodal U, Lidin-Janson G, Robbins JB: Frequency of *E. coli* K antigens in urinary-tract infections in children. Lancet 1:663–664, 1977.
142. Naeye RL: Causes of excessive rates of perinatal mortality and prematurity in pregnancies complicated by maternal urinary-tract infections. N Engl J Med 300:809–823, 1979.
143. McDowell DRM, Buchanan JD, Fairley KF, Gilbert GL: Anaerobic and other fastidious nucro organisms in asymptomatic bacteriuria in pregnant women. J Infect Dis 144:114–122, 1981.
144. Harris RE, Thomas VL, Shelekov A: Asymptomatic bacteriuria in pregnancy: antibody coated bacterial renal function, and intrauterine growth retardation. Am J Obstet Gynecol 126:20–25, 1976.
145. Wiederman J, Stone ML, Pataki R: Urinary tract infections and uterine activity: effect of *Escherichia coli* endotoxins on uterine motility in vitro. Am J Obstet Gynecol 84:290–296, 1962.
146. Cavanagh D, McLeod AG: Prematurity and urinary tract infection. I. The effect of coliform endotoxin on isolated human endometrium. Am J Obstet Gynecol 96:576–578, 1966.

147. William WA, Greenwood BM: Impairment of the immune response to vaccination after malaria. Lancet 1:1328–1329, 1978.
148. Duncan ME, Fox H, Harkness RA, Rees RJW: The placenta in leprosy. Placenta 5:189–198, 1984.
149. Scott JR: Fetal growth retardation associated with maternal administration of immunosuppressive drugs. Am J Obstet Gynecol 128:668–676, 1977.
150. Miller T, Scott L, Stewart E, North D: Modification by suppressor cells and serum factors of the cell-mediated immune response in experimental pyelonephritis. J Clin Invest 61:964–972, 1978.
151. Whalley PJ: Bacteriuria in pregnancy. In: Kass EH (ed) Progress in pyelonephritis. Philadelphia: FA Davis, 1965, pp 50–57.
152. Norden CW, Kilpatrick WH: Bacteriuria of pregnancy. In: Kass EH (ed) Progress in pyelonephritis. Philadelphia: FA Davis 1965, pp 64–72.
153. Moller M, Thomsen AC, Borch K, Dinesen K, Zdravkovic M: Rupture of fetal membranes and premature delivery associated with group B streptococci in urine of pregnant women. Lancet 2:69–70, 1984.
154. Stuart KL, Cummins GTM, Chin WA: Bacteriuria prematurity and the hypertensive disorders of pregnancy. Br Med J 1:554–556, 1965.
155. Verrier Jones K, Asscher AW, Verrier Jones ER, Mattholie K, Leach K, Thomson GM: Glomerular filtration rate in schoolgirls with covert bacteriuria. Br Med J 285:1307–1310, 1982.
156. Waters WE, Elwood PC, Asscher AW, Abernethy M: Clinical significance of dysuria in women. Br Med J 2:754–757, 1970.
157. Cohlan SQ: Foetal and neonatal hazards from drugs administered during pregnancy. NY J Med 64:493–499, 1964.
158. Clark H, Ronald AR, Cutler RE, Turck M: The correlation between site of infection and maximal concentrating ability in bacteriuria. J Infect Dis 120:47–53, 1969.
159. Whalley PJ, Cunningham FG, Martin FG: Transient renal dysfunction associated with acute pyelonephritis of pregnancy. Obstet Gynecol 46:174–177, 1975.
160. Kaitz AL: Urinary concentrating ability in pregnant women with asymptomatic bacteriuria. J Clin Invest 40:1331–1338, 1961.
161. Ronald AR, Cutler RE, Turck M: Effect of bacteriuria on renal concentrating mechanisms. Ann Intern Med 70:723–733, 1969.
162. Norden CW, Tuttle EP: Impairment of urinary concentrating ability in pregnant women with asymptomatic bacteriuria. In: Kass EH (ed) Progress in pyelonephritis. Philadelphia: FA Davis, 1965, pp 73–80.
163. Elder HA, Kass EH: Renal function in pregnancy: its relationship to prematurity, acute pyelonephritis, and excessive weight gain. In: Kass EH, Progress in pyelonephritis. Philadelphia: FA Davis, 1965, pp 81–86.
164. Cunningham FG, Pritchard JA: Hematologic disorders in pregnancy. In: Bolognese RJ, Schwarz RH (eds) Perinatal medicine. Baltimore: Williams and Wilkins, 1977, pp 249–250.
165. Condie AP, Williams JD, Reeves DS, Brumfitt W: Complications of bacteriuria in pregnancy. In: O'Grady F, Brumfitt W (eds) Urinary tract infection. London: Oxford University Press, 1968, pp 148–159.
166. Turck, M, Ronald AR, Petersdorf RG: Relapse and reinfection in chronic bacteriuria. II. The correlation between site of infection and pattern of recurrence in chronic bacteriuria. N Engl J Med 278:422–427, 1968.
167. Cattell WR, McSherry MA, Brookes HL, O'Grady FW: Relation of bacteria isolated from the urethral area to bacteriuria. In: Kass EH, Brumfitt W (eds) Infections in the urinary tract. Chicago: University of Chicago Press, 1978, pp 69–73.
168. Leveno KJ, Harris RE, Gilstrap LC, Whalley PJ, Cunningham FG, Kappus SS, Nobles B: Bladder versus renal bacteriuria during pregnancy: recurrence after treatment. Am J Obstet Gynecol 139:403–406, 1981.
169. Davies PA, Little K, Aherne W: Tetracyclines and yellow teeth. Lancet 1:743, 1962.
170. Cohlan SQ, Bevelander G, Tiamsic T: Growth inhibition of prematures receiving tetracycline: a clinical and laboratory investigation of tetracycline-induced bone fluorescence. Am J Dis Child 105:453–461, 1963.
171. Odell GB: The dissociation of bilirubin and albumin and its clinical implications. J Pediatr 55:268–279, 1959.

172. Wade A: Chloramphenicol in Martindale: the extra pharmacopocia, 27th edn. Pharmaceutical Press, 1977, p 1108.
173. British National Formulary no. 8, British Medical Association and Pharmaceutical Society of Great Britain, 1984, p 206.
174. Anderson JD, Aird MY, Johnson AM, Ree R, Goresky D, Brumwell CA, Percival-Smith RKL: The use of a single 1 g dose of amoxycillin for the treatment of acute urinary tract infections. J Antimicrob Chemother 5:471–483, 1979.
175. Brumfitt W, Hamilton-Miller JMT, Franklin INS, Anderson FM, Brown GM: Conventional and two-dose amoxycillin treatment of bacteriuria in pregnancy and recurrent bacteriuria: a comparative study. J Antimicrob Chemother 10:239–248, 1982.
176. Anderton KJ, Abbas AMA, Davey A, Ancill RJ: High dose, short course amoxycillin in the treatment of bacteriuria in pregnancy. Br J Clin Pract 37:212–214, 1983.
177. Bailey RR: Bacteriuria during pregnancy. MD thesis, University of Otago. Quoted by Bailey RR (1979) Single dose antibacterial treatment for uncomplicated urinary tract infections. Drugs 17:219–221, 1970.
178. Williams JD, Smith EK: Single-dose therapy with streptomycin sulfametopyrazine for bacteriuria during pregnancy. Br Med J 4:461–463, 1970.
179. Little PJ, De Wardener HE: Acute pyelonephritis: incidence of reinfection in 100 patients. Lancet 2:1277–1278, 1966.
180. Whalley PJ, Cunningham FG: Short-term versus continuous antimicrobial therapy for asymptomatic bacteriuria in pregnancy. Obstet Gyecol 49:262–265, 1977.
181. Furness ET, MacDonald PJ, Beasley NV: Urinary antiseptics in asymptomatic bacteriuria of pregnancy. NZ Med J 81:417–317, 1975.
182. Harris RE, Gilstrap LC: Prevention of recurrent pyelonephritis during pregnancy. Obstet Gynecol 44:736–641, 1974.
183. Bailey RR, Abbott GD: Treatment of urinary tract infections with a single dose of amoxycillin. Nephron 18:316–320, 1977.
184. Lenke RR, James MD, Van Dorsten P, Schifrin BS: Pyelonephritis in pregnancy: a prospective randomized trial to prevent recurrent disease evaluating suppressive therapy with nitrofurantoin and close surveillance. Am J Obstet Gynecol 146:953–957, 1983.
185. Harris RE: The significance of eradication of bacteriuria during pregnancy. Obstet Gynecol 53:71–73, 1979.
186. McFadyen IR, Eykyn SKJ: Diagnosis of urinary-tract infections in pregnancy. Lancet 1:1348, 1970.

INDEX

286,60